D1376061

Massage and Aromatherapy

Massage and Aromatherapy

A guide for health professionals

Andrew Vickers

Research Council for Complementary Medicine

with contributions from

Steve Van Toller
and Caroline Stevensen

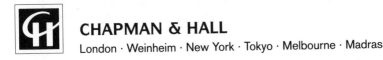

CHAPMAN & HALL

London · Weinheim · New York · Tokyo · Melbourne · Madras

Published by Chapman & Hall, 2–6 Boundary Row, London SE1 8HN, UK

Chapman & Hall 2–6 Boundary Row, London SE1 8HN, UK

Chapman & Hall GmbH, Pappelallee 3, 69469 Weinheim, Germany

Chapman & Hall USA, 115 Fifth Avenue, New York, NY 10003, USA

Chapman & Hall Japan, ITP-Japan, Kyowa Building, 3F, 2-2-1 Hirakawacho, Chiyoda-ku, Tokyo 102, Japan

Chapman & Hall Australia, 102 Dodds Street, South Melbourne, Victoria 3205, Australia

Chapman & Hall India, R. Seshadri, 32 Second Main Road, CIT East, Madras 600 035, India

Distributed in the USA and Canada by Singular Publishing Group Inc., 4284 41st Street, San Diego, California 92105

First edition 1996

© 1996 Andrew Vickers

Typeset in 10/12 pt Palatino by Mews Photosetting, Beckenham, Kent

Printed in Great Britain by Alden, Oxford, Didcot and Northampton

ISBN 0 412 57630 9   1 56593 349 4 (USA)

A catalogue record for this book is available from the British Library

Library of Congress Catalog Card Number: 95-83015

∞ Printed on permanent acid-free text paper, manufactured in accordance with ANSI/NISO Z39.48-1992 and ANSI/NISO Z39.48-1984 (Permanence of Paper).

This book is dedicated to Caroline Batzdorf, for the best back rub ever, June 1993.

Contents

Preface

This book aims to give health professionals a balanced and independent overview of massage and aromatherapy. I have written it because, despite growing interest, there is a dearth of professional literature on this subject. This book aims to cover a number of topics which are under-represented in existing publications. These include:

- scientific research in massage and aromatherapy;
- the use of the therapies in medical settings;
- the knowledge base of massage and aromatherapy;
- professional and managerial issues;
- safety.

Understanding of these subjects is essential for any reasoned evaluation of massage and aromatherapy. Yet this book is probably the first to provide information suitable for this task. At the current time of writing, almost all books on massage and aromatherapy have been written with the lay public in mind. The texts recommended to students and practitioners by the foremost schools and institutions are exactly the same as those available in health food shops as general introductions for prospective patients. Not surprisingly, such books generally fail to include in-depth discussions of professional issues.

A CRITIQUE OF MASSAGE AND AROMATHERAPY

I am broadly supportive of massage and aromatherapy. In researching this book I have been impressed by the experiences of patients and their practitioners. Health professionals who have worked alongside practitioners have generally been extremely positive and the scientific evidence, discussed at length in Chapters 4 and 5, does seem to lend at least some support to current practice. That said, I do not believe that everything practitioners claim is correct. Moreover, I do not believe that the therapies are beyond improvement. The current state of knowledge in massage and aromatherapy is likely to fall short of the optimum. This is something which could and should be said of any therapy: presumably no-one believes that doctors are always correct or that conventional medicine is perfect and could not possibly progress any further.

I will be offering a critique of massage and aromatherapy in this book and it is possible that some of what I write will upset practition-ers. For example, in Chapter 3, I analyse the writings of a number of leading aromatherapy authors and argue that much of what they say is incoherent. Authors make claims which are unusual, or simplistic, or just plain inaccurate, and there is profound disagreement between texts as to the properties and indications of the essential oils. It is worth re-stating that the rationale of the book is to provide a reasoned exam-ination of massage and aromatherapy written by an independent observer. It is quite definitely not my intention to debunk massage or aromatherapy. But neither is it my intention to offer them unqualified support. When I say that I offer a 'critique' of massage and aromather-apy, I use this word in the sense of analysis rather than in the sense of denigration.

I do hope that practitioners will not take this book as an 'attack' on massage or aromatherapy. On the contrary, I see the aim of this book as aiding the progress and development of the therapies. There can be no progress without constructive criticism: we not only need to generate new ideas, we also need to evaluate them. I hope that this book will help kick-start the process of critical evaluation in massage and aro-matherapy.

HOLISM AND INDIVIDUALISM

The very process of writing this book has involved going against two principles emphasized by practitioners of massage and aromatherapy. Firstly, that it is misleading to look at symptoms out of context of the whole person (holism) and secondly, that each whole person is a unique individual (individualism). So while I am tempted to agree that conventional distinctions between mind and body are often simplistic, it has sometimes been necessary to use those distinctions in order to write coherently. I have used conventional health-care language in the main because I am aiming to communicate with people who under-stand that language.

The main aim of this book is to help identify the role and scope of massage and aromatherapy. This has often entailed identifying the health problems that patients, practitioners and others have reported to be helped by treatment. If those problems have been predominantly psychological (for example, in cancer) it seems worth saying so, regardless of whether this may entail a 'false' distinction between mind and body. Similarly, though I agree that health care should pay particular regard to the unique characteristics of the individual, some individuals do have similar health problems. Generalizations do only go so far, but they can be a useful guide.

During one interview for this book, I asked a practitioner to talk about some of the general issues involved in work with people who had HIV and AIDS. She sighed repeatedly and claimed that 'it was difficult to say': after all, 'every patient is unique and it all depends on the individual'. While I do regret the use of generalizations, particularly those in which individual symptoms are perhaps taken out of context, health professionals do need more information than simply 'it all depends'.

METHODOLOGY

This book contains information on the scientific literature of massage and aromatherapy, the published work of leading authorities on the therapies and the activities of practitioners.

The scientific literature

The research in Chapters 4 and 5 is not presented as a systematic literature review. This is because I aim to give a broad general overview of the research base of massage and aromatherapy rather than to answer specific questions about specific issues. However, the methodology of the review did incorporate a number of standard techniques of systematic review as an attempt to overcome avoidable reviewer bias. The initial data for the literature search was obtained from the Research Council for Complementary Medicine's CISCOM database. CISCOM is widely regarded to be the most comprehensive and sophisticated bibliographical database on complementary medicine research, containing over 30 000 references to research published worldwide since the early 1960s. Supplementary searches of MEDLINE and EMBASE were conducted and the reference lists of major textbooks and journal articles consulted. All clinical papers were subjected to standard systematic review procedures (Vickers, 1995). Readers should be aware that I have no formal experience of appraising sociological or laboratory-based research. It is possible that papers I have referred to contain flaws that I would not recognize.

Textbooks of massage and aromatherapy

It was not my original intention to analyse the massage and

aromatherapy literature for this book. Early in the project I read a number of the major textbooks as background reading. What was written in these books surprised me and I decided to incorporate an analysis of the literature as part of the overview of practice. It strikes me that it would be difficult to understand the professional worlds of massage and aromatherapy without an examination of the views of leading authorities. Moreover, practitioners read standard textbooks when they train and refer to them when in practice. An analysis of the literature is therefore a good starting point for understanding the beliefs of practitioners. I located books by searching the catalogue of the British Library and by asking leading practitioners and organizations to recommend the most important and valuable texts. Each book was read with the intention of drawing out a limited number of themes. These themes were then compared across different texts.

Practice

Chapters 6–9 contain an account of the use of massage and aromatherapy in orthodox health settings. Chapter 10 discusses the management issues associated with such practice. Researching these chapters presented perhaps the most serious methodological difficulties. This is because it would have been impractical to conduct rigorous qualitative research on all aspects of practice. I decided early in this project that any discussion of the clinical use of massage and aromatherapy – their scope, effects and management – could never constitute a definitive statement. I could only hope to sketch out a rough 'first draft', intending to be informative and, hopefully, to provoke others into more rigorous and more narrowly defined research. The statements made in Chapters 6–10 are based on impressions gained from discussions with patients, carers, practitioners and other health-care staff. They are general in nature, reflect my own understanding and are not intended as knowledge claims. Not all aspects of practice are covered and I am willing to accept that some statements may be incomplete, inaccurate or misleading. However, I have shown material from this book to a number of experienced clinicians and there has been widespread agreement on the general thrust of the text. I do expect the material in Chapters 6–10 to be broadly accurate. I also expect that it will be informative, provocative and a useful basis for practical-decision making about massage and aromatherapy.

Terminological note: In the chapters 6–9, a number of references will be made to conditions which have both a medical and a colloquial usage. These include anxiety, depression and fatigue. For example, the common expression 'I feel anxious' has little to do with a clinical diagnosis of anxiety. I will be using the colloquial sense in these chapters because this is what tends to be used by patients and complementary practitioners. Mention of the use of massage or aromatherapy for anxiety, depression or fatigue in chapters 6–9 does not therefore indicate treatment of clinically diagnosed case of one of these diseases.

Andrew Vickers
London, 1995

Acknowledgements

Far more people have helped with this project than can be listed here: to all of those who have shared personal experiences or who have offered help and advice, many thanks.

Special mention must go to: Jo Campling and Helen Sanderson for getting me in involved in the first place; Catherine Walker for early support and encouragement; Jonathan Monckton for the same; Caroline Stevensen for on-going support and advice; Grace Laffan, Clare Harrison, Doreen Isherwood, Richard Ashrowan, Daniel Tangway, Peter Nixon, Jan Woolsley, Norma Nolan, Jane Watson, Adrian Tookman, Wendy Jackson, Greg Finn, Sheila Reynolds, Peter Fermie, Mary Ashwin, Liz Ropschwitz, Sylvia Baker, Jody Wells, Dione Hills, Caroline Harding, Peter Mackereth, Sue Pembury and David Peters, for either helping to prepare material for Chapters 6–10 or for commenting on early drafts; Shirley Price for writing back (!); the staff of the Science Reference and Information Service of the British Library; Ulrich and Caroline Batzdorf for helping me at UCLA library.

For help with translations I would like to thank Caroline, Tim, Beata, Nora, Ellen and Siggy.

Special mention should be made of Hands On: Thomas, Janice, Steph, Daphne and Scarlett.

Finally, for a superb job of editing (and a wonderful weekend in Wales) particular thanks must go to Rebecca and Saul. The witty editing remarks award goes to Rebecca.

PART ONE
Introduction

Introduction to complementary medicine

1

WHAT IS COMPLEMENTARY MEDICINE?

The existence of a plurality of healing methods and systems may pre-date human history. About 500 years ago, a subset of medical practices became associated with the state. It was at this point that health care first split into conventional and unconventional practices.

The concept of 'complementary medicine' is still heavily informed by this split. To many, the term 'complementary medicine' means little more than 'not conventional medicine'. Pietroni (1992) points out that talking about complementary medicine is a little like talking about foreigners: you can't say what they are, only what they are not. In this view, 'complementary medicine' is merely a convenient label for a number of disparate techniques, grouped together merely because they remain outside standard medical practice. For example:

- acupuncture originated in China thousands of years ago and is based upon traditional Oriental views about health;
- homoeopathy was founded in Europe in the late 18th century and is now used by conventional physicians in many parts of the world;
- massage has been used in almost all cultures throughout history;
- yoga was first practised in India in ancient times.

Pietroni believes that the only similarity between piercing the skin with needles, prescribing low dose pills, manipulating the soft tissues of the body and the use of special postures is that these techniques are not routinely taught to medical students.

On the other hand, at least some workers believe that complementary medicine is indeed a meaningful term. This meaning is seen to derive from systematic similarities between the complementary therapies. According to this view, if one was to write down every characteristic of every therapy – conventional, complementary or whatever – one would find that therapies would fall into natural groups. Complementary therapies are said to share the following characteristics.

- *Natural healing.* This is the belief that the body has an inherent ability to heal itself and that the aim of treatment should be to stimulate and enhance this capacity. This is often contrasted with the approach said to be characteristic of conventional medicine, which is to remove or destroy disease organisms or diseased tissue, or to inhibit the biochemical states or processes associated with disease. For example, conventional treatment of cancer focuses on destroying cancerous cells by radiation or chemicals, or by the surgical removal of tumours from the body. The alternative approach would be to start from the observation that the immune system of a healthy person is able to locate and destroy cancerous cells. The purpose of cancer treatment would then be to restore this function.
- *Holistic medicine.* There are various ways of viewing the cause and treatment of disease. It is held that conventional medicine locates all disease in the physical body: even emotional distress is viewed as a biochemical disorder that requires biochemical intervention. Holistic medicine seeks the roots and treatment of disease not just in the individual's body but also in their mind, family, environment and community. In cancer, for example, it has been claimed that an individual's temperament (Eysenck, 1988) and social and family links (Reynolds *et al.*, 1994) affect the onset and course of disease.
- *Non-invasive medicine.* It is held that some therapeutic procedures are gentle, and even pleasurable: massage is a classic example. Such techniques tend to carry a low risk of adverse side-effects.
- *Time, touch and talk.* Traditionally, one of the most important roles of the healer has been to offer to comfort those in ill-health. One common criticism of modern medicine is that this role has been lost; a consequence, at least in part, of the emphasis on curing disease. In particular, modern medicine is seen as having forgotten the significance of time, touch and talk, the basic tools of comfort-giving. This loss is seen as particularly grave by those workers who emphasize the importance of the relationship between health practitioner and patient: the 'therapeutic partnership'.
- *Patient participation.* Patients often become passive recipients of medicine. Many therapies, such as surgery, often preclude an active patient role. Perhaps more importantly, it is alleged that patients often play no part in making decisions about their treatment. ('Doctor knows best.') To become an active participant in medicine, patients may be asked to make diet and lifestyle changes, to practise physical and mental exercises and, above all, to play the central role in making decisions about their treatment.
- *The role of science and established knowledge.* Every society has a set of beliefs about what there is in the world, and how to find out about it. Systems of medicine also presuppose a certain view of the world

and this may or may not sit squarely with that of the society in which the therapy is practised. The world view of countries such as the UK and US is largely scientific. Some forms of medicine are characterized by the fact that they involve beliefs which are not found in the textbooks or practices of science.

That said, many of the characteristics of complementary medicine outlined above are also found in conventional practice.

- Many doctors are keen to avoid interventions wherever possible and to leave the patient's self-repair systems to bring about healing.
- A holistic approach to health care is increasingly common in conventional medicine, particularly in general practice.
- Many conventional health practices are non-invasive: physiotherapy and speech therapy are two examples.
- Increasing numbers of doctors are rediscovering the importance of building up a relationship with their patients. Many are learning new skills and organizing new methods of delivering health care so that more time is spent listening and interacting with patients.
- One of the most notable recent changes in medicine has been the rise of self-help, and the increased willingness of doctors to share information and decision-making with patients.

Moreover, it is clear that, in practice, complementary medicine does not always exhibit characteristics such as holism or patient participation. For example, many complementary practitioners are content to think that holistic medicine is somehow inherent in their therapy, rather than being a function of the way in which the therapy is practised. There is evidence that some practitioners do practise unholistically (p. 56).

There are those who say that many of the so-called characteristics of complementary medicine are simply the characteristics of good medicine. As conventional medicine continues to change and progress, it is likely that it will continue to incorporate philosophies aspects such as holism and patient participation, something which will have the effect of blurring the line between conventional and complementary practice.

In short, the answer to the question 'What is complementary medicine?' appears to be somewhat paradoxical. Complementary medicine is anything which is not conventional medicine. Complementary therapies share some common characteristics. Many of these can also be found in conventional medicine.

One solution is to use a sociological rather than a philosophical perspective. Instead of answering 'What is complementary medicine?' in the abstract, in terms of criteria and characteristics, it can be answered empirically, by looking at society and seeing what society describes as complementary medicine.

The result of doing so is to find that what determines whether or not something is 'complementary medicine' is the therapy being used. Acupuncture used non-holistically by a conventional doctor in a hospital setting is seen as complementary medicine. Aspirin prescribed by a herbalist is seen as conventional medicine. Chiropractic manipulation is complementary medicine. Physiotherapy manipulation is conventional medicine.

Therefore one answer to 'What is complementary medicine?' is merely a list of therapies, as given in the section below. It is clear that, as a group, these therapies have only limited philosophical and practical cohesion, something which limits generalities about 'complementary medicine' as a whole. This has two important corollaries. Firstly, massage and aromatherapy need to be evaluated independently, as individual therapies, rather than as a part of 'complementary medicine'. Secondly, it would seem worth seeking new ways of describing the differences between therapies: see, for example, Vickers, 1994a.

A BRIEF INTRODUCTION TO THE COMPLEMENTARY THERAPIES

Massage

Massage is technically described as the therapeutic manipulation of soft tissue (p. 16).

Aromatherapy

Aromatherapy is the therapeutic use of aromatic substances derived from plants (p. 27).

Reflexology

This is a type of foot massage in which certain areas of the foot are believed to correspond to areas of the body: stimulation of the foot is believed to bring about healing. As a massage-type technique, reflexology is covered in detail on page 20.

Healing

More widely known as spiritual healing, or the laying-on of hands, this therapy does not, in fact, require a religious context. For example, some nurses in the US practise a form of healing, known as 'thera-peutic touch', as part of their daily hospital work.

The common belief of all healers is that a human being can induce healing solely by an effort of will. The details vary, but a common idea is that the healer channels healing energy to the person in need. This is often done through the hands, with the healer placing the palms of their hands on or near the person being healed. The majority of healers say that they can sense energy around a person and that where they place their hands depends on whether this energy is depleted or in excess in different parts of the body. Some healers try to assess and correct the energy at specific places which they call 'centres' or 'chakras'; others are more concerned with the state of energy in general.

For the patient, healing is a very soothing and relaxing experience. In the hospital setting it has been used for anxiety, depression and pain. Healing has been said to be effective for improving an individ-ual's general sense of well-being, a typical response to healing is 'the pain is still there but it doesn't bother me so much'. Healing has also been used to promote communication between patients and health professionals. For example, some nurses have reported that patients find it easier to talk about their fears and worries after a session of healing (Payne, 1989). Some practitioners of massage and aromather-apy incorporate healing in their work.

The metamorphic technique

Perhaps best thought of as a special type of healing (see above), meta-morphic technique involves a gentle stroking of the feet and hands.

Acupuncture

Acupuncture is the insertion of fine needles into the skin at special points. Traditional acupuncture is based on the principles of Chinese medicine (TCM). In TCM, the workings of the human body are seen to be controlled by a vital force or energy called chi, which circulates between the organs along set channels called meridians. There are 12 meridians, each of which corresponds to the major functions or organs of the body, and chi energy must flow in the correct strength and qual-ity through each of these meridians for health to be maintained. Energy imbalances, which are associated with illness, can be corrected by a number of means. In acupuncture, needles are placed at special points on the meridians and, depending on how the needle is manip-ulated (for example, it may be gently twirled in place), the energy is either drawn to the meridian or dispersed from it. Herbs, diet and exercise can also be used to modify the energy state of the meridians. TCM diagnosis is an attempt to assess each patient's individual state of energy. This is done by taking an extended case history, making observations of the colour and quality of the skin and tongue and by 'pulse diagnosis', a special technique whereby the energy of the meridians may be assessed by feeling the strength, rhythm and quality of the pulse.

Some practitioners of acupuncture, particularly Western health professionals, dispense with traditional Chinese philosophy and work entirely within a scientific framework (Baldry, 1993). The acupuncture points are seen to correspond to physiological and anatomical features, for example, peripheral nerve junctions, and diagnosis is made in purely conventional terms. This form of acupuncture is called 'Western' or 'scientific' acupuncture and is the predominant form practised in conventional health settings.

Acupressure and shiatsu

Some practitioners stimulate acupuncture points by using their fingers to apply pressure. As massage-type techniques, acupressure and shiatsu are covered in detail on page 22.

Osteopathy and chiropractic

Osteopathy and chiropractic are therapies of the physical structures of the body: practitioners work with bones, muscles and connective tissue, using their hands to diagnose and treat abnormalities of structure and function.

Typically, treatment will involve a 'high-velocity thrust' or manipulation. This is a short, sharp motion designed to free up structures that are adhering to one another. Practitioners also use mobilization, a form of stretching; soft-tissue manipulation (p. 25) and functional techniques. These can best be described using the example of a stiff shoulder. In manipulation the practitioner osteopath would use a forceful manoeuvre to improve the mobility of the joint; in functional work, the arm might be gently moved within the shoulder joint's range of motion. The goal of functional techniques is for the body to respond to the practitioner's touch in such a way as to rectify abnormalities of its own accord.

One of the most important functional techniques is cranial osteopathy, or cranio-sacral therapy as it is sometimes known. Cranial osteopathy focuses on the nervous system. Practitioners place their hands on the skull bones (the cranium) and the flat bone at the base of the spine (the sacrum) of the client and feel for a rhythm which they say it is possible to detect. By working with this rhythm, and by gently handling the bones of the skull, osteopaths say that they can balance physical disturbances and distortions in the nervous system.

Rolfing

As a massage-type technique, Rolfing is discussed in greater detail on page 24.

Alexander technique

The principle of the Alexander technique is that 'use affects functioning': how we use ourselves in everyday life – how we sit, stand and move – affects the working of our bodies. To use a rudimentary example: sitting slouched in a chair at the office all day can not only lead to back pain, but possibly also to headaches and a general lack of vitality.

Rather than instructing clients in specific postures or movements, practitioners of the Alexander technique are more interested in the principles of good use. Simply speaking, they say that movement should involve a lengthening and widening of the body and the absence of unnecessary muscle tension, particularly in the neck. Teachers of the Alexander technique are particularly interested in helping their pupils identify the habits that interfere with the body's natural functioning and coordination. Helping a person to recognize and 'inhibit' these habits is seen as one of the main purposes of an Alexander session.

Feldenkrais

The principle of Feldenkrais is that the body has an inherent ability to organize itself into movement. The aim of Feldenkrais treatment is to facilitate this process. Practitioners say that if the nervous system is allowed to experience various different forms of movement in subtle variations it will recognize for itself the most appropriate and efficient way of moving. The general aim and scope of Feldenkrais is similar to that of Alexander technique.

Homoeopathy

Homoeopathy is based on the principle that 'like should be cured with like'. Homoeopaths use small doses of a substance to treat symptoms that the substance would cause if administered in large doses. For example, the homoeopathic remedy *Apis* is derived from the sting of the bee. Bee stings cause pain, stiffness and inflammation.

This is exacerbated by pressure but improves on cooling. *Apis* is typically prescribed to patients with rheumatological conditions, especially if they respond well to cold packs but are particularly sensitive to direct pressure on the joints.

Homoeopathy is one of the most problematic complementary therapies. Many of the remedies that homoeopaths use are so dilute that it is unlikely that a single molecule of the original substance remains. If homoeopathy works, it clearly poses a considerable number of questions about the nature of biological substances and the action of pharmacological agents.

Naturopathy

Naturopathy is a therapeutic system, rather than an individual therapy. It is based upon the principle of Hippocrates, 'vis medicatrix naturae', the healing force of nature. Naturopaths believe that all organisms have an inherent capacity to heal themselves but that this capacity may become compromised, often by the build up of 'toxins'. The classic nature cure consists of mineral baths, massage and fasting in an attempt to purify the body and thereby promote self-healing. Naturopaths have also traditionally stressed the importance of diet, believing that optimal nutrition is necessary for the self-healing systems of the body.

Modern naturopathy relies less upon baths and spas and more upon a range of therapeutic modalities, including nutritional therapy, osteopathy, herbal medicine, exercise and acupuncture.

Herbal medicine

Herbs have been used to treat disease by almost all cultures throughout history. Many modern pharmaceutical drugs are based on herbal remedies. Herbal medicine is distinguished by the preparation of medicaments directly from plant matter and by idiosyncratic systems of diagnosis and treatment. Practitioners of traditional Chinese medicine, for example, diagnose disease in terms of chi, the five elements and so on (see above). They use herbs according to properties conceived of in similar terms. For example, certain herbs are said to have the property of 'destagnation' and will be used when a practitioner diagnoses a stagnation of chi energy.

Modern medical herbalism, as practised in the UK, tends to have a naturopathic orientation. Great emphasis is placed on the digestive and eliminative systems of the body. As such, the prescription of a diuretic herb for an arthritic complaint would not be unusual.

Nutrition

Though nutrition is generally thought of as complementary therapy, there is little reason why it should not form an integral part of conventional medicine. For example, fatty acid supplementation, a common nutritional therapy, is now understood in terms of a single agent and a single biochemical pathway.

There are three basic aspects of nutritional medicine. The least controversial is that of ensuring adequate, but not excessive, dietary intake of protein, fats, vitamins and minerals. Nutritionists may also attempt to change a patient's diet on the grounds that individuals may be 'intolerant' to certain foodstuffs and that this may cause disease. Perhaps most controversial is the use of high-dose vitamin and mineral supplements for the treatment of specific conditions.

Hypnotherapy

Hypnotherapy is a two-stage process, the induction of a hypnotic trance and the use of specific therapeutic suggestions. Though hypnosis can be used as a psychotherapeutic technique with which to explore the unconscious, it may also be used for the treatment of physical symptoms. In the treatment of irritable bowel syndrome, for example, patients may be placed in trance and asked to imagine a smoothly flowing river. In pain clinics, suggestions of coolness and numbness may be used.

Self-regulation techniques

Self-regulation techniques are those undertaken by patients themselves, typically on a daily basis, for the purpose of improving physical and mental functioning. Relaxation is a typical aim of many such techniques. Meditation and relaxation techniques are normally learned at a class and practised daily. However, relaxation techniques can also be used as a therapeutic procedure. Some health professionals employ relaxation as an immediate measure for reducing anxiety in situations such as preoperative care, hospice care and labour. Yoga combines meditation and breathing exercises with special postures which are thought to improve the functioning of the body. Tai Chi is a gentle movement exercise which originates from China. The most well-known part of tai chi is the 'solo form', a series of slow and graceful movements which follow a set pattern.

COMPLEMENTARY MEDICINE AND HEALTH CARE

SPECIFIC AND NON-SPECIFIC EFFECTS OF TREATMENT

The range of different techniques and therapies described as complementary preclude a blanket discussion of the effects of complementary medicine on health. However, in understanding the effects of complementary therapies, it is worth introducing the distinction between specific and non-specific effects. A useful analogy is that of a set of six building blocks placed in a line. One might use a narrow instrument, such as a pencil, to push one of the blocks forward an inch or so. This would be to produce a specific effect on the blocks. Alternatively, one might use a broad instrument, such as the side of a ruler, to push all six of the blocks and thereby produce a non-specific, or generalized, effect. In this analogy, the blocks may be thought as systems of the body and the instruments as medical techniques.

Certain interventions have predominantly specific effects. An example would be a fungicidal ointment for athlete's foot. This may have a profound effect on a localized area of skin, and on feelings of pain or itching, but should have little effect on the rest of the body. Other interventions have predominantly non-specific effects. Following a course of treatment a patient may experience general feelings of well-being, relaxation and calmness. There may also be an improvement in motivation and attitude, often expressed as 'the pain is still there but it doesn't bother me so much'.

The distinction between specific and non-specific treatment effects overlaps with, but is not identical to, the distinction between objective and subjective treatment effects. Many specific effects, such as the elimination of a fungal infection, are objective, just as many non-specific effects, such as general feelings of well-being, are subjective. However, a physician may use a drug with a known and specific action to elicit a subjective change: take, for example, the treatment of pain or depression. Likewise, generalized effects of treatment may include objective changes such as lowered blood pressure or a decreased frequency of respiratory infections.

The effects of many complementary therapies, massage and aromatherapy among them, are predominantly non-specific in nature. Patients may comment that 'I feel generally better in myself', or report that they are less bothered by their health and feel calmer and more positive about life. They may also point to relief from symptoms unrelated to their presenting complaint. Often, patients may be unable to point to particular symptoms which have improved.

The distinction between specific and non-specific effects is of particular importance for two reasons. Firstly, it is central to the organization of this book. Certain techniques of massage may be used to elicit specific changes in particular tissues. An extreme example would be cardiac massage, the aim of which is to stimulate the heart muscle to resume beating. However, many practitioners use massage of the whole body to bring about non-specific improvements. The main focus of this book will be this latter type of massage. Secondly, the specific/non-specific distinction provides us with a useful intellectual tool for examining the claims made by practitioners of massage and aromatherapy. Specific treatment effects are often seen as more 'scientific' and perhaps as a result, at least some authors (p. 43) emphasize specific treatment effects and downplay the more general effects of massage and aromatherapy.

THE PRACTICE AND STRUCTURE OF COMPLEMENTARY MEDICINE

Many practitioners of complementary medicine do not have conventional medical qualifications. Typically a practitioner will have undergone a 2- or 3-year training at a special school and become registered with a suitable professional organization after qualifying. The practitioner will then start up a practice, often converting a room in their own home for this purpose.

Generally speaking, complementary medicine is private medicine. The schools and registering bodies do not receive state support and must survive on the fees they are able to generate. Moreover, unlike those working on the NHS, practitioners must be paid directly by their clients for the services they provide.

Practitioners of complementary medicine are not subject to the same laws and regulations as their conventional counterparts: for example, whereas only those registered with the General Medical Council may describe themselves as medical doctors, anyone at all, regardless of skills and training, can set themselves up as an acupuncturist or homoeopath.

There is no single governing body for all practitioners of complementary medicine, in fact, there are often several governing bodies for each therapy. Practitioners can train in a number of different schools and these schools vary in the length and intensity of the course offered, the approach of the teaching and the method of qualifying. In addition, certain complementary techniques have sub-disciplines and competing styles. As a result, practitioners doing essentially the same kind of work may have different qualifications and be registered by different organizations.

Various organizations have been established in order to regulate the field of complementary medicine. The Institute for Complementary Medicine (ICM) was established in 1982 to ensure that 'high standards of practice and training in natural health care were available to the public'. In the late 1980s they initiated the British Register of Complementary Practitioners, the aim of which was to provide members of the public with access to a list of vetted practitioners. However, the ICM remains hugely unpopular within the professional world of complementary medicine. They are perceived as wishing to dictate and rule complementary medicine and have been notorious for their lack of willingness, or ability, to work and liaise with other professional organizations. Moreover, only insignificant numbers of practitioners are registered in each of the main therapies (osteopathy, chiropractic, herbalism, homoeopathy and acupuncture). The British Complementary Medicine Association (BCMA) similarly claims to represent all groups within complementary medicine. Again, this is despite the fact that most of the major professional organizations do not wish to be associated with the BCMA.

It is apparent to many of those working within complementary medicine that the activities of the BCMA and ICM have damaged both the image and the professionalization of complementary medicine. For example, the BCMA's claim to speak for all complementary practitioners has been taken on trust by a surprising number of organizations, including the executive of the National Health Service. This is presumably because the non-unified nature of complementary medicine and the haphazard state of regulation within the field often goes unrecognized.

The future would appear to lie in statutory self-regulation of therapies on a therapy-by-therapy basis. Osteopathy and chiropractic have already succeeded in gaining statutory recognition (including protection against the use of the title 'osteopath' or 'chiropractor' by unqualified practitioners) in bills which passed in 1993 and 1994 respectively. It seems highly unlikely that massage or aromatherapy will become subject to statute in the near future. For more on the professional structure of massage and aromatherapy, see page 37.

SUMMARY

Massage and aromatherapy are often classed as forms of complementary medicine. This could be taken to suggest that they share a single body of knowledge with other complementary therapies. However, it is often argued that complementary medicine is not a unified professional discipline, rather, it is a term of convenience to group together a disparate collection of different therapies. The lack of philosophical and practical cohesion of the complementary therapies limits generalizations about 'complementary medicine' as a whole. This is reflected in the practice and organization of complementary medicine, in which a number of different governing bodies compete for recognition and status. Similarly, the medical role and scope of complementary therapies must be determined on therapy-by-therapy basis. Massage and aromatherapy should be judged on their own merits, not as part of complementary medicine.

Introduction to massage and aromatherapy

2

INTRODUCTION TO MASSAGE

Massage may be the only therapy which is instinctive: we hold and caress those we wish to comfort; when we hurt ourselves, our first reaction is to touch and rub the painful part. Almost all cultures throughout history appear to have used massage as a form of health care. Massage is part of traditions such Ayurvedic, Unani and Chinese medicine and is a routine maternal behaviour in many parts of Asia, Africa and the Pacific.

There is also a long tradition of massage in Europe. Hippocrates, famously, stated that 'The physician must be experienced in ... rubbing. For rubbing can bind a joint that is too loose and loosen a joint that is too rigid'. That said, European massage has popularly been associated more with spas and sports than with medicine. Traditional techniques were systematized in the early 18th century by Per Henrik Ling, creator of what is now known as Swedish massage. Ling felt that vigorous massage strokes could bring about healing by improving the circulation of the blood and lymph. Swedish massage has been adopted by physiotherapists, the alternative healing professions and practitioners of recreational massage. It is still in common usage.

In the past 20 years or so, complementary practitioners have adapted Swedish massage so as to place greater emphasis on the psychological and spiritual aspects of treatment. Rather than concentrating on say, stiff joints and lymph circulation, practitioners have focused on the feelings of 'wholeness', calmness and relaxation which are said to follow a good massage. One of the most prevalent ideas is that a massage of the whole body helps a person to feel 'connected' and more in touch with his or her body. Treatment has become more gentle, flowing and intuitive and now takes place in rooms specially designed for their peaceful atmosphere. The comfort of the patient has been given precedence and it is not uncommon for patients to fall asleep during a massage. This is in some contrast to the vigorous massage given in the noisy and busy environment of a 19th-century public bath.

Sensuality is also an important aspect of modern massage. One of the prime criteria for choosing a particular stroke is that of pleasure: if it feels good, it is worth using. Inkeles (1977) has pointed to the links between massage techniques and predominant social attitudes towards touch and the body. In Victorian texts, for example, great emphasis is placed on the physical benefits of massage. Absolutely no indication is given that massage is a pleasurable experience. With the advent of more liberal attitudes towards the body in the second half of the 20th century, modern massage has incorporated, and celebrated, the pleasure-giving aspects of touch. These newer forms of massage are often described as 'holistic' or 'intuitive' massage.

MASSAGE IN PRACTICE

A typical massage given by a complementary practitioner in private practice takes anywhere between 45 minutes and an hour and a half. The patient is treated, unclothed, on a specially designed massage couch. This normally incorporates soft but firm padding and a hole for the face. Without the hole, patients would have to twist their head to one side when lying front side down: this causes tightness in the neck muscles and necessitates regular changes in position. The treatment room is kept warm and quiet. Soft music may sometimes be played.

Practitioners generally treat the whole body, a typical treatment sequence being: head and neck, chest, arms and hands, front of legs, feet, back of legs, buttocks, back. A moderate amount of oil is used to help the practitioner's hands move over the patient's body. Oils widely used in massage include sweet almond, soya and safflower oil. Practitioners of aromatherapy describe these as 'carrier' oils because they provide the vehicle for the small amount of active essential oils used in aromatherapy but are themselves relatively inert.

After initial case history taking and physical preparation – undressing, towels, lying on the couch – a typical massage starts with the practitioner gently placing warmed hands on the patient's back or forehead for a minute or two. Oil is then applied to the area to be massaged first and the massage commences. Practitioners use a variety of strokes during the massage. These include: effleurage, gentle stroking along the length of a muscle; petrissage, deeper pressure applied across a muscle; kneading; friction, deep circular motions of the thumbs or fingertips and hacking, the light karate chops commonly seen in movie massage. Many strokes, however, appear to be adaptations to specific parts of the body and defy categorization.

Practitioners tend to increase the degree of pressure applied to a muscle gradually. They will start by light stroking, move on to firm pressure and perhaps use deep strokes, or special stretches, on specific areas of tightness or tension. Lighter strokes may then be used to complete work on an area of the body. Practitioners follow a number of guidelines in their use of massage strokes. These include maintaining an evenness of speed and pressure; using weight rather than muscle force to apply pressure; moulding the hands to the contours of the body and maintaining physical contact throughout the massage.

Work in particular health settings, or with particular patients, may require variations in this basic form. Time constraints often prevent the giving of full body massage and, in any case, this might embarrass or cause physical discomfort for some patients. There may also be physical limitations, such as impaired mobility, or the presence of drips and electronic monitoring equipment, which would interfere with a full body massage. Moreover, the use of certain strokes, such as deep massage, may be inappropriate in certain patients, such as those who are elderly or frail. Massage in conventional health settings therefore often consists of more limited work on the head, hands, feet or back. Massage may also take the form of a neck and shoulder rub given through clothes with the patient sitting in a chair.

DEFINITION AND INCLUSION CRITERIA FOR MASSAGE

Massage is technically described as the therapeutic manipulation of soft tissue. As such, almost all health professionals use massage in one form or another. For example, cardiac massage is a form of artificial resuscitation in which a burst of firm pressure is applied to the sternum with the heel of the hand. Similarly, massage of the carotid sinus, which causes a reflex drop in blood pressure, is used for treatment of cardiac arrhythmias in certain cases.

Soft-tissue manipulation is also a common means of treating musculoskeletal disorders. It is widely used in physiotherapy, orthopaedic medicine, chiropractic and osteopathy. Some individuals who describe themselves as practitioners of massage may use some of these specific soft-tissue techniques.

It is not the aim of this book to describe massage in all its forms. The main criterion for inclusion of a massage use or technique in this book is whether the aim of treatment is to bring about specific or non-specific effects in a patient. The book's main focus will be where massage of whole areas of the body are used to bring about non-specific improvements, such as relaxation and general feelings of well-being. Soft-tissue manipulation of a specific part of the body employed to bring about a specific effect, such as the treatment of musculoskeletal injury, will not generally be described.

As an example, compare the following two quotes. The first is from James Cyriax, a leading practitioner of physical medicine who developed a form of spinal manipulation that is named after him. The second quote is from George Downing, a teacher of massage at the Esalen growth centre in California and author of a book popular among complementary therapists.

> The site of the minor tear in the ligament should receive some minutes friction. The purpose is to disperse blood clots of effusion there, to move the ligament over subjacent bone ... and to numb it enough to facilitate movement afterwards.
>
> *Cyriax, 1985*

> Massage [brings] flowing peace and aliveness ... to the body. When receiving a good massage a person usually falls into a mental-physical state difficult to describe. [Massage conveys] trust, empathy and respect, to say nothing of a sheer sense of mutual physical existence.
>
> *Downing, 1974: 7*

The distinction between massage for specific and non-specific ends is certainly not a hard and fast one: there is obviously considerable overlap in the practices of individual therapists. That said, the distinction does correlate broadly with, on the one hand, the massage practised by physiotherapists, osteopaths and chiropractors and, on the other hand, that typically practised by complementary practitioners, nurses and occupational therapists in the settings described in this book. Sometimes, of course, this second set of practitioners will use a special technique on a limited area of the body to bring about a specific effect. Firm pressure on 'knots' in muscle tissue would be a good example. These techniques would be part of a massage covering different areas of the body, the overall aim of which would be non-specific. A patient with stiff shoulders and neck visiting a practitioner of non-specific massage would not commonly be treated by receiving firm pressure on a few particular areas of knotted tissue. It is more likely that they would receive a general body or back massage, part of which may include attention to specific areas of tension. This is in some contrast, say, to the osteopaths' traditional dictum of 'Find it, fix it, leave it alone'. In sum, the massage techniques which form the focus of this text are those which are principally non-specific in nature.

SPECIAL MASSAGE THERAPIES

Many practitioners of massage use an eclectic range of techniques. Some of these may be used to bring about specific changes in a patient, for example, for treatment of musculoskeletal pain or even asthma. As pointed out above, though such techniques will not be the main focus of this book, they will be briefly described for general information and interest.

REFLEXOLOGY

In reflexology, areas of the foot are believed to correspond to the organs or structures of the body. Damage or disease in an organ is reflected in the corresponding region, or reflex zone, of the foot. On palpation, the patient experiences pain or pricking, no matter how gently pressure is applied. Practitioners say that the particular reflex zones affected by a disease are idiosyncratic. One patient with asthma, for example, may exhibit disordered reflex zones corresponding to the endocrine system, whereas in another, these might correspond to the kidney. Reflexology treatment consists of massage of the disordered reflex zones (Figure 2.1).

Though reflexology treatment is generally very relaxing and calming, practitioners also claim to be able to elicit specific improvements in health. Successful case histories given in the classic reflexology text (Marquardt, 1983) include ataxia (muscle incoordination), epilepsy, frozen shoulder and osteoarthritis. Practitioners also claim that patients often experience symptoms said to be associated with healing in complementary medicine – diarrhoea, sweating and increased passage of urine – in the first few days and weeks after initial treatment. This is ascribed to increased activity of the elimination systems of the body and is seen as a positive sign.

The research base of reflexology is extremely narrow compared to that of most other therapies (p. 87). The basic claim in reflexology – correspondence between areas of the foot and the body – is unsubstantiated by scientific research at the current time. The effects of reflexology might well be ascribed to the relaxation afforded by a gentle foot rub. Alternatively, reflexology might be explained as a form of inadvertent acupressure (see page 22). Whatever the mechanism of reflexology, practitioners seem to have at least some therapeutic success.

Though practitioners of reflexology claim that the therapy has a range of application similar to that of say, acupuncture or homoeopathy, standards of training and qualification vary widely. The therapy remains professionally diffuse, with a large number of different teaching and registering bodies.

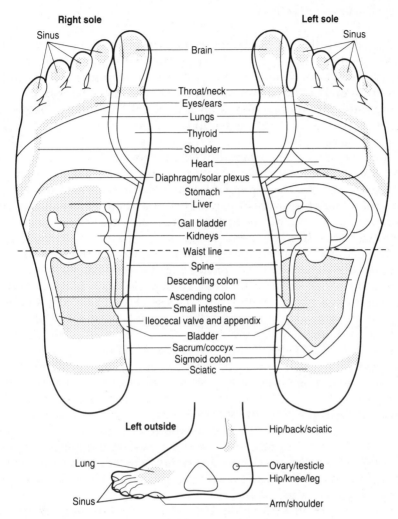

Figure 2.1 A diagram showing some of the reflex zones of the feet.

That said, a large number of physiotherapists have trained in reflexology and the technique is now recognized by the Chartered Society of Physiotherapy. Reflexology is perhaps most likely to be practised in health service settings by physiotherapists, many of whom have also trained in massage and aromatherapy and who employ reflexology whenever they feel it is clinically indicated. Similarly, some nurses and complementary practitioners specializing in massage and/or aromatherapy use reflexology techniques with selected patients.

ACUPRESSURE AND SHIATSU

Acupressure is the manipulation of the acupuncture points with the fingers. Its basic concepts are those of traditional Chinese medicine (see the section on acupuncture, p. 7). As in acupuncture, health is seen to depend on the correct flow of chi energy through the body. The acupressure practitioner makes an individualized energy diagnosis and treats particular points depending on perceived imbalances in the patient's energy flow.

There are several important differences between the two therapies. Firstly, because fingers replace needles as the primary means of affecting the flow of chi, the experience of acupressure is much more personal than that of acupuncture, with the practitioner more intimately involved in treatment. A further difference is that whereas an acupuncturist will needle perhaps four or five locations during a session, an acupressure practitioner will generally cover the whole body, though a few particular areas may be given special attention.

In many ways, acupressure may be regarded as a halfway house between massage and acupuncture: the use of touch and the involvement of the whole body are important elements of massage; the concepts of meridians and chi and the use of special points on the body to bring about specific changes are principles found in acupuncture.

In the UK, most acupressure practitioners practise what they call shiatsu. This is a Japanese system of acupressure and incorporates the principles and practices of traditional Japanese medicine. For example, diagnosis takes place on the stomach (hara diagnosis). Shiatsu treatment takes place on a thick mat on the floor, with the practitioner using the fingers, thumbs, knees and the heel of the hand to apply pressure to the *tsubo*, or acupuncture points. The practitioner may also move the patient's limbs and body during treatment, stretching a limb along the path of a meridian.

Few practitioners describing themselves primarily as masseurs or aromatherapists practise shiatsu or acupressure. This may be because training is relatively lengthy, due, no doubt, to the complexity of oriental medical philosophy. That said, many massage practitioners incorporate acupressure techniques in treatment using, for example, pressure on a few specific points if they feel that this would be of benefit.

Acupressure and shiatsu have a somewhat unusual scientific status because, though the therapies remain almost entirely unresearched, many of the underlying principles have been extensively studied. There are a number of trials that appear to demonstrate that the concepts of traditional Chinese medicine have at least some validity. Moreover, there is evidence that manual pressure to an acupuncture point may elicit specific physical changes. Research on shiatsu and acupressure is discussed on page 89.

CONNECTIVE TISSUE MASSAGE

Connective tissue massage (CTM) was developed by Dicke *et al.* (1978) after a self-cure from a serious illness. Originally known as *Bidegewebsmassage* the therapy is based on the principle that particular regions of the back correspond to the organs and structures of the body.

Massage of the back is used both diagnostically and therapeutically. Strokes use the little, middle and ring fingers of one hand and are applied slowly, and relatively deeply, perpendicular to underlying structures so as to create traction between the cutaneous and subcutaneous tissues. No lubricant is used. The strokes may cause a painful sensation, often described as 'cutting' or 'scratching'. This is said to indicate a pathological condition in the organ corresponding to the part of the back being massaged. Though all parts of the body may be treated, CTM always begins with the lumbosacral region of the back. The patient is treated either standing or sitting in a specially designed chair.

CTM has been said to be of benefit for patients with conditions as diverse as osteoarthritis, asthma, angina, migraine, musculoskeletal injury and intermittent claudication (Ebner, 1985). Like reflexology, CTM is not scientifically substantiated at the current time of writing, though there is a considerable body of speculation as to its mechanisms. Ebner (1985) claims that links between the superficial tissues of the back and the organs stem from the embryological development of the nervous system. CTM is also said to act by improving blood circulation, decreasing muscle spasm and improving the elasticity of the connective tissue.

CTM has been reported to be widely used by European physical therapists to treat both musculoskeletal and visceral disorders (Reed and Held, 1988). However, its use in the US and, especially, the UK, has been limited. The patient's sitting posture, the relatively strong and painful strokes used and the focus on a limited part of the body reduce CTM's similarity with other types of massage. This should be borne in mind when considering the research on CTM in Chapter 4.

BODYWORK

A number of specialist therapies involve idiosyncratic techniques of soft-tissue manipulation. These are often described as 'bodywork' therapies. Typically, each therapy is practised by a relatively limited number of individuals. Some practitioners combine different techniques into their own personal system of treatment.

Though bodywork practitioners do treat individuals with musculoskeletal complaints, many of their clients are actors, musicians and sports professionals seeking to enhance performance. Those without particular health problems may also visit for the purpose of general health and well-being, sometimes described in psychological terms. In the words of one practitioner, 'the goal … is to help us rediscover the essence of who we are' (Wooten, 1994).

An example of a classic case study gives an insight to the therapeutic ends of bodywork practices. Ida Rolf, the founder of a technique called 'Rolfing' (see below), has compared the footprint of an Aborigine to that of an American before and after treatment (Rolf, 1977). Following a course of Rolfing, the American's footprint was said to approximate to that of the Aborigine. This was used as the basis for a claim that Rolfing helps return posture and balance to a natural optimum.

Rolfing is one of the more prevalent bodywork therapies and is reasonably representative of the field. The technique uses strong pressure to reorganize the structures of the body. The aim of the therapy is to align the body in an optimal position with respect to gravity, something which allows a person to stand erect, and make other movements, with less muscular effort.

The work itself consists of a cycle of 10 hour-long sessions, each focusing on a different area of the body. Strong pressure is applied with the hands to parts of the body where muscle tendons are felt to adhere to each other, rather than sliding over one another in a normal way. The pressure used in Rolfing is firm enough to cause pain, but this is said to be accompanied by a sense of well-being and emotional release.

Rolfing is also typical in that, like many bodywork therapies, it is named after the individual who created the technique. Other body therapies include Rosenwork, Hellerwork, Trager, Bowen and Zero Balancing. Practitioners who use techniques of psychotherapy massage, or soft-tissue manipulation, may also describe themselves as bodywork practitioners. These techniques are described below.

PSYCHOTHERAPY MASSAGE

The links between psychology and muscle tone are widely recognized: 'tense' can be used to describe both a muscle and a mental state. In addition, particular patterns of muscular tension (postures, facial expressions and so on) are associated with particular emotions. Attention to the body is therefore a standard technique in psychotherapy. Therapists look at how a patient is sitting, standing, talking and moving as a means of psychological insight.

Some practitioners go further and use massage-like work with the body to aid the psychotherapeutic process. This is thought to be of benefit for a number of non-specific reasons. For example, massage can help develop trust between practitioner and client and fulfil a patient's need to be touched. However, the specific aim of psychotherapy massage is what has been termed 'dearmouring' (McNeely, 1987). It is thought that persistently high levels of muscle tension can constitute a 'somatic defence system' that prevents access to the unconscious in a similar manner to the conventional concept of psychological resistance. Work on the body to release muscle tension is said to be of general benefit, reducing 'somatic resistance' to psychological growth. In simple language, when we are relaxed, we tend to open up more. Practitioners also claim that specific areas of tension correspond to specific psychological difficulties: for example, release of particular areas of tension is said sometimes to result in 'flashbacks' to early childhood trauma. Practitioners may also work with the body as a direct means of exploring the unconscious: a patient might be encouraged to adopt a certain posture and asked to reflect on any feelings or memories that the posture evokes.

An important proponent of psychotherapy massage is Lowen, whose *Bioenergetics* (1976) and *The Language Of The Body* (1971) remain influential works. Lowen proposes that the body can express the unconscious. The general concept is surely not one that many would seriously contest, even though it is often crudely articulated by Lowen: take, for example, 'a weakness in the backbone must be reflected in serious personality disturbance. The individual with sway back cannot have the ego strength of a person whose back is straight' (Lowen, 1971: 102). Lowen also proposes that inappropriate muscular tension can prevent proper psychological functioning. This is linked to an idiosyncratic model of psychology in which a individual's 'core' is surrounded by various levels of physical and psychological defences. Work on the physical body is said to help break down these defences and promote better physical and psychological health. For more on the links between massage and psychotherapy, see pages 74, 207 and 217.

SOFT-TISSUE MANIPULATION

Some massage practitioners treat musculoskeletal disorders – for example, back or neck pain – by using specific techniques of soft-tissue manipulation on specific parts of the body. Many of these techniques were originally developed by osteopaths, chiropractors and physiotherapists and have been adopted by massage practitioners keen to extend their therapeutic repertoire. A number of soft-tissue techniques will be described below. Practitioners tend to be eclectic and may incorporate many different techniques in the treatment of one patient (Chaitow, 1988).

Stretching

Practitioners may use a variety of muscle-stretching techniques. The patient may either be passive or may be asked to contract certain muscles at the same time as the stretch (active techniques). Stretching is thought to relax contracted muscle in a number of different ways: increasing pressure on a tendon can cause a reflex relaxation of a muscle; alternatively, stretching a muscle can cause inhibition of its antagonist (reciprocal inhibition). Stretching is also claimed to increase circulation and stimulate hypotonic (flaccid) muscle in some instances. Some practitioners use a stretching technique knows as 'myofascial release'. To treat hip pain, for example, the practitioner would apply a gentle, prolonged pull to the leg while slowly rotating it in the hip joint. If the practitioner detects a restriction of movement, however slight, the leg is held at the point of restriction until 'release' occurs. This is described as a 'softening' or 'letting go' of muscle tissue.

Soft-tissue lesions

A number of different techniques involve identification and treatment of soft-tissue lesions. These generally use deep pressure on what are variously described as 'contractions', 'congestions', 'nodules' or 'knots'. It is thought that application of pressure causes the 'release' of restricted tissue. Rolfing is one of the most well-known techniques and is described above. Neuromuscular technique (NMT) is a systematic series of thumb strokes of the soft tissues of the whole body. The practitioner feels for an area of contraction and gradually increases pressure until the contraction is released. Some practitioners also pay attention to what are known as trigger points. These are tender spots on muscles or tendons which can cause referred pain. The presence of trigger points is also said to shorten and weaken a muscle. Deep manual pressure directly on the point causes pain but can used to 'deactivate' the lesion. Trigger points can also be deactivated by acupuncture. For more on this subject, see Baldry (1993).

Muscle energy techniques (MET)

MET involves using the patient's muscular effort in combination with that of the practitioner. It is best explained by example. Take the case of a patient who cannot turn his head to the left due to spasm in the muscles of the right side of the neck. The patient moves the head slowly leftwards to the point of resistance, where pain and restriction of motion would normally occur. The practitioner then uses isometric force (equal and constant pressure so that there is no movement) against the patient's attempt to turn further. Alternatively, the practitioner may attempt to turn the patient's head to the left as the patient uses isometric force to resist. The therapeutic effect of MET is thought to result from relaxation of the contracting muscle, or its antagonist, following the period of isometric contraction. Other terms used to describe MET include 'post-isometric contraction', 'proprioceptive neuromuscular facilitation' and 'contract–relax/hold–relax'.

Strain/counterstrain

This technique involves the identification of tender points in soft tissue. Treatment occurs by positioning of a joint so that pressure on the tender point no longer causes pain. The joint is held in this position for approximately 90 seconds and then moved slowly back to a neutral position. This is thought to interrupt a positive feedback cycle in which pain increases neuronal activity and vice versa.

INTRODUCTION TO AROMATHERAPY

Aromatherapy may be defined as the therapeutic use of aromatic substances extracted from plants. The most important class of these substances is known as the essential oils. These are generally extracted from plant material by distillation, though some oils are extracted by physical expression. 'Concretes' and 'absolutes', which are extracted by chemical solvents, are also used, albeit relatively rarely, by some aromatherapists. For the purposes of this text, 'essential oil' will be used as the generic term to denote all active preparations administered in aromatherapy.

The essential oil yield of plants varies widely, but is generally low. Many hundreds of kilograms of plant may be required to produce a litre of essential oil. The oils are therefore extremely expensive and sold in small amounts, generally 10 ml.

Essential oils are made up of many component substances and these have numerous uses in the food, fragrance and pharmaceutical industry. Aromatherapists, however, only use whole essential oils from a single botanical source. These are named after the plant from which they are extracted. A list of some typical oils used by aromatherapists is given in Table 2.1.

Table 2.1 Some common oils used by aromatherapists

- Basil (*Ocimum basilicum*)
- Bergamot (*Citrus bergamia*)
- Black pepper (*Piper nigrum*)
- Cedarwood (*Cedrus atlantica*)
- Clary sage (*Salvia sclarea*)
- Roman camomile (*Anthemis nobiles*)
- Ginger (*Zingiber officinale*)
- Juniper (*Juniperus communis*)
- Lavender (*Lavendula angustifolia*)
- Lemongrass (*Cymbopogon citratus*)
- Neroli (*Citrus aurantium amara*)
- Peppermint (*Mentha piperita*)
- Rose (*Rosa damascena*)
- Rosemary (*Rosmarinus officinalis*)
- Sandalwood (*Santalum album*)
- Savory (*Satureja montana*)
- Tea tree (*Melaleuca alternifolia*)
- Ylang ylang (*Cananga odorata*)

Essential oils are commonly adulterated by the addition of alcohol, isolates from cheaper essential oils and synthetic chemicals. In addition, some oils, melissa in particular, may be chemically fabricated. Aromatherapists believe that unadulterated natural oils are the most effective. Consequently, they are keen to ensure good quality control and accreditation of the source of an oil.

Aromatherapists administer essential oils by a number of routes. The most widely used form of administration in the UK and US is massage. A few drops of one or more essential oils are added to the 'carrier' oil used as the lubricant. The oils add a pleasing aroma and are thought to enter the bloodstream via inhalation or directly through the skin. However, the amounts involved are likely to be small. Tisserand and Balacs (1995:25) estimate that 5–25 ml of essential oil at a 1–5% concentration may be applied during an aromatherapy massage. Of this, only 4–25% will actually be absorbed, the rest evaporating from the surface of the skin. This gives a range of 0.002–0.3 ml or 0.05–6 drops of oil entering the bloodstream, though a typical range is more likely to be 0.025–0.1 ml (0.5–2 drops). The figures for inhalation are likely to be even smaller. Though many aromatherapists give a general, full body massage, some may give massage to specific parts of the body, aiming for optimal delivery of essential oils to the affected organ. For example, a patient complaining of menstrual pain may receive massage with essential oils to the pelvic area.

Oils may be added to baths or vaporized. Though a number of special devices exist to vaporize essential oils, simple methods include adding of a few drops to a bowl of hot water, a tissue or a pillow cover. Essential oils may also be applied topically to the mouth and throat in the form of mouthwashes and to the vagina via tampons soaked in an essential oil solution.

Oral administration of essential oils is a contentious topic in aromatherapy. While said to be used relatively widely in France, oral administration is rare in the UK and US. Though it is the simplest and quickest means of administration, and would seem to allow maximum control over dosing, oral administration is also likely to involve the greatest risk of adverse effects. It is on these grounds that many aromatherapists avoid the practice.

The general form of aromatherapy treatment is broadly similar to the massage treatment as described on page 17. The case history may take longer, because of the need for detailed information to guide the prescription of oils. In addition, patients may be offered a choice of oils to smell before treatment commences, in case they wish to express a preference. Aromatherapists may supplement hands-on treatment with oils prescribed for use by the patient at home, either by self-massage, in the bath or in a vaporizer.

PHARMACOLOGY OF ESSENTIAL OILS

The chemistry of essential oils is extremely complex. The oils consist of a mixture of a number of constituent fractions including hydrocarbons, oxygenated hydrocarbon derivatives (such as alcohols, ketones and esters), benzenoid aromatics (such as phenols) and nitrogen and sulphur compounds, though these latter two are not widely found in the essential oils commonly used by aromatherapists. A single oil may contain 100 or more different compounds, some of which will be present in low proportions, less than 0.01%.

Essential oils may be analysed in a number of different ways. One of the most important methods is gas chromatography (GC), which can be used to estimate the proportion of each compound in an oil. One particularly interesting finding (Chialva et al., 1982) is that there are significant differences between GC analysis of whole aromatic herbs and that of their essential oils. In particular, some particularly volatile compounds are found in the former but not the latter. This is of value in understanding the relationship between aromatherapy and herbal medicine (see also p. 142).

GC analysis has also demonstrated that the proportion of each compound in an oil varies according to the variety of the plant, the region where it grew and the stage in the life cycle at which it was harvested. For example, Stahl (1986) compared variations in the essential oil composition of *Thymus pulegioides* plants collected in different localities in Norway. The plants could be divided into two categories, known as chemotypes, which exhibited markedly different essential oil profiles. In one chemotype, the essential oil contained 40% carvacrol and 1% thymol; in the other, 4% carvacrol and 40% thymol. Similarly, Ravid and Putievsky (1986) found that the essential oils of two chemotypes of oregano growing wild in the east Mediterranean differed such that the thymol context was either 85% or 4% and the carvacrol content 2% or 63%. Chalchat *et al.* (1993) found that the chemical composition of rosemary oil varied depending on the country where the herb was harvested. For example, 1,8-cineole comprised 50% of the oil in samples from North Africa, 20% of Spanish samples but only 5–7% in one French batch. Similarly, the proportion of bornyl acetate is generally under 1% but reaches 10–15% in some French samples. Marotti *et al.* (1994) investigated variation in the essential content of fennel oil depending on stage of harvesting. The ratios of limonene to (E)-anethole in oils from plants harvested at three different stages were as follows: 38:47; 45:42; 81:5. The variation in the character of essential oils distilled from the same species has been recognized since at least the early part of this century (Baker and Smith, 1920).

It is interesting to compare GC analyses of essential oils from different species. Firstly, a number of compounds are found in a significant proportion of oils. These include alpha-pinene, limonene, 1,8-cineole (also known as eucalyptol), linalool and linalyl acetate. Nerol, geraniol, camphene and myrcene are also common constituents of essential oils, though these tend to be found in low concentrations (under 5%). An example of the constituents of some commonly used oils is given in Table 2.2.

It is clear from the table that many of the most popular aromatherapy oils contain relatively similar constituent compounds. Some compounds, alpha-pinene for example, are relatively ubiquitous. It is also apparent that differences between samples of the same oil collected from different sources can sometimes be as great as those between oils of different species. Moreover, some oils have relatively similarly profiles. The major constituents of clary sage, lavender and petitgrain, for example, are linalool and linalyl acetate. However, the three oils do not smell alike and they are given different properties by aromatherapists: Price (1993: 267), for example, ascribes seven indications for clary sage in genito-urinary conditions, three for lavender and none at all for petitgrain. Such indications could only be accurate if the pharmacological properties of essential oils are not predictable from their major constituents. Aromatherapists claim that this is because the properties of essential oils depend on compounds present in low

Table 2.2 Chemical composition in percentages of selected essential oils – note that not all constituents are shown and some values are estimates (data from Formacek (1982))

	Clary sage	Juniper	Lavender	Lemon-grass	Petti-grain	Rose-mary[A]	Rose-mary[B]
Alpha-pinene	0.25	70.82	1.53	0.24	0.22	10.38	24.50
Beta-pinene	0.29	13.67	0.68		1.57	0.47	2.96
Myrcene	0.20	2.67	0.29	0.46	1.96		1.71
Limonene	0.51	2.58	2.06	2.42	1.05	1.16	4.70
Delta-3-carene		0.03	0.11		0.39		0.19
Borneol			0.85			3.47	
Geraniol	0.16	0.12	0.44	3.80	2.24	1.27	
1,8-cineole	0.15		4.31			22.07	22.59
Linalool	18.62		42.44	1.34	26.62	0.38	0.47
Linalyl acetate	69.93		22.04		50.81		
Nerol	0.06		0.15	0.39	0.95		
Alpha-terpineol	0.70	0.57	1.22	0.38	5.10		
Neryl acetate	0.26				1.69		
Geranyl acetate	0.49		0.60	1.95	2.89	0.28	
beta-Ocimene cis&trans			1.64	0.13	1.81		
Terpinen-4-ol		2.19	5.39				1.01
Para-Cymene	0.06	1.39	1.06		0.07	2.41	2.61
Camphor			3.67			18.19	22.79
Camphene	0.06	0.81	0.76		0.11	9.49	7.80
Sabinene	0.06	0.33	0.13		0.30		
Beta-caro-phyllene			2.67	0.32	0.67		
Citral a&b				81.25			
No. of other compounds*	5	8	0	6	2	3	1

*Number of compounds identified by Formacek in more than trace amounts.
A and B: Samples of oil collected from different sources

proportions and, moreover, may be influenced by complex interactions between different constituents.

This last point is worth discussing in more detail. Aromatherapists say that the presence of a large number of different compounds in essential oils improves efficacy and reduces adverse effects. The first property is ascribed to the 'synergistic' action of essential oil constituents. Two agents are said to have a synergistic action if their effect when administered together is greater than the sum of their actions when administered independently. For example, co-trimoxazole, a drug used to treat pneumonia in AIDS, contains two antibiotics, neither of which is effective alone for this infection. The second effect, reduction of adverse side-effects, is ascribed to the 'quenching' action of certain essential oil constituents on others. It is said that the presence of an essential oil constituent which is, say, a skin irritant, is offset by the presence of a second component which negates this effect. There is at least some evidence that the three claims described above – importance of minor constituents, synergy and quenching – do indeed hold. This research in aromatherapy is discussed from page 143 on.

INTRODUCTION TO THE SENSE OF SMELL

Steve Van Toller, Director, Warwick Olfaction Research Group, Warwick University

In 1587, Michel de Montaigne, a French essayist, wrote: 'Physicians might, I believe, make greater use of scents than they do, for I have often noticed that they cause changes in me, and act on my spirits according to their qualities ....' Since that time, the sense of smell has tended to be relegated to the status of a minor sense in humans and has not been seen as a credible subject of scientific research. During the last decade there has been a steadily increasing number of research studies questioning the presumed minor role for the olfactory sense (Van Toller and Dodd, 1991, 1992; Serby and Chobor, 1992; Getchell *et al.*, 1991). Increasing interest in the sense of smell has also been reflected in works of fiction (Suskind, 1985; Robbins, 1991) and collections of general essays (Lake, 1989; Dorland, 1993).

There can be little doubt that smell is the predominant sense for most animals. A great deal of salient information is contained by an odour left by another animal. This is particularly true for odour communication between animals of the same species, where marking-odours are a particularly important form of information exchange. In some cases, smell has evolved as a mechanism for controlling stereo-typical behaviour. For example, an animal will mate with another animal of the opposite sex having a certain odour.

Humans have evolved as essentially cognitive or thinking animals and smell does not automatically elicit behaviours such as mating. However, this does not mean that the sense of smell is no longer significant in human behaviour. The question becomes one of working out how this process occurs.

THE BASIS OF OLFACTION

Odour molecules

The fundamental units of olfaction are odour molecules. These are volatile and are both water- and fat-soluble, in order to penetrate the mucus layer above the olfactory receptors in the nose and the cellular walls of the receptors. Humans are very sensitive to odorous molecules. For example, the average person can detect 1 gram of butyric acid, a sweaty, cheese smell (called a 'note') dispersed throughout a 10-storey building.

Odour molecules reach the olfactory receptors via the nose. The average person breathes about 8 litres of air every minute. Most people consider that the nose is the organ of smell but in fact the airways of the nose serve only to adjust the temperature and humidity of the breathed air before it is passed down to the delicate tissues of the lungs. Table 2.3, taken from Van Toller, Dodd and Billing (1985) where a full discussion can be found, shows a range of chemicals used in an olfactory study carried out at Warwick University on the effects of ageing.

The table includes aspects of the odorous molecules such as molecular weight, chemical structure, and occurrence. Normally smells are called by the object that releases them. For example, the fishy note is produced by the chemical trimethylamine which is the correct name for the smell. Similarly, a rose smell is produced by the chemical phenylethanol.

The nose and olfactory receptors

The nose can be thought of as a pyramid whose apex consists of a small chamber. The olfactory receptors are found lining the roof. The average size of the olfactory tissue in a human is that of a small postage stamp, half being located at the top of each nostril. A sniff causes an eddy of air to pass into the upper olfactory chamber where odorous molecules come into contact with receptors on the hair-like cilia at the ends of the olfactory cells. Incoming molecules fit into receptor sites and initiate an electrochemical reaction, in a 'lock and key' action. In the same way that the correct key will turn the tumblers of a lock, so the correctly fitting molecule will initiate an electrochemical event in the olfactory cell. A critical amount of stimulation by odour molecules will cause the olfactory receptor to become activated and pass a nervous impulse to the brain. The number of molecules needed to stimulate an olfactory cell varies, but with some odours it can be as low as 40. At this level of stimulation a person might be able to detect a smell but would not be able to say what the smell was.

Olfactory tissue

Olfactory tissues consist basically of four types of cell: olfactory cells, basal cells, supporting cells and mucus-secreting cells. The average life cycle for an olfactory cell is about a month. The basal cells grow

Table 2.3 Examples of odourant molecules

Name	Mol. wt	Chemical structure	Odour	Occurence
Trimethylamine	59	$(CH_3)_3N$	Fishy	Fish
1–valeric acid	102	COOH	Sweaty Cheesy	Sweat Foods
Phenylethanol	122	$CH_{20}CH_{20}OH$	Rosewater	Rose flowers
2-acetyl pyrazine	126		Roasted popcorn	Roasted foods
Menthone	154		Minty	Essential oils
2-isobutyl-3-methoxy-pyrazine	166		Green	Green peppers
Dodecyl mercaptan	202	SH	Petrol-like	Petroleum oils
5-α-androst-16-en -3-one	272		Urinous	Urine sweat
Musk ketone	294		Musky	Perfumes
Acetic acid	60	CH_3COOH	Vinegar (trigeminal)	Vinegar

and mature into functional olfactory cells to replace the old cells which decompose and are broken down. The olfactory nerves gather together and pass through the cribriform plate, a bone at the base of the brain, through tiny holes arranged like a 'pepper-pot'. This arrangement makes the olfactory nerves very vulnerable to blows on the head. The tiny olfactory nerves then enter the olfactory bulbs, which lie on the underside of the brain. Inside the olfactory bulbs the information from individual nerves is collected together and amplified into electrochemical signals that are passed to the brain.

Brain circuits of the olfactory system

The point at which the olfactory nerves become integrated with general brain activity is known as the limbic system. The old name for this part of the brain was the rhinencephalon, or the nose-brain. The limbic system is a complex inner area of the brain concerned with emotion and motivation. The system makes rapid parallel decisions integrating the brain with parts of the body. For example, the limbic system directs bodily motor output in eating, sexual activity and fighting. It also controls the autonomic nervous system and certain hormones (Van Toller, 1979). The limbic system has specific areas that govern moods and it directs non-verbal speech. It is constantly active but vulnerable to dysfunction and the action of drugs.

A crucial point concerning the limbic system relates to its lack of verbal functions. Speech requires involvement of cortical areas of the brain found on the outer surfaces of the left hemisphere. Most people find it easy to say if they like an odour, or recall if an odour evokes a forgotten memory yet often find it difficult to name or describe a smell.

In sum, the part of the brain associated with olfaction is intimately connected with the part associated with motivation, emotion and non-verbal thought. It may be that we can manipulate these basic functions by using the sense of smell. This possibility underpins contemporary interest in the therapeutic use of odour.

SUMMARY

- Massage may be defined as the therapeutic manipulation of soft tissue.
- A wide variety of different techniques may be described as 'massage'.
- Traditional European massage is often described as 'Swedish massage' and tends to emphasize the physical benefits of treatment.

- Recently, attention has also focused on the spiritual and emotional aspects of treatment: in particular, it is thought that a massage treatment should generally be relaxing and pleasurable. This is often described as 'holistic' or 'intuitive' massage.
- Practitioners may use elements of other complementary therapies such as reflexology, shiatsu or healing.
- Practitioners may also incorporate techniques specifically designed to treat musculoskeletal disorders.
- This book will not cover all techniques in depth and will focus primarily on non-specific massage treatment.
- Aromatherapy is the therapeutic use of aromatic substances extracted from plants.
- Most commonly, essential oils, which are produced by distillation of a single type of plant, are applied in dilute form by massage.
- The oils may also be added to baths or vaporized. They are rarely taken by mouth in the UK and US.
- Essential oils contain a large number of organic compounds, some of which are present in extremely small quantities.
- There may be great variation in the proportion of constituent compounds found in a particular essential oil, depending on the variety of the plant, where it was grown and when it was harvested.
- There may be significant similarities in the chemical make-up of different essential oils.
- If the pharmacological properties of essential oils are as aromatherapists claim, they are not predictable from the major constituent compounds. This is said to be because these properties are affected by compounds present in trace amounts and by complex interactions between different constituents.
- Olfactory nerves become integrated with general brain activity in the limbic system. This part of the brain is concerned with emotion, motivation, the autonomic nervous system and the regulation of certain hormones. This raises the possibility that these functions can be manipulated by using the sense of smell.

Massage and aromatherapy: an overview of practice

3

WHO PRACTISES MASSAGE AND AROMATHERAPY?

Massage and aromatherapy are widely, perhaps predominantly, practised in non-professional contexts: it is common for friends or relatives to exchange back massages and the home use of essential oils, for example, as bath additives, appears to be growing. This chapter will concentrate on the use of the therapies by health professionals.

Data on the numbers and demographic characteristics of massage and aromatherapy practitioners is extremely hard to come by. This is because the two disciplines are relatively unregulated and there are no central bodies through which appropriate data can be reliably collated. One of the few estimates in circulation is that of the Aromatherapy Organisations Council who claim that their associated schools have trained some 5000 practitioners in the UK. One reason why it is impossible to use this figure to estimate the level of practice in the UK is that a significant proportion of those who undertake training in massage and aromatherapy do not become full-time therapists. For many this is a voluntary decision: some receive training out of general interest and do not intend to practise professionally; others do not wish to practise full-time. Moreover, building up a practice remains a significant problem and many practitioners appear to work part-time because of a lack of clients. As an illustration, in 1991, the secretary of the Association of Massage Practitioners was a librarian who retained his day job for fear of being unable to generate sufficient massage work.

A further complication is that the many nurses and other health professionals who learn massage or aromatherapy frequently do not do so through established schools. Few join representative bodies after completing their courses and the proportion who go on to use massage and aromatherapy in practice can only be guessed at.

Perhaps the most reliable means of estimating the extent of aromatherapy practice is through population-based surveys. In a pilot study, Thomas *et al.* (1993) found that from a sample of just over 700 UK residents, 33 had visited an osteopath in the previous 12 months. Only one individual reported visiting a practitioner of aromatherapy; three had received massage. Given that there are some 2000 registered osteopaths in the UK, it would be reasonable to conclude that there are probably, at most, no more than the equivalent of say, 400–500 full-time masseurs or aromatherapists practising in the UK. However, this estimate is relatively unreliable because the sample size of the study was fairly small.

In short, the sociology of massage and aromatherapy is a subject almost completely devoid of workable information. A few general observations based on anecdotal evidence may, however, be of interest.

WHERE DO PRACTITIONERS TRAIN?

Practitioners of massage train in all manner of settings. A small proportion may have received no training at all and practice intuitively, perhaps having learnt 'on the job' or from friends or relatives. At the opposite extreme, a small number of practitioners have received extensive training in disciplines such as osteopathy or physiotherapy and have decided to utilize that training to practise massage.

Many practitioners of massage learn from small, informal training institutions. These are often established by only one or two practitioners and are generally located in the practitioners' own home or clinic. A typical course might take place one weekend a month over an 8-month period. Practitioners may take separate classes in anatomy and physiology, often as part of a general certificate, such as that of the International Therapy Examination Council. Such courses are sometimes given rather grandiose titles such as 'Diploma Course in Therapeutic Massage'. Students successfully completing the course are eligible for registration with any number of small governing bodies.

There are a number of more formal teaching institutions which, for example, hold regular courses, or have rooms set aside specifically for the teaching of massage or aromatherapy. These institutions tend to offer longer and more in-depth courses often leading to registration with some form of regulatory body, typically one associated exclusively with that college. For example, the Massage Therapy Institute of Great Britain only registers individuals successfully completing a course at the Clare Maxwell-Hudson School of Massage.

Courses in aromatherapy are generally, but not always, longer and more structured than massage courses, simply because more information needs to be taught. An aromatherapy course might typically consist of 200 hours of lectures and practicals spread over a number of weekends. Usually, a little less than half of the course is dedicated to essential oils. Teaching of massage and bodywork – often involving a large number of different techniques: acupressure, joint mobilization, soft-tissue massage and cranio-sacral therapy – may comprise a further 75–100 hours with the remaining 50–75 hours consisting of instruction in anatomy, physiology and clinical science.

There are perhaps three points worth making about the teaching of massage and aromatherapy.

1) Teaching standards vary

There is no single set of standards applicable to all schools. Most teachers have their own favourite horror stories of bad practices taking place in 'other' institutions. Essentially, this is the discourse of quackery: poor teaching is always taking place somewhere else. As Sharma (1991) has pointed out, quacks in modern day complementary therapy have a similar property to witches in medieval times: everyone presumes they exist but it is difficult for an independent investigator to locate one with any ease. That said, the current variation in the teaching of massage and aromatherapy is widely recognized to be a problem. It is likely to remain that way if the professions remain as fragmented and unregulated as they are at the time of writing.

2) Most courses are relatively short

Even the most comprehensive aromatherapy courses involve only about 200–300 hours in-class training. This is equivalent to a term or at most, a term and a half, of a standard academic training, such as that received by doctors, physiotherapists or chiropractors. Given that massage techniques and the use of essential oils form a significant part of any training, courses typically leave only 50–75 hours for teaching in anatomy, physiology and clinical science. Few, if any, schools have entry requirements such as scientific qualifications, and requirements for continuing professional education are limited. It is therefore probable that many practitioners of massage and aromatherapy practise with only an extremely limited understanding of basic medicine and science. Moreover, because of the condensed nature of these courses, little more than the basic techniques and principles of therapy are taught. What is being offered is a training: the courses offer sparse opportunity for the development of critical, reflective and interpretative abilities. Original research, one of the most fundamental elements in higher education, is almost entirely absent. The status of massage and aromatherapy schools as training establishments, rather than educational institutions, is seen by some to be the major obstacle to the development of the therapies as fully fledged professions.

3) Most courses teach within the context of an unconventional world-view

Massage and aromatherapy are often explicitly linked to specific and unconventional beliefs about medicine, food and life in general. The precise nature of this medical world-view, as expressed in the aromatherapy literature, is discussed below. What is worth stressing here is that, rather than a pragmatic approach to the role of massage and aromatherapy within health care, the therapies are often taught as part of a package of beliefs.

For example, at a weekend course on massage for nurses, the tutors began the day by teaching some yoga-like postures and stretches. In introducing these exercises, the tutors made references to acupuncture meridians and to chi, the life force postulated in traditional Chinese medicine. Photocopied instructions were then handed out to each nurse and it was explicitly suggested that they should practise the exercises every morning as an aid to good general health. During the day, the tutors were not adverse to disparaging conventional medicine – one even going so far as to describe oncologists as the 'cut, burn and poison brigade' – and reference was frequently made to the importance and utility of other complementary therapies, such as reflexology and aromatherapy.

There are those who welcome this approach to the teaching of complementary therapies. The emphasis on personal well-being, on becoming a 'living example for the therapies you promote', has been hailed as a radical and positive shift away from traditional therapist and patient roles. The doctrine of holistic medicine is also invoked to support the sort of teaching discussed above. However, there are those who wonder why the learning of a simple, useful technique such as a relaxing foot massage need be linked to a wider set of beliefs about health.

WHERE AND HOW IS MASSAGE AND AROMATHERAPY PRACTISED?

The practice of massage and aromatherapy by conventional health professionals is covered in detail in Part Two. Practice by non-medically qualified practitioners is also covered in this section, in so far as this practice occurs in conventional health settings.

A significant proportion of massage and aromatherapy practice takes place in private clinics in the community. Many practitioners establish treatment rooms in their own homes. They generate custom through the professional registers and advertisements in local health stores and the health press though, generally, most patients hear of practitioners through word-of-mouth. Practitioners may do 'out-calls' and visit clients in their own homes. Treatment is a private business transaction between practitioner and client and the number and length of sessions is by mutual agreement.

Some practitioners also rent rooms from natural health clinics. These clinics are rarely anything more than a number of individual practices with each practitioner working in effective isolation from the others. Space, bills, advertising and reception areas are shared: health care is not. Patients organize treatment with individual practitioners, and though there may be informal cross-referrals, no package of care is offered by the clinic.

Hotels, health clubs, gyms and beauty parlours may also offer massage and aromatherapy. Many practitioners are extremely disparaging about such practice. Typically, they claim that standards of training are low in such settings. Though this might well be the case, one might also see some practitioners' aversion to 'health and beauty' massage as an attempt to distance themselves from such practice and thereby locate themselves firmly within a medical context.

There is evidence (Eisenberg *et al.*, 1993) that most individuals using private complementary health services in the community do not inform their primary care physician that they are doing so. It is likely that massage and aromatherapy, as practised privately in the community, comprises a fragmented part of a piecemeal pattern of care.

CORE BELIEFS IN MASSAGE AND AROMATHERAPY

A large number of books have been published on massage and aromatherapy. These books provide one useful starting point for understanding the professional world of the two therapies.

BOOKS ON MASSAGE

The literature of massage is distinguished from that of aromatherapy by the lack of a distinct medical orientation. It is difficult to find mention of medical conditions – apart from occasional references to the role of stress in hypertension, ulcers, insomnia and the like – and certainly massage is rarely associated with the treatment of specific diseases. Moreover, the effects of massage therapy are not often discussed in medical terms. This is in contrast to the aromatherapy literature, in which essential oils are said to be antiseptic, analgesic, sedative, diuretic and so on. Discussions of mainstream medicine are also virtually non-existent in massage books, something which is again in distinct contrast to the literature of aromatherapy.

The larger part of most texts on massage consists of detailed instructions as to how to give a massage. The parts of the body are covered in turn, with a number of different strokes recommended for each. As such, massage books tend to be heavily illustrated.

One of the main themes of the massage literature is that the physical body is a reflection of a person's psychological health. Emotional tension may be expressed as muscular tension, often leading to characteristic postures. Indeed, many books have descriptions or photographs of postures said to be associated with tension, depression or fatigue. Some even describe postures associated with personalities such as 'the intellectual', 'the macho' or 'the stoic'.

> Your body constantly mirrors every aspect of yourself. Your personality, emotions, attitudes, and how you relate to the world and others: all are apparent in your body.
>
> *Lacroix, 1991: 14*

> Tension ... is a stiffness or tightening of the muscles and the connective tissue ... its origin is mostly ... emotional.
>
> *Downing, 1974: 140*

Massage of the body is said to relax muscles and habitual postures and thereby improve both mental and physical health. Improvements in the latter are often described in rather esoteric terms. For example, massage may be said to result in the release of fear. Alternatively, it may generate a feeling of 'rootedness' or of being open to change.

Massage may also be said to improve sleep, vitality and perceived well-being and to treat minor aches and pains. Reference may sometimes be made to general physiological effects of massage, such as increased circulation or improved muscle tone. However, great emphasis tends to be placed on massage as an end in itself. As a pleasurable, social activity, the massage literature often promotes massage as an enjoyable part of everyday life, just as to fish, walk or cook is promoted as a rewarding activity in books on angling, hiking or food. In sum, massage is often seen not so much as a medical therapy, but a means of pleasure and enjoyment, and possibly also of personal growth and development.

Massage books for the health professional

A small number of books have been published which are aimed at practising massage therapists or other health professionals. These include Hollis (1987); Wood and Becke (1981); Licht (1963); Tappan

(1978); Beck (1988); and Chaitow (1988). Though, like the popular 'how to' guide, these texts consist primarily of detailed instructions on giving massage, some do also make medical claims. These are often imprecise and unsubstantiated. For example, Beck (1988) states that:

> Massage encourages the nutrition and development of the muscular system by way of stimulation of its circulation, nerve supply, and cell activity. Regular and systematic massage causes muscles to become firmer and more elastic.
>
> *Beck, 1988: 200*

> Massage benefits the circulatory system by: helping to develop a stronger heart, improving oxygen supply to cells, decreasing blood pressure, increasing circulation of lymph.
>
> *Beck, 1988: 334*

There are four problems with claims such as 'massage decreases blood pressure'.

- *Origin of the claim.* Is the claim the author's own personal belief? Or substantiated by good quality research? Or a consensus among massage practitioners? Unless we know how the author arrived at this statement we will not be able to judge the likelihood that it is true.
- *Specificity of technique.* Do all types of massage reduce blood pressure? How many treatments are required? How long does each treatment have to be?
- *Specificity of patients.* Does massage reduce blood pressure in all patients? How about those with hypotension, the very old, babies or people who are severely ill?
- *Clinical value.* By how much does massage reduce blood pressure? For how long? Do these changes really benefit patients?

There is currently no text book on massage for health professionals which adequately addresses each of these four issues for even a small proportion of the claims made. Most books make no reference to the medical effects of massage at all. As such, the professional literature on massage remains in its infancy.

BOOKS ON AROMATHERAPY

There is a burgeoning literature on aromatherapy. At the close of 1994, the British Library catalogue listed over 60 books on aromatherapy published in the UK. A unique feature of these books is that they are aimed at both practitioners and at the general public. The very same texts which are recommended for students and practitioners are widely available in bookstores and health food shops. Most appear to be written for a lay audience. This is in marked distinction to conventional medicine, and to other complementary therapies such as chiropractic, where the literature can be divided into two separate categories: technical books for practitioners and general introductions for the public. It is worth speculating on both the causes and effects of the lack of such a distinction in aromatherapy: it may be that the knowledge base of aromatherapy is insufficiently developed to warrant a specialist literature.

Dualism in the aromatherapy literature

Analysis of the aromatherapy literature reveals a demarcation of two sharply distinct approaches to medicine, food and life in general. On the one hand, there is all that is natural, organic, spiritual, healthy and holistic. On the other, there is all that is synthetic, chemical, unhealthy and mechanistic. Massage, aromatherapy and other complementary health techniques are placed in the former category. Conventional medicine is placed in the latter category, often alongside cars, pollution and 'the stress of modern living'.

> In large cities ... we are ...trapped in confined spaces ... [with] cars, automatic washing machines, desk jobs ...we are under constant bombardment from radiation ... [and] traffic with its noise and pollution ...aromatherapy [gives] back the environment ... of the trees and flowers which would naturally surround us in the country.
>
> *Ryman, 1984: 36–37*

> It is because essences are organic that they tend to work in harmony with the body ...organic substances ... do not have the violent, calculated, impersonal action of drugs.
>
> *Tisserand, 1977: 47*

> Computer screens ... are responsible for many illnesses .... Drugs ... lower[] the immune system, other factors include: antibiotics; stress; VDUs; excess sugar; stimulants such as coffee ... television .... Things which strengthen the Immune System: massage, nutritious food; love; vitamin C; zinc; positive thoughts; spiritual openness; reflexology; and, of course, essential oils.
>
> *Tisserand, 1990: 70–71*

Sometimes, a direct antagonism to conventional medicine is expressed.

> Quite a number of American dollars have been spent in research to find the right drug to kill the cold bug. So far those erudite

Yankee brains have failed to come up with anything.

Tisserand, 1977: 75

This routine use of anti-coagulants [in the treatment of myocardial infarct] must stop. The author demands that patients should not be subjected to this inefficient and dangerous treatment.

Valnet, 1980: 59

Uncritical support for complementary medicine is common.

Dr Edward Bach [inventor of the Bach Flower remedies], a physician of great spiritual insight, wrote ... 'rigidity of mind will give rise to those diseases which produce rigidity and stiffness of the body'.

Tisserand, 1977: 95

The right form of treatment – chiropractice or osteopathy, acupuncture, Alexander technique, massage with or without essential oils – needs to be carefully chosen in relation to the source of the back pain.

Davis, 1988: 47

Note the omission of physiotherapy and orthopaedic surgery from the list of potential treatments for back pain. This apparent bias towards complementary medicine is such that it is extremely rare to find any critical appraisal of a complementary therapy, no matter how unusual.

It is not essential for every physician to be an astrologer, but greater account should be taken of it than is done at present.

Tisserand, 1977: 37

Dowsing is also used extensively to check on foods for allergy sufferers. This is a really useful 'spot check' ...when eating out or shopping.

Davis, 1988: 111

Touch for health practitioners ... [are] able to detect disease before the patient is actually aware of any symptoms.

Martin, 1989: 65

Similarly, many aromatherapy texts are extremely accommodating towards historical herbalism. This is often part of an attempt to link aromatherapy – a discipline first described early this century – to an ancient empirical tradition.

The history of the application of essential ... oils to the human body must be almost as old as history itself.

Arnould-Taylor, 1992: 6

Tisserand (1988) has a chapter entitled 'Nothing New' in which he describes the use of 'aromatics' in ancient civilizations such as those of Egypt, Greece and India. However, the link between the religious use of incense (thought to result from the need to mask the smell of the sacrificial altar) and the application of essential oils to treat disease must be seen as weak, at best. Moreover, Tisserand is not unusual in failing to demonstrate causal links between the historical activities described and modern aromatherapy. In what sense did the use of herbs in mummification help to bring about modern aromatherapy? Without causal links, history is reduced to a catalogue of analogous events, devoid of meaning as a whole.

It is also interesting that many of the practices that are so enthusiastically described in aromatherapy texts are exactly those which are often used as examples of the relative ignorance and powerlessness of early medical practitioners. For example, the works of Culpeper are often quoted:

> To make the breasts decrease or grow less: The juice of hemlock mixt with camphure and layd on makes them less; also white frankincense with navel-wort and sharp vinegar, hinders their growth.
>
> *Tisserand, 1977: 37 quoting Culpeper*

> [Culpeper's] book is of far more than historical interest, and any aromatherapist can find in it useful indications on the properties and uses of many oils.
>
> *Davis, 1988: 100*

> Every aromatic substance available seems to have been used ... to combat the Black Death ... it has been widely reported that those in closest contact with aromatics, especially the perfumers, were virtually immune.
>
> *Tisserand, 1977: 39*

The Black Death is easily treated with antibiotics, but killed a third of a population dependent on aromatics. Reference to this disease as a historical validation of aromatherapy can only be seen as bizarre.

Some authors underpin their vision of the world, and in particular the natural/synthetic duality, with the concept of 'life force'. Natural substances have life force, unnatural substances do not and this explains the health-giving properties and safety of natural medicines and foods.

> Over-refined food (white flour, white sugar, etc.) is sadly lacking in life force .... If [our medicines] are natural, organic and

untreated they will work in harmony with the healing forces within us, helping that healing power to restore harmony to the body.

Tisserand, 1977: 52

Essential oils. ... have a life force, an additional impulse, which can only be found in living things. ... the comparative harmlessness of organic substances [is because] they are natural.

Tisserand, 1977: 66

I believe that plants are living beings, each possessing its own energy potential which, according to the laws of nature, may be transmitted to us.

Ryman, 1984: 37

The concept of life force is itself based on a particular metaphysic.

There is an underlying truth towards which every school of thought is working. ... Surely the universe was created and is sustained on one set of principles, so there can only be one truth. If it were based on several contradictory ideas how could it possibly exist?

Tisserand, 1977: 45

Unconventional cosmology and science

Another source for the natural/synthetic dualism found in many aromatherapy books is unconventional cosmology.

We are attracted to certain colours because they have the same vibrational energy as our auras and are repelled by other colours because of a difference in wavelength.

Martin, 1989: 66

Sometimes this cosmology shades of into what is at best, naive, and at worst, plain inaccurate, science, medicine and history.

Louis Kervan is credited with the discovery that plants and animals transmute elements, although it was known to the ancient Chinese, who also knew that, in humans, it took place primarily in the liver ... chickens can transmute potassium. ... plants can thrive, producing a number of elements and compounds, from nothing but distilled water.

Tisserand, 1977: 57

To early man, smell was essential for both individual survival and the survival of the clan, and the race. Scent led hunter/

gatherers to their dinner ... smell gave the first warning of preda-
tors, or rival clans, waiting to attack, and smell was involved in
finding a mate.

Davis, 1988: 226

A model plane ... discovered in a tomb [in] Egypt ...[and] reck-
oned to be at least 2200 years old ...would seem to indicate the
existence of the real thing ....Could such planes have been used
for transporting blocks of stone for pyramid building?

Tisserand, 1988: 16

Hence the need of an extraction which respects these electronic
links [between atoms in an essential oil] and hence the need of
suitably diluted doses which will promote and reinforce ioniza-
tions favourable to chemical processes within the body.

Lautié and Passebecq, 1979: 8

Organic acid + alcohol gives ester + water [in a reversible re-
action]. This is why I said above that acids are found 'in a
combined state' in essential oils – it is possible that an inter-
change can be going on all the time. Perhaps this may be why
esters are good balancers.

Price, 1993: 46

On at least some occasions, statements made in aromatherapy texts
are demonstrably inaccurate.

In arthritis, uric acid is deposited as crystals in joint spaces.

Davis, 1988: 35

Over-indulgence of refined starch ... may help to bring on ...
coeliac disease.

Tisserand, 1977: 57

The immune system ... is also known as the lymphatic system.

Tisserand, 1990: 71

Yet, interestingly, many aromatherapy books make repeated appeals
to science, often hinting that what is stated as fact has been rigorously
researched, whereas in some areas, more research needs to be conducted. A particularly common approach is to make mention of
impressive sounding research without providing any data or references by which claims can be evaluated.

Essential oils ... are in fact known to stimulate leucocytosis.
Rovesti [no reference given] talks of 'recent experiments of considerable importance regarding the stimulating action, and the

increase of white blood corpuscles caused by essences in general'.

Tisserand, 1977: 83

The results of Dr Girault's experiments have been set out in scientific publications [no reference given]. The evidence was impressive enough to undermine the scepticism of ... the head of test laboratories.

Valnet, 1980: 42

Despite this 'appeal to science', most aromatherapy books contain vast numbers of unsubstantiated claims. A selection of these are given in the text box.

EXAMPLES OF UNSUBSTANTIATED CLAIMS IN THE AROMATHERAPY LITERATURE

Ti-tree is ... one of the most powerful immuno-stimulants we know.

Davis, 1988: 173

Juniper has a special affinity with the urino-genital tract, being tonic, purifying, antiseptic and stimulant.

Davis, 1988: 190

Some oils, like calamus, cause dilation of the splenic vessels, thus producing a reduction of blood pressure ... calamus reduces body temperature, and combats experimental auricular fibrillation in dogs.

Tisserand, 1977: 82

Lavender is good for ulcerative lesions of the cornea. It produces arterial hypotension, and decreases the surface tension of the blood.

Tisserand, 1977: 247

Essential oils of garlic and hyssop both have a normalizing effect on blood pressure .... Bergamot or geranium oil ... will either stimulate or sedate according to the needs of the individual.

Tisserand, 1990: 69

We do know that rosemary is a nervous stimulant and various studies have shown that it stimulates heart action, respiration, digestion, kidney function, liver function, gall bladder function, blood circulation and the adrenal glands.

Tisserand, 1990: 184

[Cypress's] locally constricting action on capillaries makes it invaluable for treating haemorrhoids .... Postnatally, it helps heal over sore perineal areas.

England, 1993: 126

[Neroli] will calm and relieve ... laboured breathing, insomnia, mental fatigue, irritability and stomach upsets.

England, 1993: 133

Syphilitic sores and chancres are cured by the application of deterpenated essence of lavender.

Valnet, 1980: 52

Essential oils are especially valuable as antiseptics because their aggression towards microbial germs is matched by their total harmlessness to tissue.

Valnet, 1980: 44

Essential oil of rosemary has an affinity with the liver. On reaching the liver ... the essential oils needed will be dissolved into the tissue fluid.

Martin, 1989: 31

Essential oils ... promote healthy new cell growth.

Martin, 1989: 31

Rosemary [is a] cardiac stimulant, [and an] anti-rheumatic useful in treatments of obesity.

Arnould-Taylor, 1981: 38

Because of [sage's] affinity for muscle fibres, [it] is useful in cases of fibrositis.

Arnould-Taylor, 1981: 38

[Tangerine] improves the circulatory system, especially the peripheral circulation.

Arnould-Taylor, 1981: 38

Cypress ... relieves fluid retention and cellulite ... reduces swelling in rheumatism ... can help to staunch a haemorrhage or excessive blood loss.

Price, 1991: 66

[For] menstrual pain ... clary sage and true melissa are a good combination since the former is anti-spasmodic, the latter stimulating, and both are hormone regulators.

Price, 1991: 81

Aldehydes are anti-inflammatory, anti-infectious, tonic, hypotensive, calming to the nervous system and generally temperature reducing.

Price, 1993: 43

Tea-tree oil is antiviral ... many of its attributes, including its immunostimulant effects, are no doubt due to its extremely powerful bactericidal properties. Applied before radiotherapy, it has been proved to protect the skin from the deep burning effects.

Price, 1993: 81

[Cardamom] is also an effective diuretic and is even better when used with other essences such as juniper which reinforces its action.

Ryman, 1984: 27

Most essences are stimulants. They galvanize the adrenal cortex into action, which leaves you better able to cope with stress ... [essential oils] work so fast and effectively ... because ... they act directly on the limbic portion of the brain.

Ryman, 1984:160

Lemon works on the autonomic nervous system, acting as a sedative when needed, or as a tonic.

Worwood, 1991: 13

Geranium is very effective for menopausal problems, diabetes, blood disorders, throat infections and as a nerve tonic ... [it] has many applications, from frostbite to infertility.

Worwood, 1991: 25

Rose [is a] uterine relaxant. Helps ligaments to soften ... and to regain elasticity after birth.

Worwood, 1991: 277

Miscellaneous issues

The nature of the aromatherapy literature may have implications for public health. Many of the aromatherapy books explicitly encourage self-treatment of serious conditions and often fail to mention basic precautions such as seeking medical advice or consulting an experienced practitioner. For example, the back cover of Price (1991) states that:

> [This] book shows you how to apply ... essential oils to treat a
> wide range of ailments including high blood pressure, sex-drive
> problems ... hair loss, headaches.

Finally, it is worth mentioning that at least a proportion of aromatherapy books venture into distinctly non-medical territory.

> We shall look at the oils and formulas which will bring you sexual well-being and help you realize your true sexual potential.
> Aromantics is a journey of adventure in nature's garden of
> delights and it is there you will discover the Aromantic you!
>
> *Worwood, 1987: 31*

> If you feel threatened at any time by psychic attack, you might
> try ... rubbing a little of the [fennel] essential oil on the solar
> plexus chakra.
>
> *Davis, 1991: 205*

> Libra ... Autumn can be compared with the twilight of life ... its
> light has ... delicate vibrations that reflect the energy of the beautiful, slow-growing Rosewood. ... Rosewood offers a station
> along the road, a stopping-off point to revive one's spirits and off
> load unnecessary luggage.
>
> *Grayson, 1993: 89–91*

It is of note that the book from which this last quote was taken was reviewed by a leading aromatherapy journal (Aromatherapy Times, 1994;1(23): 16) with the comment: 'will be regarded by many aromatherapists as one of their favourite non-technical solace reads'.

THERAPEUTIC RECOMMENDATIONS IN AROMATHERAPY LITERATURE

Most aromatherapy books contain lists of the properties of a variety of essential oils and a 'therapeutic index', in which specific oils are recommended for specific diseases. Analysis of these lists reveals three features in particular: firstly, the wide range of different properties ascribed to each essential oil; secondly, the range and severity of conditions thought to be amenable to aromatherapy treatment; and thirdly, the lack of consistency between different texts.

Properties of essential oils

Tisserand (1977: 239) states that essential oil of juniper has 17 different properties, ranging from aphrodisiac to carminative to 'sudorific' and sedative. Over 30 separate indications are given including 'blenorrhoea' (discharge of mucus from the genitals), diabetes, kidney stones and external ulcers. Oil of rosemary (p. 280) is given 21 properties (adrenal cortex stimulant, 'cephalic', diuretic and 'nervine' among them) and 37 uses, including baldness, diarrhoea, fainting, jaundice and scabies. Valnet (1980: 103) gives roman camomile 20 properties – including mild nerve sedative, anti-anaemic and improvement of bile secretion – and 27 indications, ranging from gastric ulcers to herpes to 'fevers of nervous origin' and convulsions.

Some recent texts are more moderate in the range of properties ascribed to essential oils. For example, Martin (1989: 78) gives sandalwood only seven properties, including aphrodisiac, soporific, decongestant and 'benefits for dry ... and oily skin alike'. Ryman (1984) tends to give each oil only four or five properties. Nonetheless, in one recent text, Price (1991: 58) gives geranium some 33 properties and indications including depression and anxiety, mouth ulcers, sterility, herpes simplex and stretch marks. In a later work (Price, 1993: 267) this is increased to 45 properties and indications.

Range and severity of conditions treated by aromatherapy

Valnet's (1980) therapeutic index includes a large number of conditions which may not, at first sight, be thought of as appropriate for primary treatment with essential oils. These include diabetes, poor sight, snake bites, tapeworm, obesity, apoplexy and arteriosclerosis. Price (1991) includes throat infections, constipation, hair loss, chronic bronchitis, palpitations, asthma and herpes simplex in her therapeutic index. Tisserand (1988) includes asthma, laryngitis, impotence and liver problems among indications for individual essential oils.

Inconsistency between texts

The extent of inconsistency between different aromatherapy texts is demonstrated by Table 3.1, which cross-references the oils recommended for specific conditions by various different authors. It is notable that in only one case do two authors give exactly the same remedy for the same disorder.

Considerable inconsistency is also found in the properties ascribed to individual essential oils. For example, Valnet's properties and uses for neroli (1980: 169) are as an antispasmodic (cardiac spasm, palpitations, dyspepsia, diarrhoea) and sedative (insomnia, 'nervous sensibility'). Ryman (1984: 32) claims that neroli is 'beneficial to the nervous system' such that it has effects on anxiety and depression. She also mentions that neroli is a 'natural blood cleanser' which may help alleviate premenstrual tension. While agreeing that neroli has all of the properties ascribed by Valnet and Ryman, Fischer-Rizzi (1990: 145)

Table 3.1 Some selected examples of therapeutic recommendations in the aromatherapy literature

Author	Hay fever	Thrush	Gingivitis	Alopecia	Diabetes	Hypertension	Acne	Dysmenorrhoea	Impotence
Davis (1988)	Lavender, eucalyptus, camomile, melissa	Lavender, myrrh, tea tree	Fennel, mandarin, myrrh, sage, thyme	Lavender, rosemary, thyme	Not listed	Lavender, marjoram ylang ylang, camomile, bergamot, neroli, rose frankincense	Bergamot, geranium, lavender, neroli, rosemary	Camomile, lavender, marjoram	Clary sage, jasmine, neroli, sandalwood
Lautié (1979)	Indications for, rhinitis: eucalyptus, lavender, niaouli, thyme	Camomile, geranium, rosemary, sage, thyme	Clove, lavender, lemon, thyme	Lavender, sage, thyme	Geranium, juniper, onion	Garlin, lemon, sage, ylang ylang	Cajeput, juniper, lavender	Anise, camomile, caraway, clove, cypress, juniper, lavender, lemon, mint, rosemary, sage, tarragon	Cinnamon, clove, mint, onion, pine, rosemary, sandalwood savory, ylang ylang
Price (1993)	Not listed	Indications for vaginitis: German camomile, clary sage, lavender, niaouli, red thyme, sweet thyme	Clary sage, juniper, lemon, sage	Not listed	Clary sage, eucalyptus, geranium, juniper, lemon, pine, red thyme, sweet thyme, vetiver, ylang ylang	Sweet basil, juniper, lavender, lemon, sweet marjoram, ylang ylang	Benzoin, cajeput, German camomile, cedarwood, clove bud, geranium, juniper berry, lavender, neroli, bitter orange, patchouli, petitgrain, rosemary, sweet thyme, vetiver	Aniseed, basil, German camomile, cinnamon bark, clary sage, fennel, peppermint, rosemary, sage, tagetes, sweet thyme, vetiver	Aniseed, black pepper cinnamon bark, ginger, peppermint, pine, rose otto, savory, sweet thyme ylang ylang

Tisserand (1977)	Eucalyptus, rose	Myrrh	Camomile, myrrh	Lavender, rosemary	Eucalyptus, geranium, juniper	Clary sage, hyssop, lavender, marjoram, melissa, ylang ylang	Bergamot, camphor, cedarwood juniper, lavender, sandalwood	Camomile, clary sage, cypress, juniper, marjoram, peppermint, rosemary	Clary sage, jasmine, rose, ylang ylang
Valnet (1980)	Hyssop	Geranium, lemon, sage	Lemon, sage	Lavender, myrrh	Eucalyptus, geranium, juniper, onion	Garlic, lavender, lemon, marjoram, ylang ylang	Cajeput, juniper, lavender	Aniseed, cajeput, camomile, cypress, juniper, rosemary, sage, tarragon	Aniseed, cinnamon, clove, ginger, juniper, onion, peppermint, pine, rosemary, sandalwood, savory, thyme ylang ylang
Worwood (1991)	Camomile, eucalyptus	Camomile, yarrow, marjoram, cajeput, eucalyptus, lavender, geranium, rosemary, tea tree, myrrh, thyme, patchouli	Thyme, eucalyptus, camomile, pepper-mint	Thyme, rosemary, lavender, carrot, sage	Eucalyptus, geranium, cypress, lavender, hyssop, ginger	Lavender, melissa, nutmeg, hyssop, marjoram, clary sage, lemon, rosemary	24 different oils in three separate stages	Camomile, cypress, geranium, lavender, sage, thyme, nutmeg, peppermint	Not listed

claims that neroli is also effective for skin conditions, headaches and broken veins. Price (1993) gives neroli's properties as anti-infectious, bactericidal, 'balancing', hypotensive, relaxant and nerve tonic. Davis (1988: 236) states that neroli is an 'antidepressant, antiseptic, antispasmodic ... aphrodisiac and a gentle sedative' and that it is 'particularly valuable in skin care'. Arnould-Taylor (1981: 35) grants only that neroli is 'bactericidal, calming [and] improves skin-elasticity'. Worwood (1991) claims that neroli is indicated for depression, anxiety, hysteria, diarrhoea, nervous tension, menopausal problems and dermatitis (p. 517); also that the oil inspires confidence, facilitates easy breathing and is antiseptic (p. 277). England's (1993: 133) combination of properties for neroli is that it will calm and relieve laboured breathing, insomnia, mental fatigue, irritability and stomach upsets. Hopkins (1991: 104) says that neroli is calming, a digestive, that it lowers blood pressure and is effective for acne, eczema, insomnia, depression, shock and dermatitis. Authors also disagree as to the species of orange tree from which neroli is extracted, each giving one or more of *Citrus bigaradia*, *Citrus vulgaris* or *Citrus aurantium*. Such variation is remarkable given the emphasis that aromatherapists place on authorities such as Valnet and Culpeper.

PSYCHOSOCIAL AND ENVIRONMENTAL INFLUENCES ON HEALTH IN THE AROMATHERAPY LITERATURE

Given that aromatherapists claim that theirs is a holistic discipline, it is particularly noticeable that so little reference is made to social and environmental influences on health. Texts do sometimes include environmental factors, such as pollution, when discussing the harm caused by all that is artificial (see above) but rarely is mention made of the effects of poor housing, unemployment, social pressures, discrimination or family stress. In addition, social models of disease and disability are rarely articulated in the aromatherapy literature. Patients are generally seen in relative isolation from their social and physical environment with their problems viewed exclusively in medical terms.

For example, in a chapter entitled 'The Holistic Approach', Price (1993) includes only individual influences on health. Emotional factors (p. 176) are articulated in terms of positive and negative emotions ('negative emotions are self-inflicted wounds which effectively close down the immune system ... smiling and laughing have a positive effect on health'). 'Social Lifestyle' (p. 186) discusses only smoking and drinking which, like lack of exercise (p. 186) and nutrition (p. 182) are considered to be unaffected by any factor other than individual will. Similarly, Tisserand (1988: 96) comments on a case where verrucae were treated by aromatherapy massage and application of oils directly to the infected skin. The case is said to illustrate 'the importance of the holistic approach' on the grounds that treatment focused on stimulating the patient's immune system rather than killing the verrucae. Furthermore, from dozens of case histories given in *A Textbook of Holistic Aromatherapy* (Arnould-Taylor, 1992: 72–89) only two or three mention any social influence on health and none involve interventions other than massage and aromatherapy. In sum, aromatherapists appear to be using the term 'holistic' without reference to social or environmental pathology or intervention.

More worrying, perhaps, is a marked naiveté in the approach to psychology found in aromatherapy texts. There are grounds for describing the aromatherapy literature as at best unconventional and at worst dangerously simplistic, in four main areas.

1) Categorization of psychological disorders

Psychological disorders referred to in the aromatherapy literature include anxiety, depression, alcoholism, impotence, frigidity, anorexia and hyperactivity. By far and away the greatest emphasis is placed on the first two of these disorders. For example, several disorders are listed in the therapeutic index of Price (1993) but only anxiety and depression are discussed in the text. Even in a book entitled *Aromatherapy and the Mind* (Lawless, 1994b) only one psychological disorder other than anxiety and depression is listed in the index.

Moreover, virtually no distinction is ever made between different forms of anxiety or depression. Acute, long-term, organic, reactive, mild, disabling, cyclical, complex: all varieties are treated as a unitary disorder. Though some authors do emphasize the need to match oils to individuals in states such as depression (Davis, 1988: 105) variations in the disease itself are rarely mentioned. Price (1993: 267), for example, lists 20 different oils as indicated for the single state 'anxiety'.

Aromatherapists apparently do not have a conventional understanding of psychological disorders. It could be argued that this is a positive feature of aromatherapy; after all, users of mental health services have long campaigned for the end of what they perceive as destructive labelling. However, there is evidence that aromatherapists' approach to the categorization of psychological disorders stems less from a radical and liberal approach to mental health than from a basic poor understanding of psychological distress. For example, Davis (1988: 27) claims that: 'An anorexic girl is afraid of growing up, and cannot come to terms with her own potential sexuality and having an adult woman's body. Rose oil cries out to be used here. It relates to a woman's sexuality on every level'. Lawless (1994b: xiii) describes hyperactivity as a form of stress; similarly, Wildwood (1992: 116) includes anxiety, depression and insomnia under the rubric 'stress related'. Moreover, there is little evidence that aromatherapists do use social models of emotional distress, such as those that examine cultural prejudices about behaviour.

2) Treatment of psychological disorders

States such as anxiety and depression, it is implied, can be successfully treated merely by the use of essential oils. Though reference is sometimes made to the need for psychotherapy, discussion of appropriate medication or of social interventions such as family or marital therapy is almost entirely absent. Aromatherapy is seen as a stand-alone intervention which deals with psychological disorders without any need for the psychosocial and environmental causes of the symptoms to be addressed.

Tisserand (1988: 141–144) gives three successful case histories of patients with anxiety and/or depression. In all three cases, improvement was brought about by essential oils and massage. For example:

> I decided to use camomile [as] it would counteract … a slightly unhealthy interest in the sensual pleasures and would help to put him more in touch with his emotions. [This was] combined with sandalwood and ylang-ylang, both of which would help to slow him down and relieve anxiety.

Only in one case does Tisserand mention a non-aromatherapy intervention. A woman said to be 'lacking in confidence' was encouraged 'in a very simple way, to be more assertive and self-confident'.

3) Psychological effects of essential oils

Essential oils are said to have simple, direct effects on the psyche. Mention is only rarely made of the mediating effects of suggestion, expectation, initial mood, classical conditioning or concurrent medication.

A famous demonstration of the effects of social psychology on the effects of medication is the 'odd one out' experiment (Rose, Lewontin and Kamin, 1984: 192). Two groups of 10 individuals are placed in separate rooms. In one room, nine are given a sedative barbiturate drug and one a stimulant amphetamine; in the second room, nine receive amphetamine and one barbiturate. In each room the odd individual out, rather than behaving in a way appropriate to the drug taken, behaves like the majority. This is no more than a robust demonstration of the well-known phenomenon that people who are sober can act intoxicated in situations where are others are drinking. Similarly, suggestion may mediate the psychological effects of medication. Reilly (1994) describes an experiment in which medical students experienced psychological changes after taking placebos when it was suggested that the pills contained medications that might have sedative or stimulant actions. Such phenomena are rarely reported in the aromatherapy literature. Perhaps the only exception is Lawless (1994b), who discusses possible mediating influence on the psychological actions of essential oils but fails to follow the argument through and instead goes on to give a standard list of properties and indications.

One further interesting feature of the psychological actions of essential oils given by aromatherapists is that many seem somewhat contradictory. For example, neroli is described by Davis (1988) as both a sedative and an anti-depressant. Such apparent contradictions are quite common in aromatherapy literature: most of the oils indicated for anxiety in the therapeutic index are also indicated for depression. Wildwood (1992: 116) even goes so far as suggest that all oils used to treat anxiety can be used to treat depression. Similarly, most of the oils listed by Wildwood, Price, Davis and others as treatments for anxiety are listed by Lawless (1994b: 81) as stimulants. Lawless (1994b: 117ff) goes on to give 'key qualities' of 53 different essential oils, about a dozen of which have at least some apparently contradictory actions, such as being soothing and reviving, or refreshing and sedating or comforting and stimulating.

It is not immediately apparent how a sedative would be of benefit to an individual with severe, endogenous depression or how a stimulant would help someone suffering from recurrent panic attacks. Some authors (Lawless, 1994a: 80) claim that oils automatically adapt to the needs of the individual, stimulating or sedating as necessary, but there is no evidence for this belief. Others (Tisserand, 1977: 87) state that many essences have both calming and uplifting properties. This may be true in an everyday sense – just as going for a walk is calming and uplifting – but it does not entail that a single essential oil can be a useful treatment for what can be very opposite psychological states. Furthermore, it remains to be explained why aromatherapists give oils specific properties and indications if they really do have such a broad range of application.

4) Role of psychology in physical disorders

There are a number of reasons why psychology can play an important role in ostensibly physical disorders. Firstly, psychological adjustment to disability – for example, the development of suitable coping strategies – can be the primary factor influencing the effects of a disease on an individual's daily life. Secondly, psychological factors can adversely influence the course of treatment. Recovery from, say, chronic back pain, may involve a patient losing a disability pension and needing to seek employment or having to re-establish sexual relations with a partner. These are potentially frightening and can compromise a patient's desire to become well. There is also evidence that the psyche can have a direct influence on the body through an endocrinological mechanism: it is claimed that emotional states affect the functioning of the nervous system and that this leads to altered secretion of hormones into the bloodstream (see for example, Calabrese *et al.*, 1987; Endresen *et al.*, 1987; Fernandez, 1988; Schelinger and Yoidfat, 1988).

The problem is that these ideas are often presented extremely crudely in the aromatherapy literature.

> Always search diligently to see if there is a further emotional cause [for ill health] ... maybe you were once hurt at a new school by children who made fun of [your accent] .... If you believe there may be an[] emotional reason, get to work with positive thinking to negate it.
>
> *Price, 1993: 179*

> If you feel your health problem may be due in part to lack of self-confidence, loneliness or fear ... enrol on an evening class or join a theatre or music club.
>
> *Price, 1993: 187*

> The major part of [eczema] is within the personality of the sufferer. The 'eczema personality' is hypersensitive and like the cancer victim tends to repress his emotions.
>
> *Wildwood, 1992: 139, 10*

There are four problems with statements of this nature. The first is that they are unsubstantiated. Is it really true that all cases of eczema are primarily caused by personality, or that positive thinking can negate an emotional cause of an illness? If so, how do we know? Has Wildwood systematically compared the personalities of a large cross-section of people with eczema to healthy individuals or those with other diseases? Secondly, the statements are so vague and general as to be applicable to almost anyone. Just as 'repressing emotions' is common enough in England to be described as a national characteristic, so almost everyone could remember at least one adverse emotional event which could be seen as the cause of illness. Are many people **not** teased at school? Thirdly, the statements are extremely simplistic. The interplay between mind and body is complex and it is unlikely that merely willing oneself better, or joining a theatre club, fully encompasses the psychology of healing. Finally, assuming such crude and simplistic links between mental and physical health appears to 'blame the victim': if you have eczema, it is because you are hypersensitive; if you are ill, it is because you are not thinking positively enough.

THE ORIGIN OF AROMATHERAPY KNOWLEDGE

An important idea in the philosophy of science is that the reliability of a belief will depend upon the reliability of the method used to generate that belief. To give a simple example, say that a friend claimed, 'There is enough food in Caroline's fridge for us to eat lunch here.' Imagine that we asked our friend how they arrived at this belief. If they said, 'I just looked and saw for myself,' we would probably be feel confident that they were correct. This is because opening a fridge and looking inside is a reliable means of checking its contents. If, on the other hand, they said 'Caroline likes eating in' we might not be so confident, simply because an evaluation of an individual's likes is not always a reliable method of predicting whether their fridge is well-stocked. So the reliability of the belief-forming method is a good estimate of the reliability of the belief.

Answering the question 'Where does knowledge about essential oils come from?' might therefore help evaluate the reliability of the knowledge base of aromatherapy. If knowledge about aromatherapy comes from reliable sources, it will probably be accurate. If the sources of aromatherapy knowledge are not so reliable, we should approach it with caution.

The origin of aromatherapy knowledge: what do leading authorities say?

It is extremely hard to obtain information on the origins of aromatherapy knowledge. As part of the research for this book, the authors quoted in the text box on page 49 were contacted and asked how they had arrived at the given statements. They were also asked whether they saw such statements merely as useful information, or whether they believed they constituted firm facts.

Arnould-Taylor sent a handwritten letter in which he said that he knew Maury and Valnet personally. He claimed to have nothing to add to his published writings and said that time pressures prevented him from entering into correspondence. Replying with reference to his first book, Tisserand claimed that though 'it is not always easy to remember back 18 years ... the statements ... are all based on individual ... [scientific] papers, rather than other books or personal experience'. He went on to say that, as he was unable to provide original material, he did not think that the statements constituted firm fact. Tisserand was sent a further set of unsubstantiated statements from his second and more recent book. He declined to reply. Davis sent a handwritten letter stating that she refused to cooperate. Martin, English and Ryman failed to answer.

The refusal or inability of so many leading figures within aromatherapy to engage in critical discourse must surely be taken as a serious failing. The only exception was Price, who did reply at some length saying that 'statements made ... are based on my experience, that of clients and staff and also letters received from hundreds of people who buy our essential oils ... and tell us how delighted they are with the results'. She went on to say that this is 'as near to fact as anyone is likely to get' due to the costs and difficulties of 'true documented research'. In another communication, she pointed out that basing practice purely on the results of rigorous trials would effectively end the use of aromatherapy in health care.

Price's point seems to be that, in the absence of firm data, it is better to use forms of information gathering (such as case histories) which do not lead to reliable generalizations (such as that tea-tree is antiviral) than to use nothing at all. This is no doubt a valid argument. But if data comes from case histories or personal experience, this should be stated in the text. Readers should be told the origin of a claim so that they can assess the likelihood that the claim holds. If the information in Price's books does come, as she says, from personal experience, she could choose to refrain from making statements such as 'Tea-tree oil ... has been **proved** to protect the skin from the deep burning effects [of radiotherapy]' (my emphasis).

Though most leading authors are not prepared to state how they arrived at statements made in their books, the tone of their statements is that of fact. No leading aromatherapist appears to be content to come out publicly and say that the beliefs held in aromatherapy should be seen as contingent and open to change as more reliable knowledge is acquired. Instead, the empirical nature of aromatherapy is obscured by the language of scientism – 'experiments'; 'test laboratories'; 'proof'; 'chemical analysis'; 'ketone' – and the use of the objective impersonal.

Davis (1991) states that, though her book was based primarily on personal experience, some was 'directly channelled', presumably from extraterrestrial or historical sources. Though few other authors are as candid, personal experience is clearly an important source of beliefs in aromatherapy. One might imagine that a practitioner gives a successful treatment for complaint x with a treatment y, and therefore concludes that y is effective for x. Arnould-Taylor (1981: 14) admits as much when he claims that 'if ... the patient's symptoms disappear ...

then it may reasonably be assumed that the treatment was a success'. Also illuminating is a story given by Price (1993: 122–123). Pointing out that insufficient research has been conducted to ascertain 'every possible health problem each essential oil is capable of helping', she claims that 'serious' writers on aromatherapy may discover new properties of essential oils. She goes on to describe how an aromatherapy teacher returned home from work because of the start of 'what she thought was flu'. She used an oil not indicated for respiratory infections yet 'could not believe how well she felt the next morning'. Needless to say, a single case of recovery from presumed flu is not a reliable basis for ascribing a property to an essential oil. But then neither would 10 cases, or even 100: it is difficult to deduce a property of an essential oil from personal experience simply because the experience of a specific individual is often a misleading basis for claims about people in general. For those wishing to investigate this point further, information on the reliability of and biases inherent in different kinds of evidence can be found in a variety of textbooks (see, for example, Keeble, 1995a, b; McConway, 1994).

Justifying claims in the aromatherapy literature

Instead of stating that their texts are based on personal experience, aromatherapy authors cite a wide variety of sources and concepts to justify their claims. As stated above, a major belief is that of the inherent health-giving properties of natural products, something which is often coupled with the concept of 'life force'. Historical herbalism is generally an important influence. Aromatherapists have also used ideas from fringe cosmology (auras, vibrational energy), both conventional and unconventional medicine and both mainstream (in vitro studies) and fringe science (Kirlian photography).

On occasion, the poor quality of arguments used to support claims becomes clear, particularly when appeals to the scientific literature are made. Tisserand (1988: 59–60) reports Sims' (1986) study of massage in cancer, claiming that 'massage led to a significant improvement in fatigue and concentration … [this] supports my own claim that massage leads to an increase in energy levels'. What he does not report is that the results of the study were not statistically significant and that the author specifically stated that the degree to which the results of the study could be generalized were limited. Tisserand appears to have no problem with using a small negative study, in which one practitioner massaged six patients with a one specific condition, to support general claims about the nature of massage. Tisserand (1988: 61) goes on to claim that 'we now have some real evidence that massage decreases stress in stressed adults'. There follows one quote from one doctor who has introduced massage for his patients. Nothing in this quote can be taken as 'evidence' for massage.

In a similar vein, England (1993: 112) claims that 'Dr Jan-Helge Larsen has **demonstrated** the success of ... belly massage for [infantile colic]' (my emphasis). Though no reference is given, the original paper can be located (Larsen, 1990). It consists of a discussion of the use of massage by one Danish general practitioner. There is no report of any research, and the paper is couched in only the most general of terms. Tisserand is also fond of using terms such as 'demonstrated' or 'scientific research', yet his references are frequently to populist journals such as *Omni* or to other aromatherapy texts. For example, in *Aromatherapy for Everyone* Tisserand makes the claim that: 'We know ... that [essential oils] are able to stimulate tissue regeneration. In the case of skin burns [they] stimulate the growth of new healthy skin resulting in very rapid healing' (Tisserand, 1988: 51). In support of this important claim, Tisserand gives two references, one to Valnet (who presents no data) and one to his earlier text *The Art of Aromatherapy*. Price (1993) supports statements about research with references that include: 'Research Institute of Fragrance Materials, various monographs'; 'Dr George Bennett, lecture notes on holistic health' and 'D.L.J. Opdyke, Food and Cosmetics Toxicology Vol. 14'. The statement 'It is also a proven fact ... that the effects of two or three oils together is greater than the sum of their individual effects' (p. 155) is given the reference 'Scottish Agricultural College, Deans and Svoboda'. Inadequate referencing makes it impossible to follow up these citations so as to obtain and evaluate the original data for oneself.

In a more recent text, Price (Price and Price, 1995) makes considerable attempts to ensure accurate and comprehensive referencing. However, the references do not always support the claims being made. For example, Price cites Gershbein (1977) to support a statement that 'essential oils containing ... menthol and thujanol-4 seem to be beneficial to liver function' (p. 68). Gershbein injected very high doses of essential oils and essential oil fractions into rats after partial removal of the liver and measured the rate of liver regeneration. Thujanol-4 and menthol were not tested and peppermint, which contains menthol, was found to have no effect. None of the oils which were found to increase liver regeneration contain significant amounts of thujanol-4 or menthol. Even if these substances were found to have potentiated liver regeneration in high doses, it is unclear whether it is possible to conclude, as Price seems to do, that aromatherapy treatment is 'beneficial to liver function'. A further case where a reference is given adequately, but which turns out not to support the claim being made is Lawless (1994a: 97), who quotes Dale and Cornwell

(1994) to support a suggestion that lavender is of benefit for perineal healing after childbirth. However, Dale and Cornwell found no difference between lavender and placebo (p. 138). These two cases reconfirm both the importance of proper referencing and the inadequacy of many of the arguments used to support claims about aromatherapy.

But to concentrate on individual cases such as these would be to ignore the wider issue of a general lack of rigour and detail in the arguments found in aromatherapy books. For example: certain essential oils are claimed to contain oestrogen-like substances and, on these grounds, they are said to be indicated for menstrual problems; essential oils are claimed to be harmless because they are natural; because stress is thought to cause disease, and because aromatherapy is said to be good for stress, it is concluded that aromatherapy is good for disease; essential oils have sedative properties, it is claimed, so aromatherapy is good for anxiety and depression; olfactory nerves terminate in parts of the brain where certain neurochemicals are concentrated therefore aromatherapy can modify mood, sexuality and pain.

It is worth speculating whether such non sequiturs are inevitable when these authors attempt to build a case for aromatherapy from such a wide and haphazard range of sources, especially when aromatherapy itself, whatever its clinical benefits, is such a new and under-researched discipline.

Critical discourse in aromatherapy

There is, perhaps, a wider issue than examining the origin of knowledge claims on a case-by-case basis. Authors of textbooks on aromatherapy are simply not subject to the same professional constraints that operate upon other health practitioners. It is highly unlikely that even the most extreme, controversial and unsubstantiated statement made by an aromatherapist will be exposed to critical examination. In fact, it is not clear whether this is even possible: it is doubtful whether there exists a discourse within which aromatherapists can evaluate knowledge claims. How, for example, could an aromatherapist dispute any of the statements quoted in this chapter? What evidence or method of argumentation could be brought to bear? Unless a critical discourse develops within aromatherapy, it is likely that leading aromatherapists will remain completely free to make any statement they choose, regardless of its accuracy, validity or utility. This is unlikely to be in the best interests of patient care.

JOURNALS OF MASSAGE AND AROMATHERAPY

At least some insight into massage and aromatherapy may be gleaned from the journals typically published by and for practitioners. Perhaps the most remarkable feature of these journals is the radical change in emphasis which has taken place in the last 5 years or so. *Aromanews*, the newsletter of the Shirley Price aromatherapy organization in the late 1980s and early 1990s, provides a useful example of the style of early aromatherapy journals. A typical feature in the journal was the 'Case Histories' section, which published short letters from aromatherapists describing successful treatments. Almost all letters follow the same form: symptoms, single treatment regimen, cure. Failures or complexities in treatment are rarely hinted at.

> My mother has incredibly thin skin thanks to 20 years on steroids. It bruises at a touch and look as if they have been slowly roasted. Treatment: White lotion 50 ml with 5% calendula, geranium – 5 drops, and lavender – 5 drops. Result: Skin more supple, bruising less evident and instant appearance of shins is pinker (less roasted).
>
> *Aromanews, February 1990: 9*

Aromanews was also characterized by a general antipathy towards conventional medicine, big science and the food industry. For example, articles included 'How to survive your medical treatment'; 'Irrelevant and immoral: the real value of animal experimentation is exposed' and 'Do you really want to eat polyphosphates?', an article on the meat trade. The following is an excerpt from an article entitled 'Sound Off'.

> I wonder how many people are banging their heads against the wall and saying 'Why won't someone listen to me!' Either about themselves or a loved one who is on drugs which gives them terrible side effects! I could write a book on the side effects which doctors tell us are only in the mind! There must be many people walking around with side effects which are worse than the original illness and people won't listen to them.
>
> *Aromanews, February 1990: 6*

Advertisements for unusual therapies were also common.

> This course [is] based on the work of Dr F Fox, BA, PhD, and MD (Med. Alt.) … consists of the following:
>
> 1) Electro-acupoint testing for diagnostic purposes and to identify the essential oils to be used as antidotes to the toxins discovered.
> 2) Magnetic antidote testing and dynamic magnet therapy.
> 3) Detoxification by chemical hygiene of the entire body, using

special deep lymphatic drainage together with indicated essential oils.

Aromanews, July 1990

The new style of journal

The *International Journal of Aromatherapy* is typical of the newer-style journals in its attempt to ensure high-quality presentation and content. Though, like any professional journal, it promotes and celebrates the practices of its readership, 'doctor bashing' is avoided and care is taken to emphasize at least some of the difficulties and complexities of health care. For example, one article, written by a French doctor, urges a liberal interpretation and application of aromatherapy.

> It is high time to take a broad perspective ... we can remain true to our own concept of aromatherapy, while accepting and respecting those of our colleagues who have a different approach.
>
> *Int. J. Aromather., 1991; 3(3): 16*

Also laudable is the *International Journal of Aromatherapy*'s positive attitude to research (Balacs, 1991) and its attempt to publish clinical studies (Hardy, 1991; Mitchell, 1993) even if these have been of poor quality (p. 131). *Aromatherapy Quarterly, Aromatherapy World, Aromatherapy Times* and the *Aromatherapist* (the new journal of Shirley Price aromatherapy) are also notable for their presentation and more balanced approach. For example, one paper in the *Aromatherapist* (1994;1(2): 30–35) calls for a greater understanding of the conventional point of view when considering implementation of aromatherapy on the NHS. A number of general issues are pinpointed, including clarification of language, improved postgraduate training and caution with therapeutic claims. An article in *Aromatherapy World* (Spring, 1994: 26) warns against over-zealousness and calls for a balance between the rational and intuitive aspects of aromatherapy.

Similarly, *Massage: News, Views and Updates*, the journal of the Massage Therapy Institute of Great Britain, is well written and presented. The journal takes care to avoid any view of massage, or complementary medicine, as a 'cure all' and its sister journal, *Health Review*, is notable for the fair spread of news and reports. For example, the Summer 1993 edition of *Health Review* discusses, without judgement, a new advance in cancer chemotherapy, a ban on a herbal remedy and a study negative for evening primrose oil.

Two American journals, *Massage Therapy Journal*, the journal of the American Massage Therapy Association, and *Massage* are worth discussing in more detail. Both have exemplary standards of writing and presentation and feature well-argued papers discussing, for example, touch deprivation, the problem of terminology in massage or career paths for massage practitioners.

> Unlike the word 'massage', the word 'bodywork' at first glance seems broad enough to cover the great variety of disciplines .... However, just because a word seems broad enough ... [this] is no justification for adopting it. I argue that there are a number of ... reasons against using this word.
>
> *Massage Therapy Journal, 1994; 33(4): 49*

That said, the newer-style journals, particularly the British aromatherapy journals, have not completely overcome their general antipathy towards conventional medicine and they do tend to take a markedly uncritical approach to complementary therapies. For example, unusual health practices are often promoted. A common interest appears to be colour healing:

> In colour healing ... ... violet treats shame, restores dignity. Blue reduces blood pressure, anxiety, asthma, angina, migraine. The spine has ... four sections of mental, emotional, metabolic and physical. Within the four spinal sections the rainbow pattern of eight colours is repeated on each of the eight vertebrae. The practitioner assesses the energy level of each vertebra by dowsing.
>
> *Aromatherapy Times, 1994;1(23): 12*

> Sometimes an association can be made between the colour of a stone and the 'colour' of an aroma ... we can see a relationship between the colour of [lavender] and that of Amethyst, which closely parallels many of the health properties of lavender.
>
> *Davis, 1994 reprinted from Aromatherapy Quarterly*

> Both colour therapy and aromatherapy are usually applied through the subtle anatomy of our being working via the chakra system ... [the] energetic vibrational effects [of oils] link with the energetic power of the colours physically, emotionally mentally and/or spiritually .... Orange – Spleen Chakra – Juniper ... Yellow – Solar Plexus Chakra – Rosemary ... Violet – Pituitary Chakra – Clary Sage.
>
> *Aromatherapy World, Spring 1994: 22–23*

Other journals read by practitioners

The International Journal of Complementary and Alternative Medicine (JACM) is a general journal which is popular among practitioners and is recommended by the Aromatherapy Organisations

Council. JACM is characterized by a strongly promotional viewpoint and a somewhat aggressive stance towards conventional medicine.

Mainstream scientists have always had an unfortunate tendency for what they refer to as 'clear and logical minds'. This boils down to a tendency to follow science as an end in itself without spending any time pursuing the possible moral overtones .... Already, foetuses with Down's syndrome are being routinely aborted. Gynaecologists ... often have no idea whatsoever about the quality of life experienced by people with Down's syndrome.
*JACM, 1993; **11**(9): 12*

Orthodox medicine has attempt to treat the affected part only, in the belief that by doing so illness will be eliminated .... The second concept that conventional medicine finds hard to swallow is that of polymorphism – that one type of organism can change into another.
*JACM, 1992; **10**(1): 12*

JACM's regular 'Update' section ('Reports and comments on the latest worldwide medical research ... from some of the world's leading medical journals') predominantly features items about studies which are either positive towards complementary therapies or negative towards conventional medicine. For example, five issues of JACM (Aug–Oct 92 and Jan–Feb 93) featured a total of 28 items in 'Update', 19 positive for complementary medicine, six negative to conventional medicine and three neutral. Incidentally, 'the world's leading medical journals' include the *British Journal of Acupuncture, Yoga Biomedical News, the International Journal of Aromatherapy* and *Townsend Letter to Doctors*. None of these journals are indexed on Medline, the leading medical database.

A typical advertisement in JACM contains the following copy.

Celloid® Mineral Therapy: A complete efficacious system. ... 10 benefits of Celloid® Mineral Therapy: 1. Celloid® Mineral Therapy has been successfully subjected to a double blind hospital trial. ... 4. Celloids® treat the cause of disease not just the symptoms; the individual not just the disease. ... 6. Celloids® are effective for both chronic and acute conditions. 7. Celloids®can be used to treat the very young and the elderly.

The company sponsoring this advertisement were asked to provide a reference for the 'successful ... double blind hospital trial'. Instead, they sent a copy of a document retyped from the Australian *Report of the Committee of Inquiry into Chiropractic, Osteopathy, Homoeopathy and*

Naturopathy. This was poorly presented and far from unequivocal in its findings. Moreover, the trial was community- rather than hospital-based, and it was not entirely clear whether the medicines used in the trial were the same as those promoted in the advert.

JACM also features a number of particularly unusual therapies.

> The Meridian approach is to give a basic detox course, which covers all the statistically most common toxins found in all parts of the body. The body resonates to the potencies it needs in the combinations. You can give these remedies without testing.
>
> *JACM, 1992; **10**(10): 16*

> Robert Jacobs ... uses computer-linked electromagnetic fields pulsed at frequencies that correspond to specific musical notes in order to create rebalancing resonances within the body.
>
> *JACM, 1992; **10**(1): 12*

In short, despite the laudable advances in the past few years, the journals read by many practitioners of massage and aromatherapy remain dogged by an uncritical stance towards unconventional therapies, no matter how unusual, and an often unnecessary antagonism to conventional medicine. Moreover, the journals consist primarily of case reports, general discussions and observations of practitioners. These are often used to underpin general theories about health, science and medicine. Research is presented only rarely and is generally of a low standard. For example, a trial of aromatherapy for Parkinson's disease published in the *Aromatherapist* (1993; **1**: 14–21) had no control group, a 50% drop-out rate and no outcome measures at all: patients were just asked what symptoms had improved. As yet, there is not a single research-based, peer-reviewed journal for either massage or aromatherapy. This must be seen as a sign of the relative professional immaturity of these disciplines.

CONCLUSION: WHAT ARE THE IMPLICATIONS FOR PRACTICE?

This chapter has given an overview of the practice of massage and aromatherapy, including an analysis of the beliefs of practitioners as expressed in books and journals. Some of the conclusions may be seen as damaging, particularly to aromatherapy. It has been argued that educational standards are inconsistent, and possibly inadequate; that leading aromatherapists have beliefs about health care which are almost always unusual, often simplistic and sometimes demonstrably inaccurate; that the knowledge base in aromatherapy (such as which oils have which properties) is inconsistent; that the knowledge is based on personal experience rather than reliable data; moreover, that aromatherapists attempt to keep this concealed.

To what extent do such inadequacies affect the ability of practitioners to provide a useful service to patients? It may well be that the lack of an intellectually rigorous basis for massage and aromatherapy is of only limited relevance because the two disciplines rely primarily on non-cognitive abilities. The sensitive use of touch, for example, depends on intuition rather than intellect: there are no rules, grounded in science, which can be applied to say, helping a dying patient feel at ease, or to calming a distressed child, or to comforting a bereaved relative.

Moreover, there is no necessary connection between the success of a therapy and the truth of its fundamental principles. Aromatherapy may still be a useful treatment modality even if every statement in every aromatherapy textbook was found to be false. The ancient Greeks explained the motion of falling objects teleologically, in terms of the earth element finding its natural place. The (likely) falsity of this proposition does not, however, entail that stones fly upwards. The value of massage and aromatherapy should be assessed by evaluating the patients of practitioners rather than the words of authorities.

A further point is that the picture of aromatherapy given in aromatherapy textbooks is not necessarily a fair representation of aromatherapy as practised, particularly in conventional health settings. A typical model of care described in the textbooks involves a patient, often with a relatively serious disease such as chronic bronchitis, visiting an individual aromatherapist who takes sole responsibility for treatment and aims to elicit a cure. Generally speaking, aromatherapy as practised in the settings described in this book consists primarily of palliative treatment, typically to calm and relax and possibly to treat minor secondary symptoms.

The current massage and aromatherapy literature leaves much to be desired. The therapies are unlikely to develop as professions without high quality published materials. In the case of aromatherapy, a serious re-analysis of the status of knowledge claims, a critical approach to the therapeutic index and to the properties of oils and a more realistic appraisal of psychosocial and environmental factors in health care are just three general changes which would improve the quality of textbooks. Above all, if they are to develop as professions, massage and aromatherapy need to establish a framework by which statements and knowledge claims can be critically evaluated.

That said, it is worth pointing out the quality of textbooks, journals and courses has rapidly improved in recent years. Newer textbooks and journals are more likely to mention some of the uncertainties and unknowns and to make reference to research. They are also less likely to include naive attacks on conventional medicine and science. In addition, there appears to be a growing awareness that educational standards need to be raised and to be more consistent. It is to be hoped that these trends will continue and that many of the comments and criticisms made in this chapter will become out of date as rapidly as possible.

SUMMARY

- There is a paucity of sociological data on practitioners of massage and aromatherapy.
- The number of full-time practitioners of massage and aromatherapy is unknown. It is likely that many of those trained and registered do not practise full-time.
- Educational standards vary widely. Even in the best institutions, training courses are relatively short.
- Most private practitioners work independently in the community.
- Books on massage tend to lack a distinct medical orientation. Emphasis is placed on massage as a pleasurable social activity, as a means of personal development and as an aid to general well-being.
- A small number of books on massage have been published which are aimed at the health professional. These are often make claims about the effects of massage which are imprecise and unsubstantiated.
- Analysis of the aromatherapy literature reveals: a dualism between natural and synthetic; antagonism towards conventional medicine; support for complementary therapies, no matter how unusual; reliance on unconventional history, cosmology, science and metaphysics.
- Aromatherapy books also make repeated appeals to science, often suggesting that the presented information is the product of rigorous research. However, most texts contain vast numbers of unsubstantiated claims.
- There is considerable inconsistency in different books as to the purported properties and indications of essential oils.
- The origins of knowledge claims in aromatherapy are unclear. Leading aromatherapists have been unwilling to discuss the basis of claims made in their books.
- The approach of the aromatherapy literature towards psychology is unconventional and often simplistic.
- Aromatherapy lacks a discourse by which statements can be evaluated and this may explain the vast range and disparity of claims made in the literature.

- Journals of massage and aromatherapy are often characterized by a promotional stance, antagonism towards conventional medicine and an uncritical acceptance of alternative practices and doctrine, no matter how unusual.
- The lack of intellectual rigour in aromatherapy and massage does not necessarily suggest that patient care will be compromised.
- Books, journals and educational standards seem to be improving.

Research on massage

4

This chapter will give an overview of research data on massage and touch. A systematic review (Chalmers and Altman, 1995) has not been undertaken and firm conclusions are therefore avoided. That said, considerable attention was paid to the methodological quality of the studies described. Readers unfamiliar with research techniques, and wishing to know more, are advised to consult a suitable textbook: Keeble (1995a, b) and McConway (1994) are recommended in particular.

One of the difficulties in assessing massage research is the heterogeneity of massage techniques. For example, the intervention assessed in a number of trials from the 1960s was connective tissue massage, a relatively vigorous technique which often causes pain or searing sensations (p. 23). The relevance of this research to the assessment of, say, a gentle hand and foot rub, is unclear. Many authors have been guilty of treating the massage literature as if it concerned a single, standardized intervention. Some authors (Harris and Lewis, 1994; Westland, 1993) have even gone as far as to include research on spiritual healing, stimulation of acupuncture points with ice or the use of mechanical vibrators as core elements in their assessment of massage. Others have used trials showing an effect of therapy in one particular condition as a vindication of the technique as a whole. Because the term 'massage' may be taken as referring to a variety of different techniques, and because massage therapists make a variety of different therapeutic claims, it is important to avoid simplistic extrapolations from trials of particular techniques for particular conditions.

CLINICAL RESEARCH ON MASSAGE

EFFECTS OF MASSAGE ON ANXIETY IN INSTITUTIONAL SETTINGS

Given that the most common use of massage is to calm and soothe, and that most research is conducted in hospital settings, it is perhaps not surprising that a significant proportion of massage research focuses on stress and anxiety for hospitalized patients. Though a relatively large number of trials have been published, almost all have been of poor quality and many have used inappropriate outcome measures. That said, most trials, including the two most rigorous studies, do show that massage improves mild and moderate anxiety in institutional settings. The duration of this effect has not been established.

Massage for psychiatric patients

In possibly one of the best clinical trials of massage published to date, Field *et al.* (1992) found that massage was of benefit for child and adolescent psychiatric patients. A total of 72 subjects hospitalized with either depression or adjustment disorder were randomized either to receive a 30-minute back massage or to watch relaxing videotapes. These were repeated once daily for 5 days. Outcome measures included standard psychological scales (such as the Profile of Mood States and Spielberger anxiety inventory), night time sleep, behaviour and activity ratings, and pulse rate. Samples of urine and saliva were taken to assess levels of cortisol and catecholamines. Immediate changes seen within the massage group included improvements on psychological tests and behaviour scores. For example, average anxiety scores fell from 34.7 to 27.3 between just before and 30 minutes after the first massage ($p < 0.001$). Mood scores improved from 20.4 to 16.4 ($p < 0.005$). Salivary cortisol also fell, and remained lowered at a 30-minute post-treatment follow-up, indicating a lowered stress response. The authors claim that they were not surprised by these results: they expected that, for example, a child with adjustment disorder would exhibit a reduction in anxious behaviour immediately following a massage.

Possibly less expected, and perhaps of greater interest, were the differences between massage and control groups at the end of the trial. These differences suggest that a course of massage leads to cumulative and persisting improvements. Depression scores fell from 20.4 on day 1 to 14.7 on day 5 in the massage group ($p = 0.01$) but only from 16.3 to 13.5 ($p < 0.05$) in controls. Anxiety scores improved by about 20%, but only for adjustment disorder children receiving massage. Night time sleep also improved significantly (from about 80% to 90% time asleep, $p = 0.05$) in the massage group, whereas controls experienced only minor improvements in sleep. Positive changes in behaviour were also seen, though, given that the nurses assessing behaviour might not have been blind to treatment allocation, a degree of observer bias is possible. The laboratory tests showed that urinary cortisol and noradrenaline fell significantly, though only in depressed children. Because these hormones are released in response to stress, this result suggests that massage leads to a decreasing of the stress response in depressed subjects over the 5-day period.

Field's study represents possibly the best evidence that massage reduces anxiety and stress responses in institutional populations. Apart from a possibly confusing presentation of data, and the lack of between-group statistical analysis, the trial is of exemplary quality and future workers would do well to follow Field's example.

Massage for anxiety in hospital settings

There is possibly only one other trial massage for anxiety which is of comparable quality to Field *et al.*'s psychiatry study. A total of 100 post-cardiac-surgery patients were randomized to four groups: aromatherapy massage with essential oils, massage with inactive carrier oil, a chat and no intervention (Stevensen, 1994). Patients in the first two groups received a gentle, 20-minute foot massage. Physiological changes were assessed by measurement of heart rate, respiratory rate and blood pressure. Psychological effects were measured using a modified Spielberger questionnaire (STAI) which assessed pain, anxiety, tension, calm, rest and relaxation on a four-point scale. Outcome measures were repeated on five occasions both before and after the intervention. The massage groups also received a written questionnaire at a 5-day follow-up.

The physiological effects of massage were minor and transient, the only statistically significant difference consisting of a slight fall in respiratory rate immediately following massage. However, psychological changes resulting from massage were both clinically and statistically significant. Modified STAI scores improved by 8 points during the intervention in the massage groups compared to a change of 0.7 and 1.32 points in the control and chat groups respectively. These differences remained at the 2-hour follow-up. The results of the 5-day follow-up demonstrated differences between massage groups attributable to the use of the essential oil. These data, and possible criticisms of the trial, are discussed below in the section entitled 'Clinical Research on Aromatherapy.'

Other studies have been of poorer quality, one of the most common failings being the use of small sample sizes. Fraser and Kerr (1993) investigated the effects of back massage on 21 elderly patients in a long-term care institution. Because the study design incorporated three separate groups – back massage with conversation, conversation only, and no intervention – each group consisted of only seven patients. Outcome measures were taken immediately before and after a single intervention and included a self-evaluation questionnaire, electromyography, blood pressure and heart rate. Subjects in the massage group enjoyed the greatest improvement in anxiety scores: this was statistically significant compared to the no intervention group, but only approached statistical significance when compared to the conversation group. Subjects in the massage group also experienced improvements in systolic blood pressure, EMG and self-report scores other than anxiety, though again, these were not statistically significant.

Another example of a small-scale study with positive, though statistically non-significant results, measured the effects of massage on well-being of six patients receiving radiotherapy for breast cancer (Sims, 1986). The author claims that the patients 'reported less symptom distress, higher degrees of tranquillity and vitality and less tension and tiredness following the back massage when compared with the control intervention'. However, as even the author admits, the poor methodology of the study and the lack of statistically significant results limit the extent to which the findings can be generalized.

A more recent trial of massage for anxiety and pain in cancer patients (Ferrell-Torry and Glick, 1993) is also limited by a small sample size and lack of a control group. Nine hospitalized, male cancer patients experiencing moderate levels of pain were given a 30-minute massage on two consecutive evenings. In addition to conventional back massage, deactivation of trigger points (p. 26) was used. Pain and anxiety were assessed immediately before and 30 minutes after treatment by using analogue scales and the Spielberger anxiety questionnaire (STAI). Blood pressure, respiration rate and heart rate were also measured. The results appear to indicate an effect of massage on pain and anxiety. After the first massage, visual analogue scores for pain fell from about 48% to 19% ($p < 0.01$) whereas those for anxiety fell from 64% to 32% ($p < 0.0001$). STAI anxiety scores improved from 56 to 43 ($p = 0.02$). Minor falls in psychophysiological measures were also recorded. For example, respiration rate fell from 22.6 to 19.7 breaths per minute after the first massage ($p < 0.05$). Though these results are encouraging, the study would need to be repeated with a control group before any firm conclusions could be drawn.

One aspect of standard clinical trial methodology is the use of averages. It may be that individual responses to massage vary, an effect obscured by averaging data from different subjects. Corley et al. (1995) compared a 3-minute back rub with 3 minutes of rest in 19 elderly residents of a long-stay nursing home. Physiological and psychological measures were taken after 15 minutes of rest and then immediately following treatment. There were no significant differences between groups on average changes in heart rate, respiratory rate, blood pressure, skin temperature or skin conductance. Mood ratings improved slightly more for the massaged subjects than for controls but the difference between groups did not reach statistical significance. Despite the lack of intergroup differences, individual responses varied greatly. For example, the change in systolic blood pressure following massage ranged from a decrease of 24 mmHg to an increase of 22 mmHg. Subjects were also asked to complete a questionnaire which assessed tactile aversion and tactile sensitivity. The results of this questionnaire were correlated with the physiological and psychological outcomes of the massage treatment. Though this data is not presented clearly, it seems that greater falls in heart and respiratory rate following treatment were associated with lower tactile aversion and lower reaction to touch. The authors conclude that it is important to assess individual patient preferences before undertaking back massage.

Wilkinson's (1995) study of aromatherapy in hospice care is discussed in full on page 128. Wilkinson found that massage reduced anxiety scores measured immediately before and after treatment (STAI scores fell from around 40 to about 30 ($p < 0.001$)) but had no effect on physical and psychological symptoms. The massage group in this trial were acting as controls and the absence of a no-intervention group precludes attributing the improvements in anxiety to the massage. Likewise, Corner, Cawley and Hildebrand's (1995) trial (p. 129) seems to demonstrate an effect of massage on anxiety, but not depression or symptom distress, in cancer patients. However, patients were not randomly allocated to treatment and control groups so it may be that initial differences between groups caused the apparent improvements from massage. A third trial of aromatherapy, this time in an intensive care setting (Dunn, Sleep and Collett, 1995) did involve randomization of patients to massage and control groups. There were no differences in physiological response or behavioural scores between groups. Psychological changes appear to demonstrate the superiority of massage over rest, though this did not reach statistical significance. There were a number of flaws and confounding variables in the study (see p. 129 for full details).

A study reported by Meek (1993) examined the effects of slow-stroke back massage in 30 hospice clients. Measures were taken at baseline, after 5 minutes of rest, after 3 minutes of slow-stroke back massage and after a further 5 minutes of rest. Moderate but statistically significant decreases in blood pressure and heart rate, and increases in skin temperature, resulted from massage, but not the initial rest period. For example, mean systolic blood pressure fell from 111 mm before treatment to 107 mm immediately after. Interestingly, most scores continued to decrease during the final rest period. This suggests that any relaxation induced by massage continues after the cessation of treatment, an effect which has also been described by Naliboff and Tachiki (1991) (p. 96). Despite these encouraging findings, Meek's trial is flawed by lack of a control group and the absence of clinical outcome measures (e.g. subjective anxiety scores). Fakouri and Jones's (1987) study of slow-stroke back massage for elderly nursing home residents was also uncontrolled. This represents a particular problem because treatment took place in bed just before sleep. So though the statistically significant changes in heart rate, skin temperature and blood pressure were indicative of relaxation, it is impossible to know whether this effect was due to the massage or to relaxation prior to sleep.

An uncontrolled study reported by McKechnie et al. (1983) is of interest because it is widely quoted. Five patients who presented with symptoms of tension and anxiety were treated with connective tissue massage. All five patients showed a significant response to treatment in at least one psychophysiological parameter. The authors claim that the study supports the hypothesis that each individual has a unique 'stress response pattern' and that connective tissue massage may be of benefit to at least some individuals suffering from 'anxiety states'. Given that this was a small trial, and that there was no control group, this conclusion is probably unwarranted and it is disappointing that the study is often quoted as evidence of the effectiveness of massage.

Methodological considerations

With the possible exception of Field's research on adolescent psychiatric patients and Stevensen's intensive care trial, it is not hard to find flaws with much of the research examining massage for anxiety. Most of the studies had small sample sizes and insufficient control groups. Many also contain basic errors such as failure to match groups for baseline comparability.

A particular problem is the use of psychophysiological outcome measures such as heart rate or blood pressure. A fall in heart rate does not necessarily imply a fall in anxiety levels (p. 103). Clinical outcome measures, those which assess symptoms such as pain or anxiety, may therefore be more appropriate. On the other hand, symptom scales, such as anxiety questionnaires, which are filled in by patients can cause problems of their own. Patients obviously cannot always be blinded to their treatment allocation and may have been influenced, or may have had motives, for giving an unrealistic set of answers. In general, if a health professional asks a patient: 'Did that help?', they will usually say 'Yes'. It may be, for example, that patients enjoyed the massage, wanted to ensure that they received further treatment and therefore gave an over-positive response to a questionnaire.

The timing of outcome measurement is also an important issue. In many trials, anxiety scores before treatment were compared to those taken immediately afterwards. The duration of relief from anxiety was not assessed.

In summary, research provides limited support for the use of massage to decrease anxiety in institutionalized patients. The evidence is certainly suggestive of benefit, but more carefully conducted studies are required. In particular, sample sizes need to be larger and both the nature and timing of outcome measures more carefully chosen. Overall, attention should be paid to the question being asked in research. Practitioners should try to define, as precisely as possible, what it is they are attempting to achieve in giving massage and design trials accordingly.

MASSAGE IN NEONATAL CARE

Montagu (1978) reports the story of a doctor who visited an orphanage while on vacation in Mexico in 1946. The doctor found that, though the babies were not so clean and well-fed as those in his hospital in New York – which administered the best modern nutrition in hygienic surroundings – they appeared to be healthier and happier. This was attributed to the fact that women from a local village came to the orphanage to fondle, stroke and talk to the children. The doctor is said to have implemented a similar regime in New York, with the result that death rates at the hospital fell. This story is probably somewhat romanticized: the doctor obsessed by modern hygiene and nutrition learns the simple peasant ways of the Mexican and reassesses his medical world-view. However, it also appears to contain a kernel of truth. Massage of preterm infants has been researched in great detail and there is extensive evidence that it is of benefit.

Early studies of massage and touch stimulation

In perhaps the first study of its type, Hasselmeyer (1964) found that premature infants receiving sensory, tactile and kinaesthetic stimulation were more quiescent, especially at feeding times, than unstimulated controls. Solkoff et al. (1969) seemed to confirm these findings. Five low-birth weight infants were stroked for 5 minutes every hour of the day for 10 days. Compared to a control group receiving routine nursery care these infants were more active and appeared to cry less. In contrast to Hasselmeyer, infants in the experimental group experienced greater weight gain and greater growth and motor development at an 8-month follow up. In a similar trial published 6 years later, Solkoff and Matuszak (1975) failed to demonstrate changes in weight gain, though improvements on the Brazleton scale (which assesses development) were reported.

A further replication was conducted by Freeman (1969). A total of 24 preterm neonates receiving 5 minutes of stroking, either hourly or after feeding, for the first 10 days postnatally were compared with 24 matched controls. Weight gain was higher in the handled infants, with a decreased incidence of respiratory problems in infants stimulated after feeding. Using a similar research design, White and Labarda (1976) demonstrated increased caloric intake, greater weight gain and fewer required feedings in premature infants receiving touch stimulation.

Powell (1974) compared handling by nurses and handling by mothers with a control group receiving routine care in 23 preterm neonates. The group receiving greatest touch stimulation – handling by nurses – regained birth weight faster and experienced more optimal mental scores at 4 months and behavioural scores at 6 months on the Bayley scale. However, no differences in height or weight were found at 2-, 4- or 6-month follow-ups. Rausch (1981) compared 20 premature infants receiving 15 minutes of tactile and kinaesthetic stimulation with 20 matched historical controls. Statistically significant improvements in caloric intake and stooling frequency were observed in the experimental group. Weight gain was also higher, though this difference did not reach statistical significance. This trial is somewhat flawed by the lack of randomization and by insufficient blinding.

These and other early studies of tactile stimulation were reviewed by Ottenbacher et al. (1987). A total of 19 studies were analysed. It was calculated that 72% of infants receiving touch stimulation did better than controls. However, as might be guessed from the descriptions given above, the methodological quality of many of the studies was low.

Rigorous research on massage for premature neonates

A number of more rigorous studies of tactile stimulation of premature infants have been conducted since the mid-1980s. Much of the best work has been undertaken by Tiffany Field and Frank Scafidi of the Touch Research Institute at the University of Miami and Saul Schanberg and Cynthia Kuhn of Duke University. In perhaps the most well-known randomized study (Field et al., 1986) preterm neonates were massaged three times a day for 10 days. Treatment consisted of two 5-minute periods of stroking separated by a 5-minute period in which the neonate's limbs were moved passively (kinaesthetic stimulation). Subjects had 47% greater weight gain than controls and were rated more mature on habituation, orientation, motor and range of state behaviour on the Brazleton scale. Subjects were also rated more active and alert by nurses, though, given that the nurses may not have been blind to the experimental assignment, this finding should perhaps be taken with some circumspection. Hospital stay was 6 days shorter for subjects than for controls, representing savings of some $3000 per infant. A follow-up at 8 months (Field, Scafidi and Schanberg, 1987) found superior performance on developmental assessments in the massage group.

A replication of this study was completed by the same team (Scafidi et al., 1990). In a complex and detailed clinical trial, which involved the somewhat unusual expedient of time-lapse video recording, massage was found to lead to 21% greater weight gain and to a 5-day reduction in hospital stay. Habituation scores on the Brazleton scale were also significantly improved compared to controls. No differences were found in activity level or sleep/wake behaviour, though greater activity was recorded during periods of tactile stimulation. Sympathetic nervous system activity and adrenocortical function was also assessed in this study and reported separately (Kuhn et al., 1991). Tactile stimulation was found to lead to higher catecholamine excretion. This was attributed to a greater maturation of the sympathetic nervous system. No differences were found in urinary dopamine, cortisol or serum growth hormone.

Scafidi, Field and Schanberg (1993) later attempted to determine which premature infants benefited most from massage therapy. A total of 93 infants were randomly assigned to receive either 15-minute massages three times daily or usual care. Mean weight gain was significantly higher in experimental subjects ($p < 0.01$), with 70% of massaged infants gaining more weight than the mean for the control group (i.e. the expected weight gain). Though the authors did identify certain characteristics, such as a greater number of obstetrical complications, which were associated with good outcome from massage, they concluded that massage is generally indicated for premature infants.

All neonates entered in the aforementioned trials were medically stable. Though it has been suggested (Field, 1980) that weaker neonates are likely to benefit most from tactile stimulation, research has yet to address this question and it is likely that particular care, for example, monitoring of behaviour and vital signs, should be taken if using touch stimulation with medically unstable infants. Gorski et al. (1984) conducted an observational study of touch and bradycardia (abnormally slow heart rate) in nine preterm infants. In one infant, episodes of bradycardia tended to follow periods in which touch had been used. These findings reconfirm the importance of individual assessment in programmes of neonatal stimulation.

Wheeden *et al.* (1993) showed that massage is also of benefit to preterm infants exposed to cocaine *in utero*. Using a similar methodology to Field *et al.* (1986), 30 infants were randomly assigned to either 3, 15 minute massages a day for 10 days or to no intervention. Compared to controls, massage lead to a 28% greater average weight gain ($p < 0.01$) despite no difference in caloric intake. Massaged infants were also reported to exhibit significantly fewer postnatal complications and stress behaviours and to demonstrate more mature motor behaviour on the Brazleton scale at the end of the study period.

Multimodal stimulation of the premature infant

A number of studies have examined multimodal programmes of stimulation of which touch is one component. Rice has developed a special programme of stimulation, now known as RISS, which includes massage, talking, eye contact and rocking. In an early study, Rice (1977) assessed the effect of massage and rocking administered four times a day by mothers. Improvements in weight gain and various measures of maturation were reported at some, but not all, follow-ups. White-Traut and Tubeszewski (1986) compared RISS with usual care for a group of 36 premature infants. Trends for increased weight gain were found, though these missed statistical significance. The trial was somewhat flawed in that there were variations in the number of treatments given to each infant. The lack of statistical significance might also result from the relatively small number of subjects and the lack of post-discharge follow-up.

In a further trial, the RISS programme (White-Traut and Nelson, 1988) was taught to a group of mothers. Compared to a control group, and a talking only group, the experimental group scored significantly higher on measures of mother–infant interaction on discharge. This result may have been confounded by the greater number of multiparous mothers in the RISS group. It is of interest that the mothers were primarily young (21 years), single and of low socio-economic status. It is possible that the RISS programme constitutes a form of training in mothering skills which may be lacked by this particular subject group.

The safety of RISS was assessed by White-Traut and Goldman (1988). RISS treatment was found to lead to slight decreases in body temperature and slight increases in heart and respiratory rates. These changes were transient and measures returned to baseline within 15 minutes. It was concluded that, though care should be exercised in selecting infants for RISS, and though vital signs and behavioural responses should be monitored during RISS, it was unlikely that the minor physiological changes reported would lead to adverse effects.

Kattwinkel *et al.* (1975) reports that rubbing the extremities of premature infants produced a significant decrease in the frequency of apnoea, both during and shortly after the period of stimulation. Scarr-Salapatek and Williams (1973) found that regular visual, auditory, tactile and kinaesthetic stimulation followed by social worker visits after discharge led to improvements in weight gain and maturity scores. Helders, Cats and Debast (1989) compared the effects of a multimodal stimulation programme, which included massage, to a control group in very-low-birth-weight infants. Increased weight gain and improved scores on some aspects of a psychomotor development profile were found at 1 year. Rose and Bridger (1979) studied the effects of three daily sessions of 20 minutes of body massage, rocking and talking. At 6 months, preterm infant performance on a visual recognition memory task was indistinguishable from full-term infant performance. As performance on the visual recognition memory task has predictive value for childhood IQ, this finding, like that of Helders, Cats and Debast (1989) and Field, Scafidi and Schanberg (1987) suggests that supplemental tactile stimulation of preterm neonates may have long-term effects on development.

A number of authors have also studied non-massage forms of touch stimulation. These have included non-nutritive sucking, rocking, mechanical rocking and the use of oscillating waterbeds. Most of the studies have demonstrated a beneficial effect of stimulation such as improved weight gain and greater maturity as measured by appropriate scales. These studies have been reviewed by Field (1980).

Mechanism of massage for premature infants

Touch stimulation of premature and low-birth-weight infants seems to be of benefit either as a stand-alone intervention or as part of a multimodal programme of therapy. However, there is disagreement as to why touch stimulation is of benefit. Field (1990) has reviewed the potentially stressful features of the NICU environment, including factors such as continuous, high-intensity noise and bright light. Some authors see this as sensory deprivation, others as overstimulation or an inappropriate pattern of stimulation. There is some support for the second hypothesis. Scafidi *et al.* (1986) reported that signs of stress, such as facial grimaces and clenched fists, were reduced by massage and that positive changes in sleeping patterns were produced by the touch intervention. Similarly, Acolet *et al.* (1993) measured biochemical responses to massage in neonates and found that, though levels of adrenaline and noradrenaline remained constant, levels of plasma cortisol fell, an effect possibly indicating relaxation.

That said, there remains considerable confusion as to whether tactile stimulation increases or decreases overall activity level in premature neonates. Weiss (1992) points out that whether touch sedates or stimulates will depend on the type of touch used. For example, in a simple within-subjects design, Weiss found that intense and vigorous touch of infants with congenital heart disease was found to produce greater activity, and higher heart rate and blood pressure, than other types of tactile stimulation. For a good overview and analysis of the conflicting data, see Scafidi *et al.* (1986) who concludes that the underlying mechanisms by which massage improves clinical outcome in preterm infants is unknown. Rose (1984) has suggested that the long-term effects of tactile stimulation relate to a deficit in the ability of premature infants to integrate tactile information. This deficit persists up to 1 year of age. Rose reports that, compared to full-term infants, preterm infants have difficulty in perceiving touch and in effectively using active touch to explore their world. It is suggested that tactile stimulation ameliorates preterm infants' difficulties with touch and that this has long-term consequences for development.

In sum, massage and kinaesthetic stimulation can play an important role in promoting development among premature neonates. Given the therapy's simplicity, cost-effectiveness and lack of adverse effects, the reasons for its relatively limited use, in the UK at least, remain unclear.

MASSAGE AND PAIN

A number of authors have pointed out that massage is an instinctive response to pain: if we injure ourselves, one of our first responses is to rub the affected part. One explanation often given for the pain-relieving effects of touch is the 'gate control theory', which was first proposed by Melzack and Wall (1965). Put simply, this states that only a certain amount of information can reach the brain from a particular region of the body. Stimulating a painful area, by rubbing it or inserting an acupuncture needle, can limit the number of pain impulses reaching the brain. Other workers have suggested that massage relieves pain because it leads to the release of endorphins. However, neither gate control theory or endorphin release are likely to account fully for any analgesic effects of massage: pain is a complex physiological and psychological state which is not dependent simply on some quantity of nervous stimulation or blood levels of a hormone.

Research on massage for pain is disappointing. Though practitioners are quick to claim at least some benefit, good-quality clinical studies are few and far between: there is almost no reliable evidence that massage relieves pain. In 1990, Weinrich and Weinrich published the results of a small study that indicated that massage could have a moderate, short-term effect on pain in cancer patients. A group of 14 subjects receiving a 10-minute back massage were compared to a control group who were visited for a similar amount of time. Immediately after the massage, there was a significant decrease in pain in males, with a non-significant decrease for females. No changes in pain scores were noted at 1- and 2-hour follow up. Ferrell-Torry and Glick's (1993) study is discussed on page 77. Though significant decreases in pain were found, the lack of a control group entails that the effect cannot necessarily be attributed to massage. Moreover, it may be that traditional back massage was not responsible for the improvements recorded because the practitioners in the study used trigger point deactivation as part of treatment (see Baldry, 1993). That said, reductions in pain scores were relatively dramatic and it might be argued that they were of a scale which makes discussion of placebo effects and so on rather academic.

Another study of massage for pain is of poor quality and is worth discussing for that very reason. Two trials conducted by Lundeberg (Lundeberg, 1984; Lundeberg, Nordemar and Ottoson, 1984) have been widely reported to constitute evidence for the pain-relieving effects of massage (Westland, 1993; Mackereth, 1993). Lundeberg claimed about 70% success in the short term and about 25% over the course of 12 months. However, the studies are uninterpretable due to serious methodological flaws. Not only were the trials uncontrolled, but they involved heterogeneous study populations (mixed acute and chronic pain of various types) and poorly defined outcome measures: patients were counted as benefiting from treatment if they continued to use it; moreover, outcomes such as 'reported more than 50% pain relief' were used without details of how this was assessed. Perhaps most importantly, the therapeutic modality studied by Lundeberg was touch stimulation from a mechanical vibrator placed at specific points on the body. The similarity between this technique and those generally used by practitioners of massage can only be guessed at.

Possibly the only other study which directly studied the role of massage in pain relief compared the effects of massage given by a nurse to the effects of a 'Dermapoints Massage Roller' (Naliboff and Tachiki, 1991). The results suggest that the pain-relieving effects of massage stem, at least in part, from general effects associated with skin stimulation (such as increased skin temperature), from decreased muscle tension and from stimulation of peripheral nerves (gate control theory).

Other studies have focused on the biochemical changes associated with pain relief. A number of workers have examined whether massage leads to the release of endorphins but there is little robust evidence that this occurs (p. 105) . Danneskiold-Samsoe *et al.* have studied the role of massage in the treatment of fibrositis (1982) and myofascial pain (Danneskiold-Samsoe, Christiansen and Bach Andersen, 1986). Highly significant increases in plasma myoglobin were found after massage treatment. A positive correlation was found between the degree of muscle tension and pain and the increase in plasma myoglobin. For example, five patients in the 1986 study who did not benefit from the massage also experienced no significant increase in myoglobin. Increases in plasma myoglobin following massage gradually declined with repeated treatment. This was associated with a reduction in muscle tension and pain. The authors hypothesize that massage causes myoglobin to leak from diseased muscle fibres, but that it also has a curative effect. As the two trials did not incorporate a control group, such a conclusion may be viewed as premature.

In short, there is an almost complete absence of reliable data regarding the effect of massage on pain. This is disappointing given that massage is widely reported to be of short-term benefit for pain, and that a controlled clinical trial of massage for pain should not theoretically present any great technical difficulties.

RESEARCH ON REFLEXOLOGY

Despite wide-scale practice, reflexology remains an under-researched therapy. At the time of writing, there are only four published trials in reflexology. Two of these are methodologically flawed and inadequately reported and a third failed to find a difference between the effects of reflexology and non-specific counselling in asthma. The fourth trial did find reflexology to be superior to a sham technique. However, subjects in this trial received acupressure in addition to reflexology and it is therefore unclear which modality was of benefit.

Lafuente *et al.* (1990) claimed a beneficial effect of reflexology in headache. A total of 32 patients with a variety of migraine and headache disorders were randomized to receive flunarizin (a drug) plus sham reflexology, or true reflexology plus placebo medication. Reflexology treatments were repeated 12–30 times over a 2–3 month period. The outcome measure was a diary score of headache frequency, severity and duration at the end of treatment and 3 months later. Overall, improvements were almost twice as great in the reflexology group as in flunarizin-treated patients, though this difference was not statistically significant.

A number of methodological flaws, and details missing from the trial report, preclude any confidence in the authors' conclusion of benefit from reflexology. The use of a drug or placebo represents a confounding variable which complicates the comparison between reflexology and sham reflexology. Moreover, no information was provided as to whether patients remained unaware of their treatment allocation and it is possible that patients had less faith in the sham than in the true reflexology. Finally, baseline comparisons, withdrawals and results are inadequately reported.

Another trial with intriguing results is reported by Eichelberger (1993) but, once again, methodological flaws and lack of experimental detail in the report reduce the credibility of its findings. Reflexology treatment was given to half of a group of 60 women who were catheterized after gynaecological surgery. The control group received no intervention. Only 10% of women in the experimental group, as against 40% of controls, required medication after removal of the catheter. Few other details are reported. The lack of a placebo in the control group and the choice of outcome measure constitute further flaws in this study.

A more carefully conducted and reported study (Petersen *et al.*, 1992) examined reflexology for the treatment of bronchial asthma. In this trial, 30 patients were randomized to receive 10 weekly reflexology treatments or non-specific counselling. Outcome measures included diary card symptom scores, use of medication and objective measures of pulmonary function at baseline, 3 and 6 months. No significant differences were found between groups at the end of the trial. Lung function did improve in the reflexology group, but it improved slightly more in the control group. The authors attribute the benefits of reflexology to 'a sense of security [brought about by] conversations with the therapist'.

There are a number of different conclusions that can be drawn from this trial. Firstly, the trial may have been inadequate. The use of only one practitioner in the trial makes it possible that it was the therapist rather than the therapy which was ineffective. A replication with more quality-of-life-oriented outcome measures might also be welcomed. We might also conclude that the trial is correct, that reflexology has no specific effect in asthma but that it may have benefit in other conditions. Or it could be concluded that reflexology does not work in asthma because reflexology does not work at all.

Perhaps the best evidence to refute this last claim comes from a more recent trial of reflexology for premenstrual syndrome (Oleson and Flocco, 1994). Using a particularly rigorous design, 35 women who regularly suffered premenstrual syndrome were randomized to receive eight half-hour sessions of reflexology or a placebo treatment.

The latter consisted of either 'overly light or very rough' pressure on reflexology points thought inappropriate for premenstrual syndrome. Outcome was assessed by diary scores of 38 physical and psychological symptoms taken each day for the week before menstruation.

Women in the true reflexology group showed a 45% decrease in symptom scores compared to a 20% fall in the placebo group. This difference in effectiveness was highly statistically significant ($p < 0.001$). Interestingly, the improvement was largely maintained at 2-month follow-up, symptom scores being 38% lower at the end of the trial in the true reflexology group compared to 17% in controls. Significantly, the authors reported that subjects in the placebo group believed they were receiving true reflexology, which argues against a purely psychological explanation of the findings.

Oleson's trial is of impeccable methodological quality and might well have been enough to conclude that reflexology has value greater than that of placebo were it not for its mixing of treatment modalities. Subjects in the reflexology group also received manual pressure at a number of classical Chinese acupuncture points. It is quite possible that acupressure was entirely responsible for the changes seen and that stimulation of reflexology points was not of any additional benefit. So, unfortunately, it must be recognized that there is no acceptable research demonstrating a specific effect due to reflexology.

RESEARCH ON ACUPRESSURE AND SHIATSU

The research data on shiatsu and acupressure is particularly sparse. There does not appear to be a single published controlled trial of either technique. However, the picture is blurred somewhat by research in acupuncture. Clinical trials have been conducted which seem to show that acupuncture is of specific benefit in pain (for example, Vincent, 1989; DeLuze et al., 1992) and there is an abundance of research which appears to justify the notion of the acupuncture point (see Baldry (1993) for an overview). In addition, there are a large number of trials which appear to demonstrate that manual pressure on one particular acupuncture point may have an effect on vomiting and nausea. In a typical trial, Dundee et al. (1988) randomized 350 women in the first trimester of pregnancy either to press a true acupuncture point (known as P6), or a dummy point or merely to record levels of nausea. True acupressure was very significantly more effective than either dummy acupressure or no intervention at controlling the symptoms of morning sickness ($p < 0.0005$). Severe or troublesome sickness was experienced by 56% of those in the control group, 36% of those in the dummy acupressure group and 24% of those in the P6 group.

The trial was marred by missing data in both the dummy and active treatment groups. The authors therefore conducted a 'worst case' analysis in which all non-respondents were assumed to have either severe or troublesome sickness. The superiority of acupressure remained statistically significant at $p < 0.001$. This trial is complemented by a number of others (Belluomini et al., 1994; Barsoum, Perry and Fraser, 1990; de Aloysio and Penacchioni, 1992; Gieron et al., 1993) each of which show a greater anti-emetic effect of acupressure at the P6 point than pressure at a non-acupuncture point or a placebo intervention.

Perhaps what can be concluded about shiatsu and acupressure is that their basic principles and technique – manual pressure at acupuncture points – appears to have at least some support from rigorous research. That said, their value as treatment modalities has yet to be demonstrated.

SPECIFIC TECHNIQUES OF SOFT-TISSUE MANIPULATION

The specific soft-tissue techniques used by some practitioners to treat musculoskeletal disorders are discussed on page 25. Though these techniques fall somewhat outside the remit of this book (p. 18) it would seem worth giving a quick overview of relevant studies. Interested readers are advised to consult the original papers. Though there are only a limited number of clinical studies, see page 97 for a discussion of basic research on soft-tissue manipulation.

Tanigawa (1972) found proprioceptive neuromuscular facilitation (PNF), a muscle energy technique, to be more effective than passive stretch in increasing passive straight-leg raising in subjects with limited hip flexion. Dickstein et al. (1986) did not find significant differences between PNF, Bobath and traditional exercises for the treatment of stroke. Patients were treated for 6 weeks and evaluated using a number of measures, including activities of daily living and muscle function tests. Kraft, Fitts and Hammond (1992) found that 3 months of PNF treatment did improve outcome in stroke at post-treatment, 3-month and 9-month follow-up. However, effectiveness was moderate (an 18% improvement on a muscle function test) and inferior to that achieved by two electrical stimulation techniques. In a third, but uncontrolled study of hemiplegia, Wang (1994) found positive responses to PNF. It was claimed that the effects of PNF are cumulative and, not surprisingly, that patients with hemiplegia of short duration respond to training sooner. Ries, Ellis and Hawkins (1988) randomized 45 patients with chronic obstructive pulmonary disease to PNF, exercise training or control. Both treatment groups were superior to control on some measures of muscle function but there were no differences between groups on activities of daily living, fatigue or breathlessness. In perhaps the most carefully conducted clinical trial of soft-tissue techniques, Cassidy, Lopes and Yong-Hing (1992) randomized 100 consecutive outpatients with neck pain to receive either a single intervention of either manipulation or muscle energy technique. Immediate improvements in pain were reported by 69% of those receiving muscle energy technique and 85% of the manipulated patients. Though both treatments increased range-of-motion, the decrease in pain intensity was 50% greater for the manipulated group. Flexibility therefore does not always correlate with pain and it would therefore be unwise to conclude that PNF was necessarily of value on the basis of the studies (reported in the section on basic research) showing increased range of motion in healthy volunteers.

Studies have also been conducted on Rolfing (p. 24). In an uncontrolled trial, Perry, Jones and Thomas (1981) examined the effects of Rolfing on 10 children with cerebral palsy. Though mildly impaired patients made gains in velocity, stride length and cadence, muscle strength and electromyography were not altered and the effects of treatment on range of motion were highly variable. Moderately and severely disabled children did not benefit significantly from the treatment. In a randomized trial of 32 healthy subjects selected on the basis of 'exhibiting an anteriorly tilted pelvis', Cottingham, Porges and Richmond (1988) found that 45 minutes of Rolfing decreased standing pelvic tilt. In other words, subjects stood straighter after the Rolfing intervention. No comparable changes were found in the control group. In a separate study, Cottingham, Porges and Lyon (1988) found that Rolfing increased parasympathetic tone (associated with relaxation) in subjects aged 26–41 but not in those over the age of 55.

In summary, there is a distinct lack of clinical data evaluating the effects of soft-tissue techniques on musculoskeletal disorders. Randomized controlled trials need to be undertaken to explore the possible value of these techniques.

MISCELLANEOUS MASSAGE STUDIES

Abdominal massage has been claimed to be an effective treatment for constipation. Klauser et al. (1992) measured the effect of nine 20-minute sessions of abdominal massage on stool frequency and colonic transit time in nine patients with chronic constipation and seven healthy volunteers. Bowel habit during treatment was compared with a baseline control period. Minor improvements in stool frequency (0.59 defecations per day before treatment, 0.68 afterwards) and transit times (from 126 to 111 hours) were observed in patients, but these did not reach statistical significance. Scores of well-being and stool consistency did not differ significantly during control and massage periods. Control subjects experienced no change in stool frequency or transit times. These results suggest that abdominal massage does not change bowel function and is not an effective treatment for constipation in this group of patients.

UNPUBLISHED DATA FROM THE TOUCH RESEARCH INSTITUTE

The Touch Research Institute (TRI) at the University of Miami School of Medicine has been involved in some of the most rigorous published studies on massage therapy. Many of the trials discussed in this chapter have been conducted by researchers such as Tiffany Field, Cynthia Kuhn, Frank Scafidi and Saul Schanberg, all of whom are on the faculty of the TRI. At the time of writing, over 30 studies were under way at TRI and preliminary data is available for at least some of these trials. Continuing the work on neonates, a trial on HIV-exposed infants has found that massage leads to increased weight gain and improved scores on developmental measures. Similarly, a single, daily 15-minute massage was found to improve behaviour and sleep patterns of infants born to depressed adolescent mothers. In a separate study, depressed adolescent mothers themselves received massage. Preliminary results indicated that mothers reported improvements in anxiety, depression and mood immediately after massage and that urinary cortisol levels decreased over the treatment period, suggesting relief from the effects of stress.

Other on-going TRI studies have found improved sleep and behaviour in abused and neglected children, improved communication and classroom behaviour in autistic children and decreased anxiety and depression in children with post-traumatic stress disorder following a hurricane. A study of daily massage given by mothers to asthmatic children has indicated improved behaviour, decreased anxiety and depression and increased peak flow immediately after massage. Positive results have also been reported for job stress, eating disorders and HIV, where a course of massages five times weekly for a month led to lowered anxiety and depression, increased serotonin levels (associated with better mood) and some positive effects on the immune system. Similar results have been reported for a trial on seronegative gay men. In a particularly interesting study, older people enrolled as volunteers to give massage to infants reported improved mood and self-esteem and decreased numbers of doctor visits. This trial suggests that giving massage is itself of benefit.

Clearly, it would be unwise to draw firm conclusions from unpublished data, especially as details of methodology are not available. However, were these trials to be completed and published, and were they to be as rigorous as previous TRI studies, our understanding of the clinical scope and effectiveness of massage would be revolutionized.

Readers wishing to learn more about the TRI data are advised to contact the institute at the University of Miami School of Medicine, PO Box 01680, Miami, Florida 33101, USA and/or to check bibliographical databases using the author names mentioned above.

BASIC RESEARCH ON MASSAGE

What are the physical effects of massage on the human body? Practitioners have made a number of claims about the physiology of massage (see, for example, Wood and Becker, 1981; Joachim, 1983; Beck, 1988). These have included: increased blood circulation; increased lymph flow; improvement in muscle tone and flexibility; 'sedation' of the nervous system; physiological relaxation (decreased heart rate, respiration rate and blood pressure); removal of soft adhesions; effects on skin, bone, fatty tissues and the internal organs. Practitioners have also claimed that massage leads to beneficial hormonal and enzymatic changes. Research has been conducted to evaluate a subset of these claims. Because much of this research has used physiological and biochemical end-points in healthy human volunteers or animals, it might correctly be described as 'basic research'. However, the clinical research literature in massage has also occasionally provided pertinent data.

THE EFFECTS OF MASSAGE ON THE FLOW OF BLOOD AND LYMPH

Given the mechanical action of massage, it does not seem unreasonable to suggest that it may increase blood and lymph flow. There is now accumulating evidence that this is indeed this case. Hansen and Kristensen (1973) examined the effects of diathermy (heat treatment), ultrasound and massage on the clearance rate of a radioactive tracer, xenon-133, from the human calf. The tracer is carried away from the calf muscle in the blood stream and the clearance rate is therefore thought to be a good indicator of regional blood flow. Massage was found to increase blood flow in muscle but not subcutaneous tissue. Neither diathermy nor ultrasound increased clearance rates. This finding casts an interesting light on practitioners' claim that massage leads to improved 'elimination of toxins'.

The effects of massage on the blood circulation appear to be contingent on the technique used. Hovind and Nielsen (1974) used similar radioactive tracer methodology to examine blood flow in human skeletal muscle. Significant increases in blood flow were recorded after 'hacking'. However, 'kneading' caused only transient and statistically insignificant increases in blood flow. Bell (1964) reported that 10 minutes of deep stroking and kneading of the calf increased blood flow and volume. Severini and Venerando (1967) reported that whereas superficial massage of a limb caused only insignificant physiological change, deep massage increased blood flow. This effect also occurred in the untreated limb, suggesting a systemic increase in blood circulation. See also Skoglund and Knutsson (1985) and Oliveri, Lynn and Hong (1989), who found that mechanical massage vibrators lead to increases in local blood flow.

Research has also been conducted in animals. Mortimer et al. (1990) found that massage increased lymph flow in a pig model. This effect occurred both in areas which had received massage and in those which had not, leading to the conclusion that massage has a systemic effect on lymph flow. This replicates the results of a study (Elkins et al., 1953) which demonstrated improved lymph flow after massage and passive exercises. In a short report, unfortunately lacking in detail, Shao (1990) described an animal experiment on the effects of massage on lymph flow. Ink was injected into the hind limb skin of rabbits. This was followed by 10 minutes of gentle compression as the massage intervention. Massage increased the permeability of the lymphatic system, though not to a statistically significant degree. Shao also claimed that there was increased passage of ink into lymph, though this was not fully supported by the data presented.

Wood and Becker (1981) also report a number of prewar studies of massage using animal models. In one study, ink was injected into the hind limbs of rabbits. One limb of each rabbit was then massaged. The rabbits were later killed and dissected. It was found that, whereas the ink had not passed towards the heart in the untreated limb, a great absorption of ink above the joint, and particularly in the lymphatic system, occurred in the limb which had been massaged. Similar experiments on dogs are also reported. It is difficult to obtain the original reports of these experiments and they should probably be considered to be of general, rather than scientific, interest.

A variety of clinically based studies also suggest that massage can improve the flow of blood and lymph. In early experiments, Wakim (Wakim et al., 1949; Wakim, Martin and Krusen, 1955) reported that deep stroking and kneading massage produced 'moderate, consistent and definite' increases in blood circulation in patients with 'flaccid paralysis'. Both Olson (1989) and Ek, Gustavsson and Lewis (1985) report increased blood flow from massage procedures associated with the prevention and treatment of pressure sores. Massage is also a traditional physiotherapy treatment for oedema. The study of Flowers (1988) comparing massage and string-wrapping for hand oedema is typical of the large literature on this subject. Flowers found that a combination of massage and string-wrapping was superior to either technique used alone. Such findings lend further credibility to the claim that certain types of massage improve the flow of lymph.

Ernst *et al.* (1987) found that whole-body massage led to falls in blood viscosity, haematocrit (percentage by volume of red blood cells in the blood) and plasma viscosity in both healthy volunteers and ankylosing spondylitis patients. The mechanism of this effect is thought to be haemodilution (dilution of the blood), which is postulated to result from increased capillary flow. Because capillary vessels with stagnant flow are thought to be filled with fluid which is both cell-free and of low viscosity, release of this fluid back into general circulation would lead to haemodilution. Ernst's findings therefore suggest that massage results in increased blood flow.

In summary, there is good evidence that some massage techniques can have both local and systemic effects on blood flow. There may also be an effect on lymph, but this has yet to be demonstrated convincingly.

EFFECTS OF MASSAGE ON MUSCLE TISSUE

One of the most widely discussed benefits of massage is relaxation. Practitioners have claimed that massage can bring about muscular, as well as psychological relaxation. Though a number of studies have been conducted, there is only a moderate amount of evidence that massage does reduce muscle tension. In a widely quoted study, Nordschow and Bierman (1962) examined the effects of massage on trunk flexion in 25 healthy volunteers. The distance between the subject's fingers and floor in the 'touch-your-toes' stretch was measured at baseline, after 30 minutes rest on a massage table and after a 30-minute massage of the back and extremities. Though there was no change in flexion after the rest condition, finger-to-floor distance decreased by a mean of 1.35 inches after massage. The authors concluded that 'massage elicits relaxation of voluntary muscles', a strong claim given that the trial was uncontrolled. Similar results have been demonstrated for massage using mechanical devices (Bierman, 1960; Williams, Drury and Bierman, 1961). Crosman, Chateauvert and Weisberg (1984) found that massage leads to increased range of motion of the hamstring muscle group in 34 healthy female volunteers. A 9–12-minute leg massage was found to lead to significant increases in hip and knee flexion in massaged legs compared to unmassaged controls. Wiktorsson-Möller *et al.* (1983), however, failed to replicate these results. Though a 6–15-minute leg massage was found to increase the range-of-motion of the ankle joint in eight volunteers, no effect was found on hip abduction, extension or flexion or on knee flexion. Interestingly, subjects who underwent a 'warming-up' period of 15 minutes of moderate exercise experienced reduced range-of-motion if they were subsequently massaged. Massage was also found to reduce some measures of leg muscle strength.

An alternative approach to measuring the effects of massage on muscle tissue is to use electromyography (EMG). EMG measures the electrical currents in muscle tissue and gives an estimate of muscle tone. Naliboff and Tachiki (1991) investigated the effects on EMG of a mechanical massage device known as the Dermapoints Massage Roller. This consists of a rod on which are mounted 28 12 mm wheels each containing 20 points. As the device is rolled lightly over the body, the rapidly moving points provide stimulation to the skin. Naliboff and Tachiki found that, compared to a placebo roller, the Dermapoints device led to significant post-treatment decreases in forearm EMG when massage was applied at this site. No changes in trapezius EMG were found, but this may have been due to the sitting position adopted by subjects in the study. Longworth (1982) found that back massage reduced EMG in healthy volunteers, particularly during the post-treatment period (see p. 107 for experimental details). On the other hand, Fraser and Kerr (1993) reported no differences in EMG between massage and a conversation group. However, Fraser and Kerr give no detailed results and this study is flawed by small sample sizes (p. 76).

A number of studies have examined the effects of massage on muscle by measuring what is known as the Hoffman reflex (H-reflex). This gives an estimate of the tendency of motor neurones to fire and hence contract a muscle. In a replication and extension of Morelli, Seaborne and Sullivan's (1990) study, Sullivan et al. (1991) examined the effects of deep effleurage to the back of the calf in 16 healthy volunteers. Highly significant falls in H-reflex amplitude were recorded during massage but measures returned to baseline immediately following its cessation. This suggests that motor neurone excitability decreases during a massage but that this effect is not persistent. Morelli, Seaborne and Sullivan (1991) later demonstrated that falls in H-reflex could not be explained by changes in skin temperature, nerve conduction velocity or effects on antagonist muscles, thereby confirming a direct effect of massage on spinal motor neurone excitability. Changes in H-reflex amplitude have also been found to be dependent on massage technique (Goldberg, Sullivan and Seaborne, 1992) with deep massage producing greater falls than light massage. Goldberg et al. (1994) went on to demonstrate falls in H-reflex amplitude during massage in persons with a spinal cord injury, but again, these changes did not persist after the end of the massage. These

studies suggest that massage may lead to generalized muscle relaxation during the actual treatment period.

In an unusual and many would say extreme experiment reported
by Wood and Becker (1981), Rhesus monkeys were subjected to uni-
lateral section of the sciatic nerve. One half of the monkeys were then
treated by massage and passive motion for a period of 7 minutes daily.
On later microscopic examination, the limbs of the massaged animals
showed less fibrosis and fewer soft-tissue adhesions. On the basis of
this and other denervation experiments, Wood and Becker conclude
that: 1) massage will not directly increase strength or muscle tone; 2)
massage may inhibit development of fibrosis (thickening and stiffen-
ing of connective tissue) in immobilized, injured or denervated muscle; 3) massage does not prevent atrophy (loss of muscle mass and
strength) in denervated muscle. Many of the experiments quoted by
Wood and Becker are difficult to obtain. The effects of massage on
muscle tissue remain poorly understood. Its effects on muscle tension
must be seen as largely unknown (though see 'Psychophysiological
Effects of Massage' below).

BASIC RESEARCH ON SOFT TISSUE MANIPULATION

Clinical trials of special techniques of soft tissue manipulation for
musculoskeletal disorders are discussed on page 90. These techniques
fall somewhat outside the scope of this book (p. 18) and the research
will only be covered in brief.

Sullivan, Dejula and Worrall (1992) found that proprioceptive neuromuscular facilitation (PNF) (a muscle energy technique) and static
stretching increased hamstring muscle flexibility to a similar extent.
However, orientation of the pelvis during stretch or PNF has been
found to affect subsequent hamstring flexibility. Lucas and Coslow
(1984) also found that though PNF did increase hamstring flexibility,
similar improvements were elicited by stretching. Surburg (1979) compared two different PNF techniques to weight training but found no
differences on a number of variables, including response times.
However, Etnyre and Abraham (1986a) did find that PNF was significantly superior to static stretching for increasing range of motion of
the ankle joint. Moreover, the contract–relax–antagonist–contract PNF
technique was significantly superior to simple contract–relax. PNF
was also found to increase flexibility more than stretching or no intervention by Sady, Wortman and Blanke (1982). Range of motion of the
shoulder, trunk and hamstring was increased by PNF. In addition,
treatment lead to greater consistency of flexibility scores between
days. Markos (1979) found statistically significant increases in hip
flexion in PNF-treated subjects but not in controls. Contract–relax

technique was found to be superior to hold–relax. Interestingly, PNF treatment also increased range of motion in the untreated limb. Cornelius *et al.* (1992) similarly found that PNF techniques resulted in greater hip flexion than passive stretching. In perhaps the only study to examine myofascial release techniques, Hanten and Chandler (1994) found that though myofascial release leg pull did increase hip flexion, it was inferior ($p < 0.05$) to a PNF contract–relax technique.

Studies have also been undertaken to investigate the mechanism of PNF. Moore and Kukulka (1991) recorded H-reflex responses after voluntary isometric contraction. The H-reflex was depressed by 67% at 0.05 s after contraction with maximum decrease of 83% between 0.1 s and 1 s post-contraction. Values returned almost to baseline after 10 s. Moore and Kukulka conclude that strong, but brief, neuromuscular inhibition follows isometric contraction. Etnyre and Abraham (1986b) also found that PNF produced dramatic reductions in H-reflex amplitude in the first half-second or so following contraction. H-reflex depression indicates lowered motor neurone excitability. This is thought to reduce muscle contractability and hence promote muscle lengthening under a stretching procedure. In short, these two H-reflex studies give some support to the underlying principle of PNF. However, in two trials, Osternig *et al.* (1987, 1990) found that PNF increased range of motion at the knee joint despite higher hamstring muscle tension. It may be that factors other than muscle relaxation are therefore responsible for increased flexibility after PNF.

In summary, with the exception of muscle energy techniques, there is little good quality data on soft tissue manipulation. PNF has been found to improve range of motion in healthy volunteers in some cases. There is also some support for post-isometric relaxation, the basic principle of muscle energy techniques. However, as pointed out on page 91, these effects do not necessarily imply that muscle energy techniques are of clinical value and rigorous clinical trials are required.

SPORTS MASSAGE

Massage has also been traditionally used in sports medicine to aid recovery from muscular fatigue. Though a number of trials have investigated this effect, few have unequivocally favoured massage over control treatment. Balke, Anthony and Wyatt (1989) examined the effects of mechanical and human massage on the muscle function of seven volunteers undergoing a number of different exercise tests. Muscular endurance was increased by both types of massage compared to a 'rest only' control condition. Muscular strength was unchanged. It was concluded that 'mechanical and manual massage aids recuperation from fatigue more effectively than total rest alone'.

However, there were a number of methodological weaknesses in the study. There was no statistical comparison of results and the use of subjects as their own controls entails that the results may have been confounded by order effects (in other words, the order in which the treatments were applied may have affected outcome) or by greater motivation of subjects after receiving massage. This latter flaw may also have bedevilled an experiment reported by Eltze, Hildebrandt and Johanson (1982), in which volunteers received mechanical massages or no intervention after exhaustive exercise. Though there were no differences between groups in pain or return of upper body muscular strength, there was a smaller loss in thigh strength on the first and third day after exercise. Similar results were reported by Zelikovski *et al.* (1993) who investigated the effects of a mechanical massage device used to treat lymphoedema on fatigue caused by an exhaustive exercise bout. Though use of the device did not cause any changes in serum levels of metabolites associated with fatigue (e.g. lactate), performance on a subsequent exercise task was significantly improved compared to controls. The authors discuss the possibility that this may have been due to an effect of massage on muscle tissue, for example, removal of fluid accumulating in the interstitial space, but admit that a psychological explanation – subjects worked harder having enjoyed the massage – cannot be discounted.

Cafarelli *et al.* (1990) studied the rate of fatigue resulting from exercise of the quadriceps (thigh muscle) in 12 healthy volunteers. The exercise was conducted in three stages, with intervening 5-minute rest periods, either with or without a preliminary 30-minute session of cycling. The experimental subjects received 4 minutes of percussive vibratory massage during the rest period. This intervention did not improve rate of fatigue compared to a control group. The authors concluded that 'short-term recovery from intense muscular activity is not augmented by percussive vibratory massage'. Ellison *et al.* (1992) similarly found no effects of massage on muscular strength or soreness after an exhaustive exercise bout. A further trial unfavourable to massage is that of Tomasik (1983) who, interestingly, reported that 'hydromassage' was of benefit for post-exercise recovery despite failing to show significant differences between treatment and control groups on a number of physiological and biochemical measures. In a randomized trial, Rodenburg *et al.* (1994) investigated the effect of pre-event warm-up and stretching combined with post-event massage on delayed onset muscle soreness (DOMS) after eccentric exercise. Statistically significant differences between treatment and controls were found for some measures of DOMS and for secondary outcome measures such as muscle strength and serum creatine kinase (an enzyme indicative of muscle damage). However, no differences were found on a number of other outcome measures. The authors conclude that the moderate effects of the multimodal treatment do not indicate an effect of massage on DOMS. This conclusion is also drawn by Wenos, Brilla and Morrison (1990) who, in a short report, claimed that massage had no effect on DOMS induced by eccentric exercise of the quadriceps muscle. Weber, Servedio and Woodall (1994) randomized untrained volunteers to receive massage, upper body ergometry, electrical stimulation or no intervention immediately following and 24 hours after an exhaustive bout of eccentric exercise. Measurements of soreness and muscle force taken at 24 and 48 hours showed no significant differences between groups.

Smith *et al.* (1994), however, did find that post-event massage improved DOMS after exhaustive exercise. A total of 14 untrained males were randomized to receive either 30 minutes of sports massage to the exercised arm or a placebo treatment 2 hours after completing an exercise designed to induce muscle soreness. Subjective muscle soreness, creatine kinase, neutrophils (a type of white blood cell) and cortisol (a stress hormone) were recorded at 8 hours after exercise and for the following 6 days. DOMS scores were significantly lower for massaged subjects ($p < 0.05$) than for controls with maximal scores 46% and 59% respectively. Post-exercise increases in creatine kinase were also lower in the massage group ($p < 0.05$). Serum neturophil counts were higher in massaged subjects, suggesting that massage interferes with the emigration of cells from the circulation into the tissue spaces by increasing blood flow to exercised muscle. Smith provides probably the best evidence that sports massage is of value. However, the results of this one trial must be set against the large number of studies which failed to demonstrate an effect of post-exercise massage on muscle soreness or function.

Pre-performance massage

In addition to being used after exercise to aid recovery, sports massage is used before sporting activity to improve performance. Boone, Cooper and Thompson (1991) measured the physiological responses of non-athletes undertaking a treadmill test with and without a prior 30-minute sports massage. No significant differences were found between conditions, suggesting that sports massage does not improve subsequent sporting performance. Harmer (1991) did find some increases in stride frequency in sprinters following massage but the results were equivocal and complicated by order effects: the experiment was repeated twice and all subjects, regardless of whether they received massage, did worse on the second trial. Tyurin (1985) attempted to measure the effects of massage on the 'psychoemotional state' of athletes. It was claimed that a combination of mechanical and manual massage was more effective than manual massage alone. However, it must be said that the report was poorly presented and lacks sufficient experimental detail for any firm conclusions to be drawn.

Naturalistic studies of sports massage

All the above experiments involved subjects undertaking an artificial exercise, such as lifting a weight, rather than participating in a sport. It would be illuminating to repeat such experiments in a more naturalistic setting. For example, it would be interesting to know whether a massage of an athlete, as typically used by sports physiotherapists before or after a sport, reduced soreness or improved performance on a similar task the following day. Drews *et al.* (1990) went some way towards fulfilling this criterion. Six élite cyclists performed two 4-day stage races of 100 miles per day on a computerized race simulator. Following each race, subjects received either 30 minutes of massage or diathermy treatment as a placebo. Treatment allocations were crossed over for the second 4-day race. No significant differences were found in any of a large number of performance or blood parameters. The authors concluded that 'post-event muscle massage therapy' does not enhance recovery from ultra-endurance cycling or improve subsequent performance.

In conclusion, though much of the data on sports massage is contradictory, most results are negative, with few rigorous studies showing an unequivocal, beneficial effect. However, while the claims of practitioners (for example, Beck, 1988: 334) remain unsubstantiated, good-quality trials in naturalistic settings are required before the value of sports massage can properly be assessed.

PSYCHOPHYSIOLOGICAL EFFECTS OF MASSAGE

Physiological variables, such as heart rate, skin conductance and blood pressure, are thought to be affected by psychological state. The study of this phenomenon is called, naturally enough, psychophysiology. A classic finding (see Benson, 1988) is that relaxation leads to a number of linked physiological changes. This effect is generally interpreted in terms of the action of the autonomic nervous system (ANS). Arousal leads to activation of the subdivision of the ANS known as the sympathetic nervous system, leading to increases in heart rate, respiration rate, sweating and blood pressure. Activation of the parasympathetic nervous system elicits the opposite response.

One might expect massage to lead to an increase in parasympathetic nervous activity – for example, decreased heart and respiration rate and lowered blood pressure – as this is traditionally associated with relaxation. However, research has not found this to be the case. A number of studies have shown, conversely, that massage leads to autonomic arousal. In a small study – and one unfortunately without statistical analysis – Barr and Taslitz (1970) found increases in heart rate, systolic blood pressure, sweat gland activity, skin temperature, body temperature and pupil diameter, all indicative of increased sympathetic activation. Kisner and Taslitz (1968) (connective tissue massage) and Naliboff and Tachiki (1991) (massage roller) also reported increases in sympathetic nervous activity after massage. In a study involving a battery of psychophysiological outcome measures, Longworth (1982) concluded that a 6-minute session of slow-stroke back massage led to an 'increase in autonomic arousal' (i.e. sympathetic activity). Tyler *et al.* (1990) found that a 1-minute back rub slightly increased heart rate and decreased mixed venous oxygen saturation in critically ill patients. This suggests that massage has an initially stimulating effect. Levin (1990) also found statistically significant increases in heart rate and blood pressure following 60 minutes of Swedish massage in healthy volunteers.

On the other hand, many studies have reported no effect of massage on autonomic activity. Reed and Held (1988) found that neither connective tissue massage nor placebo ultrasound affected the autonomic nervous system of healthy volunteers. Unfortunately, no data is presented, Reed and Held merely state that statistical analysis revealed no significant differences either within or between groups. Kaufmann (1964), Bauer and Dracup (1987) and Corley *et al.* (1995) similarly found no autonomic effects of slow-stroke back massage in general hospital patients, myocardial infarct patients and elderly residents of a long-stay nursing home respectively.

From the clinical trial data, Dunn, Sleep and Collett (1995) recorded no change in heart rate, blood pressure or respiration rate following massage in ICU patients. Stevensen (1994) did report statistically significant decreases in respiration rate following massage in this patient group, but these were transient. Moreover, changes in heart rate and blood pressure were indistinguishable from those experienced by the control group. Both Meek (1993) and Fakouri and Jones (1987) reported that a 3-minute slow-stroke back massage led to significant decreases in heart rate and blood pressure. However, neither trial incorporated a control group. Fakouri and Jones's trial took place just before bed and it is quite possible that physiological changes after massage were a function of rest before sleep. In another uncontrolled trial of a 30-minute massage in cancer patients, Ferrell-Torry and Glick (1993) also found decreases in psychophysiological measures. But Longworth's (1982) report of significant falls in blood pressure and heart rate following rest reinforces the difficulty of interpreting the results of studies without control groups. Fraser and Kerr (1993) are possibly the only workers to have reported a controlled trial in which decreases were found in at least some psychophysiological variables following massage. That said, no change reached statistical significance.

The physiology of psychological relaxation

The research findings on massage and autonomic activity are summarized in Table 4.1.

There are a number of comments worth making about these studies. Studies which used volunteers tended to report autonomic arousal. It is possible that individuals unused to massage would respond to a novel experience with an increase in sympathetic activity, particularly while connected to electronic measuring instruments in a laboratory setting. It is also possible that medication may have overwhelmed patient response in trials taking place in intensive care units. So there may be a case for further research to examine psychophysiological responses to massage in anxious subjects, for example, or healthy volunteers who had undergone a preliminary massage treatment. Such research should incorporate a rest-only control group and possibly a number of different massage techniques and/or durations of treatment.

That said, the current literature is clear: where psychophysiological changes do occur in massage, they often do so in a manner associated with arousal rather than relaxation. Does this suggest that massage is therefore not relaxing? On the contrary, some studies (Stevensen, 1994; Longworth, 1982; Fraser and Kerr, 1993) found statistically significant falls in anxiety scores despite failing to record parasympathetic activation. In other words, psychological relaxation can occur in the absence of physiological relaxation, or even in the presence of physiological arousal. This is a somewhat surprising result and certainly presents a challenging heuristic for psychophysiological research. However, given the nature of massage, the poor correlation between physical and mental relaxation might appear to be predictable, or even obvious. This is because the mechanical effects of massage may counteract the physiological changes usually associated with relaxation. For example, increased blood flow caused by the kneading of muscle tissue may lead to an increase in heart rate, a sign of sympathetic nervous activity normally associated with increased anxiety.

In short, it is not clear whether sympathetic nervous activity is, in fact, an infallible indicator of subjective feelings of anxiety or relaxation. Everyday experience tells us that people undertake all sorts of

Table 4.1 Psychological effects of massage

Author	Year	Technique	Length	Patients	Control group(s)	Result
Barr	1970	Back massage	20 min	Volunteers	Crossover	Arousal
Kissner	1968	CTM	20 min	Volunteers	None	Arousal
Naliboff	1991	Massage roller	8 min	Volunteers	Placebo roller	Arousal
Longworth	1982	SSBM	3–6 min	Volunteers	Pretreatment rest period	Arousal
Tyler	1990	Back massage	1 min	ICU	Pretreatment rest period	Arousal
Levin	1990	Swedish massage	60 min	Volunteers	Rest and reading	Arousal
Reed	1988	CTM	15 min	Volunteers	Sham ultrasound	No effect
Kaufmann	1964	Back rub	5 min	Hospital	Crossover	No effect
Bauer	1987	Back rub	6 min	ICU/Heart	None	No effect
Dunn	1995	Various	15–30 min	ICU	Rest	No effect
Stevensen	1994	Foot massage	20 min	ICU	No intervention and talk	No effect
Corley	1995	Back rub	3 min	Geriatric	No intervention	No effect
Fraser	1993	Back massage	5 min	Geriatric	No intervention and talk	Sedation?
Fakouri	1987	Back massage	3 min	Geriatric	None	Sedation
Meek	1993	SSBM	3 min	Hospice	Pretreatment rest period	Sedation
Ferrell-Torry	1993	Massage, trigger points	30 min	Cancer	None	Sedation

Key: SSBM = slow stroke back massage; CTM = connective tissue massage; ICU = intensive care unit vigorous activities to relax: they dance, jog and throw frisbees. Each of these activities leads to psychological relaxation in the presence of physiological arousal. The research literature on the psychophysiology of massage therefore tells us as much about psychophysiology as it does about massage.

EFFECTS OF MASSAGE ON SKIN, BONE, FATTY TISSUES AND INTERNAL ORGANS

There appears to be little research evaluating the effects of massage on the skin, bones or fatty tissue. There is also a dearth of research on the effects of massage on the internal organs. Possible the only trial of interest is that of Klauser *et al.* (1992) which is reported in full on page 91. Klauser did not find that abdominal massage affected mean daily defecations or transit time in either healthy volunteers or patients with chronic constipation.

EFFECTS OF MASSAGE ON HORMONES AND ENZYMES

Though massage has widely been reported to be of benefit for pain, this effect often appears to be short-lived. One possible mechanism could be that stimulation of the skin causes the release of endogenous opiates such as beta-endorphin and beta-lipotropin. It is known, for example, that both acupuncture and transcutaneous electrical nerve stimulation can stimulate production of endogenous opiates in certain circumstances (Peets and Pomeranz, 1978; Pomeranz and Stux, 1991; Kho, Kloppenborg and van Egmond, 1993).

Kaada and Torsteinbo (1989) reported that 30 minutes of connective tissue massage led to a statistically significant 16% mean increase in beta-endorphin levels in 12 healthy volunteers. This lasted for about an hour after treatment. However, the lack of control group in the study entails that changes in beta-endorphin cannot necessarily be attributed to the massage intervention. Day, Mason and Chesrown (1987) did incorporate a control group in a study of 21 healthy volunteers undergoing a 30-minute back massage. Levels of beta-endorphin and beta-lipotropin did rise, but only in the control group. The authors of this paper recommend that their study be repeated with pain patients, rather than healthy volunteers. In a short report, Puustjarvi, Hanninen and Leppåluoto (1986) similarly failed to show an effect of massage on endogenous opiates. It is possible that differences in the massage technique and outcome measure (combination or single assay) led to the observed differences between studies. But it is just as likely that these disparate results are simply a function of the difficulties associated with accurate assessment of endogenous opiates and the great individual variability in baseline levels. That said, endogenous opiate release following massage has yet to be demonstrated and researchers (Sanderson and Harrison, 1991; Dossetor, Couryer and Nicol, 1991) should certainly avoid assuming that this does indeed occur.

Kaada and Torsteinbo (1987) attempted to examine whether another widely reported effect of massage – vasodilatation and increased regional blood flow – could also be explained in terms of blood biochemistry. However, massage was not found to lead to increased levels of vasoactive intestinal polypeptides, a class of substances that induce vasodilatation.

Arkko, Pakarinen and Kari-Koskinen (1983) assessed a wide variety of serum values, enzyme activities and haematological parameters for nine volunteers receiving 'fairly vigorous conventional whole body massage ... for 1 h'. Findings were similar to those of Bork, Korting and Faust (1972): significant increases in activities of lactate dehydrogenase and creatine kinase were recorded 2 hours after massage and peaked at 24 hours. Rates were still elevated at 48-hour follow-up. This is explained in terms of mechanical damage to the muscle causing break-up of muscle cells and concomitant release of muscle enzymes into the blood stream. Some trends in serum hormone levels were seen – growth hormone and adrenocorticotrophic hormone rose immediately after massage; cortisol and prolactin fell – but wide individual variation entailed that the results did not reach statistical significance. Unlike Ernst et al. (1987), Arkko, Pakarinen and Kari-Koskinen did not report a significant fall in haematocrit values.

A number of studies have examined effects of massage on hormone levels as secondary outcome measures. Once more, results seem to conflict. In Green and Green's (1987) study of massage on immune function (reported below) a back rub was found to have no effect on salivary cortisol in healthy volunteers. This may have been because anxiety scores were initially low and not significantly affected by treatment. Field et al. (1992), found that a 30-minute back rub reduced salivary cortisol levels in adolescent psychiatric inpatients. Persisting falls in cortisol and noradrenaline were found in depressed subjects. Kuhn et al. (1991) found that massage of premature neonates led to high catecholamine excretion. No differences were found in urinary dopamine, cortisol or serum growth hormone. Acolet et al. (1993), reported the opposite effect: levels of adrenaline and noradrenaline remained constant but plasma cortisol fell. From the sports massage data, Drews et al. (1990) did not find any effect of postexercise massage on a variety of enzymes. Smith et al. (1994) found that massage did reduce creatine kinase relative to controls. Cortisol was reduced immediately after massage but massaged subjects exhibited higher serum levels at 6-hour follow-up.

In sum, massage does not have clear, consistent effects on hormone or enzyme levels. The many contradictory results can be explained in two ways. Firstly, they may result from experimental error: levels of hormones and enzymes vary greatly depending on the individual, the time of day and a variety of psychosocial factors. Many studies used small sample sizes – typically about 12 – and this is likely to exacerbate the effects of natural variation. It may also be that the data fails to show clear trends because the effects of massage on hormone and enzyme levels is highly sensitive to the patient group, the techniques used and the length of follow-up: Smith *et al.* (1994), is particularly interesting in that serum cortisol in massaged subjects was either higher, lower or equal to that of controls depending on how long after treatment outcome was measured.

EFFECTS OF MASSAGE ON THE NERVOUS SYSTEM

Most studies examining the effects of massage on the nervous system have done so indirectly, by using psychophysiological endpoints such as heart rate, respiration rate and blood pressure (see above). There are few experiments which directly examine the effects of massage on the nervous system. The studies on the H-reflex have already been discussed (p. 95) and seem to indicate a transient effect of massage on motor neurone excitability. Ueda, Katatoka and Sagara (1993) investigated the effects of gentle stomach massage on regression of sensory analgesia during epidural block for minor gynaecological surgery. Regression of analgesia occurred significantly faster in massaged patients compared to controls. Only light massage was used, so this effect is unlikely to be due to the mechanical action of massage on blood flow and seems to be related to stimulation of peripheral nerves.

EFFECTS OF MASSAGE ON ANXIETY IN HEALTHY VOLUNTEERS

Longworth (1982) recruited 32 healthy nursing students to examine psychophysiological responses to a 6-minute back massage. Subjects served as their own control, with measures being taken at baseline, after 10 minutes of rest, after 3 and 6 minutes of massage and after a further 10-minute rest period. Results for physiological outcomes have already been discussed. Of interest here is that Spielberger anxiety scores (STAI) fell significantly, from 34.5 to 28.1 ($p < 0.0001$). This approximates to a fall from normal anxiety scores to those associated with a relaxed state. However, because outcome was measured before and after the experimental intervention as a whole, and because this included a rest period, it cannot necessarily be concluded that massage alone was responsible for the change in anxiety scores. In a non-randomized study, Weinberg, Jackson and Kolodny (1988) compared the effects of various sports to 30 minutes of Swedish massage (40 subjects) and to a similar period of rest (56 subjects). Three psychological tests – the Profile of Mood States (POMS), the Spielberger anxiety inventory and the Thayer activation checklist – were completed immediately before and immediately after the exercise or treatment period. Anxiety scores in the massage group fell from 35.5 to 26.1 ($p < 0.001$). Beneficial changes in Thayer scores were also statistically significant at $p < 0.001$. Massage was also found to lead to improvements on all six POMS subscales (tension, depression, anger, vigour, fatigue, confusion). Except for vigour, each of these changes reached statistical significance. No similar changes were observed in the control group or in any of the exercise groups apart from jogging. This trial does seem to suggest that massage leads to reduction of tension and anxiety scores and improved general mood. Because the study was not randomized, and because subjects in the massage group did have generally higher baseline scores, it would be unwise to use this study alone to support claims about the effects of massage.

Groër *et al.* (1994) failed to find decreases in anxiety following massage, though this may be due to low baseline scores. A total of 32 healthy older adults were assigned to receive either a 10-minute back rub or 10 minutes of rest. STAI anxiety scores fell marginally in both groups, the massage group experiencing a slightly greater decrease. However, the mean pre-massage STAI scores were only 27 in the massage group. As the normative STAI score for a relaxed adult is 29, and the minimum score is 20, it is unlikely that any intervention could be shown to elicit further decreases in anxiety in such a population. The reported decrease of 2.7 points, though non-significant, might therefore be described as a positive result for massage.

To get around the problem of low anxiety levels in healthy volunteers, Levin (1990) induced stress by having subjects undertake a variety of tests, such as timed mental arithmetic and a structured interview involving questions of a personal nature. On the first day of the trial, all 36 subjects undertook the stressor tasks. Stress responses were measured using heart rate, blood pressure, STAI, POMS and the Thayer checklist. On the following day, subjects were randomly assigned to a 60-minute Swedish style massage, or to a control condition consisting of an equivalent period of reading Science Digest. Subjects then repeated the stressor tasks and retook the outcome questionnaires. STAI scores fell significantly during massage treatment, but not during the control condition. Perhaps of greater interest, is that 'the response to psychosocial stress and the recovery from stress were reduced following the massage treatment'. The massage group exhibited significantly lower physiological arousal during the stressful tasks ($p < 0.02$) enjoyed a more rapid recovery to normal functioning ($p < 0.001$) and reported significantly less state anxiety following the period of stress ($p < 0.02$).

Levin's study provides an excellent model for evaluating the effects of massage on stress in healthy subjects. The relevance of this research to say, occupational health, is obvious. So it is extremely disappointing that Levin's work has yet to be published: research of this quality surely deserves a wider audience.

In summary, massage does seem to lead to a lowering of anxiety scores in healthy subjects, except where baseline scores are low. Future research might examine the use of this effect in a naturalistic setting, for example, in a busy office or hospital. The role of massage in occupational health has yet to be examined.

EFFECTS OF MASSAGE ON THE IMMUNE SYSTEM

Groër et al.'s (1994) study is worth discussing because, at the time of writing, it is one of only two published studies apparently demonstrating an effect of massage on the immune system. In a randomized trial with healthy volunteers, mean levels of salivary immunoglobulin A (s-IgA) were measured before and after a back rub or rest period. Concentration of s-IgA increased from 28.2–45.5 mg/dl in the massage group compared to an increase from 24.9–29.1 in controls ($p = 0.004$). The rate of secretion of s-IgA also increased, though this just missed statistical significance. Green and Green (1987) randomized 50 college students to receive relaxation, visualization, massage, rest or placebo touch, in which a masseur touched the patient with one finger at a time. Though there were no differences in salivary cortisol, s-IgA concentrations increased from 15–47 mg/dl in the massage group ($p < 0.01$). Increases in the relaxation and control groups were less dramatic, though, unfortunately, no statistical comparisons were made between groups. The authors claim that salivary flow would not have decreased during treatment, so that the increases in s-IgA concentration do reflect genuine increases in s-IgA secretion.

The mechanism of this change is unknown. Both sets of authors make reference to the psychoneuroimmunological literature, suggesting that s-IgA level is linked to psychological state and can be affected by events such as a bereavement. The implication is that massage is of benefit to the immune system because it improves psychological well-being.

It is important to avoid speculating on the clinical significance of the s-IgA increases reported by Groër et al. and Green and Green.

According to the authors, levels of s-IgA correlate with resistance to upper respiratory tract infections. However, it cannot necessarily be concluded that massage improves immunity to a clinically significant degree. This is because the duration of raised s-IgA after massage is unknown. Furthermore, the effects of massage on other aspects of the immune system are yet to be researched: no generalized effect of massage on immunity has been demonstrated.

RESEARCH ON TOUCH

Substantial literature exists on the effects of touch. This literature is distinct from basic and clinical research on massage and can be subdivided into three separate categories: anthropological research on touch, animal research and clinical research on the outcome of non-massage touch as an intervention.

ANTHROPOLOGICAL RESEARCH ON TOUCH

A number of researchers have examined how humans use touch in everyday life. They have found that touch is mediated by a variety of social and cultural factors, though these are not always susceptible to simple generalizations. Researchers have also looked at the use of touch by health professionals. In general, they have found that this is determined by pre-existing social attitudes rather than by medical need.

Use of touch in everyday life

At least one aspect of the anthropology of touch is widely recognized: the extent to which people touch one another varies by culture. The English, Germans and Americans are widely thought of as non-tactile compared to the French and Latins. An interesting, but methodologically questionable experiment described by Autton (1989) provides some evidence to support this stereotype. A researcher sat in a cafe in various different cities and counted the number of physical touches occurring in one hour. The results were as follows: San Juan (Puerto Rico): 180; Paris: 110; Gainesville (Florida): 2; London: 0.

The nature and style of touch is also thought to vary. For example, in many Arabic countries, public touching (e.g. hand-holding) between men is very much more common than touch between men and women, which may even be proscribed. In Britain and the United States, the opposite is true. Gender differences in touch are also exemplified in the finding by Watson (1975) that men are less accepting of caring touch than women, unless they are very old or under extreme

stress. Touch has also been linked to social status: touching is generally initiated by the individual of higher status so that, for example, it
is the physician who initiates touch with the patient rather than the
other way around. Similarly, the teacher initiates touch with the student and the employer with the employee. Autton (1989) has commented that touch can be 'regarded as a non-verbal equivalent of call-
ing another by first name: that is, used reciprocally, it indicates
solidarity; when non-reciprocal, it indicates status'. Use of touch has
also been shown to be correlated with personality traits such as self-
esteem (Deethart and Hines, 1983; Jourard and Rubin, 1968; Larsen
and Leroux, 1984; Silverman, Pressman and Bartel, 1973). Generally
speaking, individuals with higher self-esteem are more likely to give
and receive touch than those with lower self-esteem. Studies by Fisher,
Rything and Heslin (1976), Duncan (1969), Goodykoontz (1979), Major
(1981) and Tobiason (1981) further explore cultural determinants of
touch.

However, caution is warranted in making generalizations about
touch, even when these are based on apparently plausible research. As
an example of some of the complexities of anthropological research on
touch, Stier and Hall (1984) reviewed a number of studies investigating gender differences in touch. One particular aim was to explore
Henley's (1973) hypothesis that young adult men touch young adult
women more than the other way round and that this may be explained
in terms of power relationships. While uncovering some interesting
data, Stier and Hall's main conclusion seems to be that a behaviour as
subtle and complex as touch is unlikely to be explored fruitfully by
crude techniques such as a simple counting of the number of touches
between individuals. Touch varies in quality and location and the significance of a light touch on the hand is unlikely to be similar than a
compassionate hug or, on the other hand, a punch. Moreover, it is
unlikely that touch can be related simply to single variables such as
gender. For example, though in general females tend to touch each
other more than males, teenage African-American males have higher
rates of same sex touch than their female counterparts.

Touch also appears to involve more instinctive pre-social responses.
Stack and Muir (1992) studied the effects of tactile stimulation on
adults' interactions with 5-month-old infants. This utilized what is
known as the still-face (SF) procedure in which adults pose a neutral,
still expression. It has been shown that infants decrease gazing and
smiling at adults during SF. This effect was substantially reduced
when mothers or strangers continued to touch infants actively during
SF, suggesting that touch moderates infant affect and attention during
interactions with adults. Weiss (1984) reports that parents' use of
touch is important in determining body concept at later stages of

development. Parents were asked to guide blindfolded 8-, 9- or 10-year-olds around a playroom, communicating only by touch. The activity was videotaped and the types of touch used by parents recorded. Children whose parents used strong intensity touch, and contact with a large extent of the child's body, tended to have a more sophisticated body concept. Positive body concept was associated with strong intensity touch and with touch causing discomfort. This latter finding seems surprising unless one takes into account that this type of touch – which included pulling, squeezing and grabbing – was rarely forceful enough to cause pain. Moreover, the correlation between discomfort and positive body concept was most marked for boys and for fathers. Overall, the research seems to indicate that a healthy body image in children is related to instrumental, arousing touch from the father but touch which arouses or sedates as required from the mother. Though this study does not necessarily suggest that fathers should avoid gentle or sedating touch, it does highlight the importance of tactile stimulation in development: touch can be used to arouse as well as to relax.

A number of studies have been conducted examining the effects of what is termed 'casual' or 'subliminal' touch. Examples of casual touch include a gentle touch on the arm or hand or a guiding hand on the flat of the back. Fisher, Rything and Heslin (1976) asked librarians to touch readers 'insignificantly' while returning their library card but to avoid smiling. Readers who were touched were more likely to report positively about the library and about life in general than controls. Interestingly, readers also tended to report that the librarian smiled but did not touch them.

Ackerman (1990) reports two similar studies, though no references are given. In the first study, waitresses who used insignificant touch received higher tips, although customer satisfaction with food and service was not higher. In the second study, a researcher deliberately left money in a telephone box. The money was more likely to be returned if the researcher used casual touch on the person finding the money.

Use of touch by health professionals

The anthropological studies on touch which are perhaps the most relevant for health care are those which have examined the nature of touch between practitioners and patients. These have included quantitative, observational studies as well as more qualitative work. A good example of the former is a study conducted in Texas hospitals by Barnett (1972) who categorized touch by the age, gender, race and rank of the health professional and by the age, gender, race and condition of the patient. The following groups had a high use of touch: registered nurses and nursing students; those aged between 18 and 33; Caucasians and females. Patients experiencing most touch were: aged between 26 and 33 years or between 0 and 1 year; Caucasian; female and of 'good' or 'fair' medical condition. Low use of touch were found among: interns and senior nursing students; older health professionals (66 years and over); males and Mexican-Americans. Patients experiencing least touch were those aged 6–17; those of Mexican-American race and those listed as being in 'serious' condition.

These findings suggest that the use of touch by health professionals is predominantly determined by pre-existing social attitudes. For example, female–female contact is more common than male–male or mixed-sex touch. Moreover, younger, healthier patients are touched more often than older, sicker individuals. Schoenhofer (1985) has confirmed that patients in this last group receive low rates of affectational touch. Thirty older patients in a critical care setting were observed for one hour each. The average number of touches defined as being comforting in intent was two, approximately one-third of the number of touches associated with medical procedures.

The use of massage as a therapy for premature neonates is discussed on pages 80–85. Pohlman and Beardslee (1987) undertook an observational study to determine the use of touch in 16 intensive care neonates. Each touch received by the infant was categorized as either intrusive, comforting or an activity of daily living (e.g. cleaning). Intrusive procedures comprised 69% of touch with a further 15% comprising of activities of daily living. Only 16% of touches were classed as comforting. Moreover, one child received a disproportionately high number of comforting touches from a parent who remained with her during the study. If the data from this subject are excluded, comforting touch comprised only 8% of all touches. The use of comforting touch was also found to be very much lower in severely ill neonates, a finding which echoes that of Barnett (1972). Gottfried (1984) similarly reports low levels of 'social' touching of premature neonates. He records that only 3% of an infant's contacts were with family members.

Perhaps the definitive research on nurses' views on and uses of touch was conducted by Estabrooks (1989), a model example of rigorous qualitative research. It is only possible to give the briefest outline of the findings here and interested readers are recommended to locate the original paper. In the study, Estabrooks described three different types of touch used by intensive care (ICU) nurses: task touch, caring touch and protective touch. Task touch was defined as procedures such as moving or bathing a patient or conducting more technical operations such as suctioning or taking blood. Caring touch 'has a predominantly emotional intent; that is, the dominant intent is to minister to the psyche of the patient'. A good example might be taking a patient's hand as a sign of reassurance. Protective touch is a novel concept introduced by Estabrooks in this paper. It refers to physical protection either of the patient – for example, preventing interference with intravenous lines – or of the nurse, such as preventing infection. It can also refer to touch used to protect the nurse emotionally. This type of touch was seen by the nurses in the study as a necessary means of distancing themselves from suffering and emotional involvement with particular patients.

Estabrooks distinguishes three variables which affect the patterns of touching among ICU nurses: nurse variables, daily contextual variables and patient variables. Nurse variables reflect the cultural influence, life experience and personality of the nurse and are relatively stable. Daily contextual variables include day-to-day fluctuations in mood, energy levels and work atmosphere. Patient variables reflect attributes of the patient which either facilitate or inhibit nurses' use of touch. As an example, a happy nurse on a good day is highly likely to use caring touch with a patient who he or she believes is in need of touch, for example, due to pain or anxiety. A nurse suffering professional 'burnout' on a bad day is unlikely to use caring touch, especially with a patient who is difficult or who might be considered to be culpable, such as an alcoholic.

DeWever (1977) reversed Estabrooks's question and asked patients their feelings towards touch from nurses. In the study, photographs of touching behaviours were shown to residents of a nursing home for elderly people. Patients were asked whether they would be comfortable or uncomfortable with the touch shown. Comfort with touch was found to be mediated by the age and sex of the nurse and by the invasiveness of the touch. The highest levels of discomfort were expressed with regard to touch by older, male nurses and to that where nurses placed their arms around a patient's shoulders. Though these findings are of interest, it is unclear as to what extent they may be generalized. An important variable mediating comfort towards touch might well be the patient's need for touch. This was not addressed by DeWever in the rather artificial experimental conditions of the study.

In summary, touch is mediated by a variety of social and cultural factors. Though these are often not susceptible to simple generalizations, lower rates of touch are often found in men, older people, in Anglo-American cultures and people who are sick. Touch can be used in various different ways and a distinction is often made between procedural and caring touch. Use of touch by health professionals is generally determined by pre-existing social attitudes, rather than by medical need.

Most of the studies cited above took place some 20 or more years ago. It would be interesting to know if the anthropology of touch has changed over this time. In particular, it would of great interest to assess how the use of everyday nursing touch – holding of the patient's hand or touching of the brow – changes with the increased use of massage – touch-as-therapy – on the ward.

ANIMAL STUDIES

A considerable amount of research has focused on the effects of touch on animals. There have been three main findings. Firstly, touch stimulation seems to be necessary for optimal growth and development in animals. Secondly, infants may remain near the mother primarily for touch comfort and stimulation rather than for feeding. Thirdly, gentling of adult animals can lead to lowered stress responses in some instances.

Tactile stimulation and development

From the moment of birth, a mammal is licked repeatedly by its mother. The conventional explanation for this behaviour has been that it serves to clean the newborn animal. However, Montagu (1978: 15) claims that cleaning is unlikely to explain the extent and intensity of mother–infant licking. For example, Rosenblatt and Lehrman (1963) found that rats spend about 20% of their time licking their pups. Schneirla, Rosenblatt and Tobach (1963) reported that maternal cats spent 27–53% of their time licking themselves and their young, the greatest amount of time spent on any single activity.

Montagu hypothesized that licking represents a form of cutaneous stimulation. He reports that this is supported by people with long experience of animals who, he claims, have observed that if newborn animals remain unlicked, particularly in the perineal region, they are likely to die of genitourinary or gastrointestinal failure. He reports on a number of cases, such as the breeding of Chihuahua dogs, in which human stimulation of newborn animals has been used to reduce mortality. Typically, this has taken the form of cutaneous stimulation of the perineal areas using a cotton swab.

Most published studies have investigated the effects of human gentling (petting, stroking and holding) on newborn rats. Solomon, Levine and Kraft (1968) found that early gentling exerts a beneficial effect on the immune system. Levine (1960), Weininger (1953) and Ruegamer et al. (1954) independently showed that handling of newborn rats in their early days results in significantly greater increases in weight, higher levels of activity, less fearfulness, greater ability to withstand stress and greater resistance to physiological damage. Bernstein (1957) demonstrated that rats receiving extra handling are better at learning and retention than ordinarily handled or unhandled rats. Smart *et al.* (1990) reports that artificially reared rat pups subject to an 'enrichment' programme, which included gentling, showed accelerated development compared to controls.

Altman *et al.* (1968) report that handled rats have a lower brain weight but higher cell proliferation than unhandled controls. The authors conclude that 'handling leads to prolongation of brain maturation'. This is seen as an adaptive trait which provides a longer opportunity for the exertion of environmental influences on the organization of the control mechanisms of behaviour. In a further experiment, Altman, Das and Anderson (1968) claim that handling increases the length of the cerebrum. The effect was comparable to that induced by training in a complex visual discrimination task or by raising in social as against isolated environments.

Pauk *et al.* (1986) demonstrated that tactile, but not kinaesthetic (motion) or vestibular (balance) stimulation, prevents adverse effects resulting from short-term separation of preweanling rat pups from the mother. Pups were stimulated by heavy stroking with a moistened camel hair brush, the rhythm of which was chosen to simulate maternal licking. In a clear echo of Montagu's hypothesis, the authors conclude that: 'tactile interactions between rat pups and their mother modulate pup physiology and provide experimental support for the hypothesized role of tactile stimuli on early infant development'. Schanberg, Evonuk and Kuhn (1984) reported similar findings. Stroking with a camel hair brush prevented adverse effects associated with maternal deprivation. Other forms of tactile stimulation, such as light stroking with a brush and tail pinching, were ineffective, as was nutritional support. This last finding is supported by Stanton and Levine (1984). Rat pups were exposed to an anaesthetized female rat after isolation. Four experimental conditions were created by either allowing contact or preventing touch by a wire mesh and by having either a virgin or lactating female as 'mother' animal. Corticosterone levels (associated with stress) were highest in the non-contact groups. In a second experiment, corticosterone levels elevated by a novel stimulus were reduced by contact with a female rat. Evonuk, Kuhn and Schanberg (1979) found that vigorous tactile stimulation of rat pups using a moistened brush prevented the decreases in serum growth hormone and ornithine decarboxylase otherwise associated with a period of separation from the mother rat. Again light stroking and tail pinching were ineffective. Evonuk, Kuhn and Schanberg's conclusion – that 'active [maternal] tactile stimulation is essential for the maintenance of normal physiological and biochemical function during development of the rat pup' – is also supported by Kuhn *et al.* (1978) and Smotherman (1983).

Fuller (1967) extended such experiments to dogs. Puppies were isolated from all contact shortly after birth. Those which were stroked and handled did better on emergence from isolation than controls.

Touch comfort and mother–infant bonding

Perhaps the most well-known animal experiments on touch were conducted by Harlow and Zimmermann (1958). They separated infant monkeys from their mothers and raised them in wire cages in which two model 'mother' monkeys were placed. One model – the 'wire mother' – was constructed from wire, the other – the 'cloth mother' – was covered with soft terry-cloth and heated by a light bulb. The experimenters varied which model mother 'lactated' and measured how long infant monkeys spent clinging to each. As it turned out, which mother 'fed' the infant monkeys had only a minor influence on their behaviour. On average, the infant monkeys spent 18 hours a day clinging to the cloth mother and at most 1 or 2 hours on the wire mother regardless of where they fed. This effect persisted throughout the 165 days of the experiment. Harlow and Zimmermann concluded that 'contact comfort is a variable of overwhelming importance in the development of affectational response, whereas lactation is a variable of negligible importance'. In other words, infant monkeys maintain contact with their mothers primarily for tactile comfort. The same group of investigators later went on to show (Seay, Hansen and Harlow, 1962) that tactile contact is an important mediator of exploratory behaviour. Young rhesus monkeys usually venture away from the mother on exploratory forays which end with the infant returning for a brief period of tactile contact. When experimentally denied tactile access to their mother, young monkeys immediately cease exploratory activity, even though they are still able to see, hear and smell her.

Cordland and Mason (1968) studied the heart rates of infant monkeys which habitually clung to terry-cloth towels. The absence of the towel in the room in which it was sometimes available produced the highest heart rate and the presence of the towel produced the lowest heart rate. This suggests that an object providing tactile comfort becomes associated with security to the extent that its absence produces a stress response.

Tactile stimulation in adult animals

Research has also been conducted on the effects of touch on adult animals. Roth and Rosenblatt (1965) demonstrated that licking in rats was, in addition to cleaning, a form of self-stimulation. Pregnant rats were prevented from self-licking by the use of special neck collars. The mammary glands of these rats were 50% smaller than those of a control group, who wore collars which did not prevent self-licking. Ackerman (1990) reports on an experiment conducted at Ohio University Medical School. Rabbits were fed a high-cholesterol diet so as to induce cardiovascular disease. Half of the rabbits were subject to 'tender loving care': a daily session of fondling and stroking. Mortality rates were reportedly lower in this group compared to control animals. Similarly, March and Macmillan (1987) found that gentling of chicks reduced concentrations of plasma corticosterone, a steroid hormone associated with stress.

A number of studies have examined the effects of gentling on adult rats. Hirsjarvi, Junnila and Valiaho (1990) examined the behaviour of rats to a stressful test situation (a loud noise and bright light). The response of unhandled rats after repeated exposure approximated to that of gentled rats, which showed no changes in behaviour with repetition of the test. It was claimed that gentling increases the stability of a rat's reactions to stressful stimuli. A similar conclusion is suggested by Smythe and Edwards (1992), who studied the effects of central nervous control of glucose production by subjecting rats to stress. Smythe and Edwards report that 7 days of gentling significantly reduced stress response as measured by central nervous activity and serum glucose. Van Bergeijk et al. (1990) found that gentling of adult rats improved response in various stressful test situations. However, gentling was found to have no effect either on the mass of the adrenals, spleen or thymus or on plasma concentrations of cholesterol, triglycerides, glucose or corticosterone. Park et al. (1992) reported that gentling of pregnant rats improved acceptance of surgically manipulated pups. However, Ramsey and Van Ree (1993) found that gentling of rats had no effect on cocaine self-administration in response to emotional stress.

A radically different type of animal research focuses on human–animal relationships, in other words, 'pet research'. One finding which has entered popular folk-lore is that possession of pets reduces blood pressure in elderly hypertensives. This effect is attributed to tactile interaction with the pet (Vormbrock and Grossberg, 1988; Cullition, 1987). Pets themselves appear to show a favourable physiological response to being stroked and patted (Lynch and McCarthy, 1967, 1969).

In summary, touch stimulation seems to be necessary for optimal growth and development in animals. Infants may remain near the mother primarily for touch comfort and stimulation rather than for feeding. Gentling of adult animals can lead to lowered stress responses in many instances.

CLINICAL RESEARCH ON TOUCH AS AN INTERVENTION

In the public's mind, the classic use of touch by a health professional takes the form of a gentle touch to relax and reassure: the nurse wipes the brow of the injured soldier; the doctor takes the arm of the patient on the way to the surgery door. Research has been conducted to assess the effects of these forms of touch intervention. It has been found that simple touch can lead to moderate improvements in psychological or physiological variables in some populations, but that this is mediated by the type of touch, the intent of the person giving the touch, the health status of the patient and the patient's attitudes towards and previous experience of touch. Further research is required to clarify the ways in which touch should be used as an intervention by health professionals.

Touch and anxiety

Whitcher and Fisher (1979) attempted to assess the physiological and psychological effects of touch during a preoperative teaching session, where a nurse explains a forthcoming operation to a patient by using a explanatory booklet. The touch took the form of a brief touch of the hand during the introduction and the nurse taking the patient's arm for a minute during the teaching session. The control group received an identical teaching session without touch. Compared to controls, women in the experimental group experienced lowered anxiety, more positive reactions to the nurse and improved postoperative responses such as lower blood pressure. The lack of response among males was explained in terms of a socialization both against touch and against demonstrating discomfort and dependency.

In a similar study, McCorkle (1974) examined the effects of 'gentle physical contact made by the investigator's hand at the patient's wrist'. Patients receiving the touch intervention were compared with a no-touch control group. Touch was reported to be associated with moderately more positive facial expressions and body movements. However, no difference was found in eye contact and 'general response'. The relatively small difference between groups in this experiment, especially when compared to Whitcher, may be explained by the nature of the interaction during which touch was used. In the McCorkle study, the nurse asked questions about the patient. This is generally a pleasant experience and it is unlikely that the patient would require touch comfort. A preoperative education session is a stressful and possibly unpleasant experience. Clearly, the effects of an intervention will only be measurable if there is some variable on which the intervention can operate.

Glick (1986) found that a session of hand-holding with a nurse immediately before a ward transfer elicited only minor, and statistically insignificant, reductions in anxiety in coronary patients. However, the appropriateness of the touch intervention used in this trial is open to question. In the study, the nurse approached the subject and said, 'Mr R, I'd like to hold your hand for a few minutes.' This does not appear to be a good model of the kind of touch comfort actually given by nurses in everyday practice. Another study which failed to demonstrate an effect of a touch intervention but which is open to criticism is that of Henneman (1989). A total of 26 patients being weaned from mechanical ventilation were randomized either to receive special verbal and tactile interaction or to a control condition. Though no difference was found between groups, only physiological outcome measures were assessed and, as has been pointed out (p. 103), these do not always correlate precisely with subjective anxiety levels. Another possible explanation of Glick and Henneman is that though simple touch may have an effect on anxiety, this is moderate and is likely to be overwhelmed in extremely high-stress situations such as transfer or weaning from ventilation. Such a contention is supported by Drescher, Gantt and Whitehead (1980) who found that an extremely artificial touch situation (an experimenter touched the wrist of a healthy volunteer for 30 seconds in a laboratory setting) did lead to a small but statistically significant decrease in a physiological measure (a 7% fall in heart rate). Interestingly, Drescher, Gantt and Whitehead also found that self-touch led to a slight increase in heart rate. In other words, it is the interpersonal aspect of touch, rather than tactile stimulation, which leads to a reduction in heart rate.

Lynch has undertaken a series of studies examining the physiological effects of touch in coronary care patients (Lynch et al., 1974a, b; Mills, Thomas and Lynch, 1976). Given the nature of the critical care environment, formal experimentation was impossible and so Lynch used a number of case examples. It was found that human contact could have dramatic effects on heart responses, even when patients were subjected to strong stimuli (such as tracheal suction), were comatose or were treated with drugs to prevent movement and hence unable to move. For example, heart rates were often found to decrease by 20–30 beats per minute when nurses touched and comforted patients. However, not all physiological responses to touch were favourable. For example, in one study (Mills, Thomas and Lynch, 1976) an increased number of ectopic beats were found during pulse palpation of some patients with cardiac arrhythmia. As Weiss (1986) has pointed out, touch cannot always be assumed to be an essentially positive intervention. The physiological effects of touch are mediated by a number of factors, including the physical characteristics of the touch (location, duration, intensity, etc.) the intent of the touch (comforting or procedural) the patient's health status and their attitudes towards and previous experience of touch.

Triplett and Arneson (1979) examined the use of verbal and tactile comfort to alleviate distress in young hospitalized children. Crying children were offered either verbal comfort (humming, soothing noises, talking) or verbal and tactile comfort (stroking, patting, holding). Only 12% of children in the verbal comfort group had stopped crying after 5 minutes, compared to 88% of those who also received tactile comfort. This result would probably not surprise anyone who has ever cared for a young child. That said, there are those who would argue that it is always worth conducting research on unexamined, traditional nursing measures.

Touch and labour

Another area in which touch has traditionally been used as a means of reassurance is during labour. Penny (1979) studied the use of touch and 'back rubs' in 150 women undergoing labour. Over 80% experienced generally positive feelings towards touch during labour. Negative experiences of touch were often associated with procedures such as abdominal palpation. Touch from husbands, relatives and friends was usually perceived as positive, whereas doctor touch was rated, on the whole, as negative. Nurse/midwife touch was rated as positive by two-thirds of subjects and negative by the remaining one-third. Where found to be positive, touch was felt by subjects to convey concern, caring and reassurance.

Touch and the new born child

Research on massage for premature infants is discussed on pages 80–85. Studies have also been conducted to examine whether non-massage touch may be of benefit. In a famous trial, Scott et al. (1983) randomized very-low-birthweight infants to lie either on lambswool mats or cotton sheets. Significantly higher weight gains were found in the lambswool group. As both groups experienced similar care, environment, temperature and movement patterns, improvements in weight gains were attributed to the tactile stimulation provided by the lambswool. Nelson, Heitman and Jennings (1986) found no significant change in weight gain when premature neonates were raised on Dacron (polyester) pads. It is surmised that any benefits of tactile stimulation from the pads were offset by increased sweating and irritation caused by loose filaments. The value of wool has also been demonstrated in adults by Dickson (1984) who found improved sleeping times. Schaeffer Jay (1982) examined the effects of gentle human touch on mechanically ventilated, very short-term gestation infants. A nurse placed hands on the head and abdomen of the infant for 12 minutes daily. No massage was given. Though infants in the intervention group showed some positive responses, such as lowered oxygen requirement, there was no difference in weight gain between groups. Moreover, the control group experienced fewer episodes of apnoea (cessation of breathing). The trial was non-randomized and there were a number of confounding variables. However, it may be concluded that the strokes and motions used in infant massage (p. 81) are necessary to elicit positive changes in weight gain and development and that human touch in and of itself is a minor variable.

Another interesting set of research questions concerns the role of touch in aiding the development between mother and child. The use of special programmes of intervention for premature and low-birth-weight infants has already been discussed. It is worth briefly mentioning here research which indicates that there is a special attachment period between mother and child just after birth. Kennel *et al.* (1974) examined an intervention designed to ensure extended contact between mother and newborn immediately after birth. Measurable changes in maternal behaviour could be detected, even at a 1-year follow-up. For example, mothers randomized to the extended contact group picked up and soothed their children more often when it cried and used more suitable feeding positions than controls. The interpretation of these findings, in particular the role of touch in the attachment period, is beyond the scope of this text. Interested readers are referred to the original publication and others by the same authors.

Touch and professional–patient relations

Another continuing theme in this book is the role of massage in fostering communication and therapeutic relationships. Aguilera (1967) found that use of appropriate touch, such as a handshake or a touch on the shoulder, resulted in increased verbal interaction, rapport and approach behaviour towards nurses in psychiatric in-patients. Positive changes in general attitude were also noted. However, this study was neither randomized nor blinded. Nurses' knowledge of the patient's treatment allocation may have affected their treatment of the patient in other respects and influenced outcome assessment. In a study of touch in psychotherapy, Pattison (1973) found that patients who were touched engaged in more self-exploration than those who were not. The use of touch was seen to build rapport between therapist and client. Autton (1989) gives a number of examples of the use of touch in child abuse cases claiming that 'if touch is the damaging modality … it may be the source of restoration'. That said, numerous authors have pointed out that the use of touch in a psychotherapeutic setting is fraught with difficulties. For a good introduction to the various views on the use of touch in psychotherapy see Autton, 1989. See also page 218.

Research on touch intervention has also been undertaken in the elderly care setting. Langland and Panicucci (1982) conducted a simple experiment in which elderly confused patients were asked to complete a basic task. This was accompanied in the experimental group by a light touch on the forearm from a nurse. Compared to the control group, attention, verbal response and appropriate action increased in subjects, though this improvement reached statistical significance only for attention. This result is perhaps surprising given that mental status scores were lower in the experimental group. Similarly, Greenberg (1972) reported a trend toward improvement in psychotic behaviour in 10 institutionalized elderly patients who were touched regularly during the day and Burnside (1973) found that touch in elderly patients with organic brain disease increased appropriate verbal and physical responses to a task.

Touch for people with learning disabilities

Various forms of tactile stimulation are used with people with learning disabilities (p. 189). One of the reasons given for this practice is that touch can be used to stimulate and aid physical and intellectual development. In a pilot study of 13 hypotonic (flaccid limbs), developmentally delayed children aged 1–4 years, Linkous and Stutts (1990) found that stimulation with different textured surfaces increased muscle tone. The authors concluded that such children 'should be exposed systematically to body contact with highly textured surfaces'. In contrast, a number of workers have speculated that the stereotyped, repetitive actions – rocking, rubbing and self-injury – found in many of those with learning disabilities are a form of self-stimulation which might be reduced if stimulation was provided by others. Dossetor, Couryer and Nicol (1991), Bright, Bittick and Fleeman (1981) and Wells and Smith (1983) have independently reported decreases in self-injury in patients with learning disabilities following massage or tactile stimulation. However, Brocklehurst-Woods (1990) found that a variety of activities aimed at providing tactile, proprioceptive and vestibular stimulation did not lead to clinical significant improvements in stereotypical behaviour in two adults with Down's syndrome.

RESEARCH ON MASSAGE AND TOUCH: A SUMMARY OF THE MAIN FINDINGS

Research on massage can be divided into two main categories: clinical research, in which the effects of massage are assessed using clinical endpoints (for example, symptoms) in a patient population, and basic research, in which the effects of massage are assessed by examining animals or healthy volunteers. Research on the anthropology of touch is also of interest.

CLINICAL RESEARCH

- Most of the clinical research is of poor quality, with small sample sizes and lack of control groups a particular problem.
- There is some evidence for a short-term effect of massage on anxiety in institutional settings: further randomized controlled trials would be of value.
- There is good evidence that a gentle form of massage is of benefit for premature and low-birth-weight infants. A systematic review should be undertaken to evaluate the literature more rigorously.
- Research on massage for pain is of poor quality: no firm conclusions can be drawn.
- There are two good quality trials of reflexology. Though one of these did show reflexology to be superior to placebo, the treatment regimen also involved acupressure and the positive result cannot therefore be interpreted as a validation of reflexology.
- Though there do not appear to be any controlled trials of acupressure or shiatsu as treatment modalities, there is some evidence that their underlying principle – manual pressure on acupuncture points – is valid.
- There is little unequivocal evidence that massage is of value for musculoskeletal disorders. Some techniques of soft-tissue manipulation have been evaluated. Though there is some evidence that these may increase flexibility, there is a dearth of data on clinical effectiveness.
- Use of simple, caring touch by health professionals can be of benefit. However, its effect is moderate and can be swamped by gross stimuli (e.g. extreme stress).
- The effects of touch are mediated by the type of touch, the intent of the touch and the psychological and physiological characteristics of the patient.

In sum, with the possible exception of anxiety in institutional populations and massage of premature neonates there is little evidence from well-conducted clinical trials to support the therapeutic claims of massage practitioners. However, 'no evidence of effect' should not be interpreted as 'evidence of no effect': the lack of informative research on massage is primarily a function of the practical difficulties associated with research on unconventional therapies and should not be taken as a reflection of its therapeutic value.

BASIC RESEARCH

- There is good evidence that some massage techniques can have both local and systemic effects on blood flow.
- Massage may increase lymph flow but further evidence is required to confirm this effect.
- There is some evidence that massage reduces muscle tension, but this has not always been consistent: further studies are required.
- The H-reflex is decreased during massage, suggesting decreased motor neurone excitability. The implications of this effect are unclear.
- Most of the data on sports massage fails to find it superior to control with few rigorous studies showing an unequivocal, beneficial effect. Most trials have involved 'artificial' exercise undertaken by volunteers rather than sports played by sportsmen.
- Massage has been shown to lead to reductions in anxiety scores in healthy subjects, except where baseline scores were low.
- Most studies show that massage either leads to autonomic arousal or has a neutral effect. Massage may therefore be physiologically stimulating even when it is psychologically sedating.
- There is some evidence for an immediate effect of massage on salivary immunoglobulin A. The duration and clinical significance of this effect is unknown.
- No clear, consistent effects of massage on hormone or enzyme levels have been demonstrated: it may be that such effects are contingent on the patient group, the technique used and length of follow-up.
- Cutaneous stimulation is essential for the optimal development of animals.
- Gentling of rats reduces stress responses.

In conclusion, practitioners have claimed that massage has a number of effects on the body. Many of these claims, for example, increases in blood circulation, appear to be valid; some, such as physiological sedation, do not. That said, the clinical value of such changes remains to be demonstrated. In other words, even if it is true that, say, massage increases lymph flow, it does not follow that this is of benefit to patients.

ANTHROPOLOGICAL RESEARCH ON TOUCH

- Use of touch is mediated by a variety of social, psychological and cultural variables.
- Health professionals use different types of touch. A distinction is often made between affective touch, where touch is used as a deliberate means of conveying care to the patient, and functional touch, in which touch is used as a necessary part of a medical or nursing procedure.
- Use of affective touch by health professionals is primarily determined by pre-existing attitudes rather than medical need.

Research on aromatherapy

5

CLINICAL RESEARCH ON AROMATHERAPY

THE EFFECTS OF AROMATHERAPY MASSAGE ON ANXIETY IN INSTITUTIONAL SETTINGS

The main use of aromatherapy within conventional health care is as a means of relieving stress and anxiety. Despite the publication of three clinical trials in the first 6 months of 1995, there remains a dearth of clinical research on this intervention. Most trials are of low methodological quality and the majority fail to find aromatherapy to be statistically superior to massage with plain carrier oil.

Recent research on aromatherapy for anxiety

The design of Stevensen's trial of aromatherapy following cardiac surgery (1994) has already been discussed (p. 76). What is of particular interest here is Stevensen's claims that aromatherapy massage led to an improved outcome compared to massage with a plain carrier oil. If this claim is correct it would provide evidence that the addition of essential oils in massage is of specific benefit. It is therefore worth assessing this trial in more detail.

Patients recovering from cardiac surgery received a single 20-minute foot massage with either plain oil or oil to which neroli had been added. At a 5-day follow-up, patients were given a written questionnaire asking whether they found the massage to be of benefit on any one of six dimensions: calming, relaxing, restful, reduction of pain, reduction of anxiety and reduction of tension. Patients were also asked about the perceived duration of these effects. The results, presented graphically, seem to suggest the superiority of aromatherapy oil, particularly in calming, relaxing and in reducing anxiety. Moreover, the effects of aromatherapy appear more persistent than massage for reducing pain, anxiety and tension. Because the patients were wearing oxygen masks at the time of massage, it is suggested that the difference between groups is attributable not to smell, but to the pharmacological effects of neroli oil entering the bloodstream through the skin. There is, however, a significant amount of missing data and no statistical comparison of results. The trial therefore provides only limited evidence that the use of essential oils within massage is of value.

Wilkinson (1995) overcame at least one of the problems of the Stevensen study by undertaking a statistical analysis of a trial comparing massage and aromatherapy. In this, 51 day-care or in-patients of a cancer hospice were randomized to receive three full-body plain or aromatherapy massages over a 3-week period. Subjects in the aromatherapy group were massaged with 1% roman camomile essential oil; those in the massage group were treated with plain almond oil. Outcome measures included the Rotterdam Symptom Checklist and the Spielberger State Trait Anxiety Inventory, which was taken immediately before and after treatment.

The massage group experienced improvements in anxiety but not in physical symptoms. In the aromatherapy group, anxiety scores fell from the mid-40s to the low 30s ($p < 0.001$) and there were also statistically significant improvements in physical symptoms, quality of life and 'top ten' symptoms. Perhaps of greater interest are the statistically significant differences seen between massage and aromatherapy groups for anxiety and some symptom scores. For example, STAI scores fell by an average of 16 points during treatment in the aromatherapy group but only by 10 points in the massage only group ($p < 0.05$). Improvements in physical symptoms and quality of life occurred in aromatherapy subjects but not in the massage group ($p < 0.05$ and < 0.001 respectively). Given that these outcomes were measured 1 week after cessation of treatment, this suggests that aromatherapy had a persistent effect on physical symptoms. Moreover, aromatherapy patients showed a consistent fall in anxiety scores over time, there being about a 9-point difference between the first pre-treatment score and follow-up 1 week after the final treatment. Patients in the massage group did not experience changes from pretreatment anxiety scores.

In sum, Wilkinson suggests that addition of essential oil of roman camomile to the carrier oil used for massage not only improves anxiety scores but brings about persistent, if moderate, improvements in anxiety, physical symptoms and quality of life. Though the presentation of Wilkinson's paper is sometimes confusing, the trial was well designed and provides the best (and possibly the only) direct evidence that use of essential oils during massage is of benefit. Perhaps the only significant problem with this study is one which seems inherent to aromatherapy research: could the practitioners have varied their technique when giving a treatment depending on whether they were applying aromatherapy or plain oil? It is not inconceivable that practitioners, understandably keen to show the value of aromatherapy, gave better massages when they knew they were applying essential oils. Such variations in treatment may have been unconscious and, as such, would not have been affected by the use of strict treatment protocols.

Dunn, Sleep and Collett (1995) randomized 122 patients admitted to a general intensive care unit to three sessions of one of three interventions: massage with plain oil, massage using 1% oil of lavender or a period of undisturbed rest. There were no significant differences in physiological response (heart rate, respiration, blood pressure) or behavioural scores between groups. Psychological changes along three dimensions – anxiety, mood and coping – were assessed using a simple four-point scale. These changes appear to demonstrate the superiority of aromatherapy over massage and of massage over rest, though the only statistically significant difference was between aromatherapy and rest after the first session of treatment. However, the presentation of data was rather unusual, with the main outcome variable being 'percentage of patients whose psychological assessment improved as a result of treatment'. The degree and longevity of this improvement was not recorded.

The study may have underestimated effect sizes for a number of reasons. One of the main problems was a failure to collect data if a patient was asleep following therapy. Though this would appear to indicate a positive effect of treatment, sleeping patients were classed as non-respondents. Moreover, the study design would prejudice positive findings if the benefits of massage and aromatherapy were cumulative. This is because the results of psychological assessments were compared before and after each intervention. If a patient maintained an improvement from one treatment to the next, the likelihood of further improvement is reduced. It is difficult to tell if this was indeed the case because of the rather limited and unusual data presentation. The study suffered from a number of other flaws, including the omission of baseline measures and matching. Again, it is possible that practitioners in the trial varied their massage, perhaps even unconsciously, when applying the aromatherapy oil.

Corner, Cawley and Hildebrand (1995) randomized 24 cancer patients to massage or aromatherapy massage; 18 patients unable to attend the course of massage served as controls. The sample represented a good cross-section of cancer patients including both those in remission, those with advanced disease and those receiving active treatment. Treated subjects received eight weekly half-hour back massages with either plain massage oil or an oil to which a blend of lavender, rosewood, lemon, rose and valerian had been added at a dilution of 2%. Outcome was assessed with a semi-structured questionnaire, the Hospital Anxiety and Depression Scale and a quality of life/symptom distress scale. The latter two measures were taken before every massage and 24 hours later so that the effects both of a single intervention and of the course of treatment as a whole could be measured. Unfortunately, the results of the trial are not well presented. In particular, the use of median rather than mean scores makes the outcome data difficult to interpret, as does the presentation of inference statistics when it is not made clear whether between group or before and after comparisons are being made. Nonetheless, it does seem worth concluding that both forms of massage led to a moderate improvement in anxiety scores over the course of treatment. The authors state that this effect was more pronounced in subjects receiving aromatherapy massage, but this claim is not clearly supported by the data: if anything, the opposite seems to be the case. Reductions in depression scores were small and not significant. All three groups experienced improvements on the symptom distress and quality of life scale: differences between groups are not reported. Apart from the lack of baseline data, and the aforementioned poor presentation of results, the main methodological flaw in the trial was that patients were not randomly allocated to the two groups which were the subject of the main comparison, that is, controls and combined massage groups. In short, though the trial included an element of randomization, it was not a randomized trial. There may well have been initial differences between control and massage groups which explain the apparent effect of treatment.

Other trials on aromatherapy for anxiety

Much of the data on aromatherapy is a good deal less rigorous than the four trials described above. Using an innovative research design, Buckle (1993) gave post-cardiotomy patients a 20-minute massage using oil extracted from one of two different species of lavender. Both researcher and patient were blinded to treatment allocation, thus circumventing the possibility that the massage technique may vary depending on the oil used. If differences could be shown between the two lavender oils, it would follow that the effects of aromatherapy massage were due, at least in part, to the pharmacological action of essential oils entering the bloodstream through the skin. Buckle claimed that this was indeed this case and stated that the study 'disprov[ed] the hypothesis that aromatherapy ... is effective purely because of touch, massage or placebo'.

Given that differences between the results of the two oils did not reach statistical significance, this claim must be seen as somewhat overstated. Moreover, the study's presentation can only be described as appalling: inclusion and exclusion criteria are omitted; baseline measurements are not given; the outcome measures used are not described; outcome criteria are not defined and the statistical presentation is confusing. In short, more details of the trial would need to be given before any conclusions or recommendations could be made.

Another widely quoted study is that of Hardy (1991). The sleep patterns of four long-stay elderly residents were assessed for three consecutive 2-week periods. In the first fortnight, patients received sedative medications as normal. These were withdrawn in the second fortnight. In the final third of the trial, lavender oil was diffused into the air at regular intervals by the use of an electric vaporizer. Hardy claims that, though sleep patterns deteriorated after withdrawal of medication, sleep with lavender oil was at least as good as that achieved using sedatives. However, there are several reasons why it would be unwise to regard this trial as anything more than of general interest. The small number of patients and lack of statistical analysis are obvious flaws. Moreover, sleep was assessed by simple observation: because the observers could not have been blind to the presence of lavender vapour, it is possible that outcome measurement may have been subject to bias. There is also the point that the recovery of sleeping times in the final third of the trial may not have been due to the presence of lavender. It is quite possible that the patients in the trial were tolerant to medication, that the deterioration experienced after withdrawal of medication was 'rebound insomnia' and that the improvement observed during the use of lavender was merely the recovery of normal sleeping patterns. In short, Hardy's paper is a classic example of poor-quality research. Despite its positive result, it does not lend support to aromatherapy practice.

Another study which fails to meet many standard methodological criteria is that of Mitchell (1993), who examined the effects of a simple aromatherapy intervention in 12 adults with dementia, using a randomized crossover design. Drops of lavender oil were added to the subject's bath in the morning and pillow at bedtime; melissa oil was applied to the subject's chin at midday. Grapeseed oil was used in the control condition. The outcome measure used was not a validated one: 'staff or carers' were asked to rate a patient as 'very poor, poor or satisfactory' on a variety of criteria such as functioning, restlessness and communication. Observers were not blinded to treatment allocation so observer bias cannot be excluded. Only minor differences in behaviour occurred as a result of aromatherapy treatment and these were not statistically analysed. The author makes a number of claims based on the data which are unsubstantiated. For example, it is claimed that 'the positive impact of treatment on functional difficulties was maintained after withdrawal of the oils'. Given that this effect only occurred in one group after crossover and that sample sizes were small, it seems more likely that any changes seen were the result of chance variation.

Waldman *et al.* (1993) have briefly described a trial in which 122 intensive care unit patients were randomized to receive massage, massage with 1% oil of lavender or a period of rest. No differences in physiological measures were found between groups. Psychological outcome was slightly better in the aromatherapy group, but not significantly so, and the assessments used were not described. A host of other methodological details were omitted in the report. For example, no description was given of the treatment regime. Waldman *et al.*'s study may be no more than an unusual example of publication bias: a negative trial is reported with so little detail that no critical analysis of the trial can be undertaken.

Two unpublished studies relating to the use of aromatherapy by nurses are also worth reporting. A total of 30 patients admitted to an acute psychiatric ward were given a single 30-minute massage with either plain carrier oil or oil to which either lavender or geranium had been added (Bell, 1992). A number of changes in heart rate, respiration rate and blood pressure were recorded. Falls in heart and respiration rate were greater in the lavender group than in controls, though diastolic blood pressure increased. The small sample size, the lack of a coherent statistical analysis and the possibility of unconscious variations in massage technique entail that these results should be interpreted with particular caution. Perhaps of greatest interest is that anxiety, as measured by a simple four-point scale, fell sharply in all three groups. The number of patients describing themselves as 'calm' increased from 40% pretreatment to 90% post-treatment.

Cannard (1993) reported that the use of massage and aromatherapy in a geriatric setting led to improved sleep and a decreased requirement for sedative drugs. However, the poor presentation of the study, its small sample size and the use of historical controls preclude any firm conclusions being drawn.

In summary, there is only limited evidence that essential oils have sedative actions in institutional populations. Most trials have been of extremely low quality and a significant number have either not been published, or have been reported with insufficient methodological detail. Moreover, the majority of trials fail to find statistically significant differences between aromatherapy and massage. Out of the five trials incorporating an intelligible statistical analysis (Buckle, 1993; Corner, Cawley and Hildebrand, 1995; Dunn, Sleep and Collett, 1995; Waldman *et al.*, 1993; Wilkinson, 1995) only one (Wilkinson, 1995) found significant differences between groups. Future trials need to pay more attention to the *question* being asked in research. Does the research aim to investigate whether the use of aromatherapy oils in massage is of benefit? Or assess the value of aromatherapy as a treatment? Moreover, terms such as 'benefit' or 'effectiveness' need to be defined in terms of specific symptoms and the duration of any changes elicited by treatment.

ORALLY ADMINISTERED ESSENTIAL OILS

Essential oils are only rarely administered orally by aromatherapists in the UK and US. Though trials of oral aromatherapy are thus perhaps of less interest than of trials involving other forms of administration, they do give some insight into the pharmacological action of essential oils. Pharmaceutical preparations containing essential oils or essential oils constituents have been found to be of benefit for irritable bowel syndrome and for both gall stones and ureteral stones. However, a traditional aromatherapy treatment was not found to prevent infection in elderly subjects with chronic bronchitis.

Essential oils and calculi

The use of essential oil preparations for the treatment of ureteral calculi has become widespread enough to reach the attention of the British National Formulary (Sept 1993) which states that 'a terpene mixture ... is claimed to be of benefit in urolithiasis'. Mukamel *et al.* (1987) conducted a randomized, double-blind, pilot study which indicated that a trademarked essential oil preparation, Rowatinex, led to greater stone expulsion than placebo. Engelstein, Kahan and Servadio (1992) attempted to replicate these findings with a larger group of 87 patients admitted to an emergency room with acute renal colic. Patients were randomized to receive either Rowatinex or placebo. The success rate, defined as expulsion of the ureteral stone or unequivocal disappearance of ureteral dilatation, was superior for the essential oil preparation (81% v. 59%, $p < 0.025$).

This study replicates the findings of a series of uncontrolled experiments (Bell and Doran, 1979; Doran, Keighley and Bell, 1979; Ellis *et al.*, 1980, 1984; Ellis and Bell, 1981; Somerville *et al.*, 1985) which found that an essential oil preparation known as Rowachol was of value in the treatment of gallstones. A typical result (Ellis, 1984) was that concomitant Rowachol treatment increased the dissolution rate of a standard preparation from 13.5% to 50% over 2 years. Rowachol has been reported to have a choleretic effect (stimulates bile secretion) (Ellis, 1981b) and cineol (an essential oil fraction) has been found to dissolve cholesterol stones in vitro (Leuschner *et al.*, 1987). Igima *et al.*

have reported that d-limonene can dissolve gallstones both *in vitro* (1976) and *in vivo* (1991). Leuschner *et al.* (1988) have found that menthol enhanced the effect of a standard preparation on the dissolution of gall stones.

Neither Rowachol and Rowatinex are pure distillates of plant material, rather they are mixtures of essential oil fractions. Rowachol contains menthol, menthone, pinene, borneol, camphene and cineol; Rowatinex contains pinene, camphene, borneol, anethol, fenchone and cineol in olive oil. Trials have also been conducted using pure essential oils. Elson *et al.* (1989) reported that a daily dose of 140 >mg of lemongrass oil reduced cholesterol levels in eight out of 22 hypercholesterolaemic patients ($p < 0.06$ for the group as a whole). Though no comparison group was used, a return to baseline scores was reported after termination of treatment. The authors proposed that this effect occurred because lemongrass oil is largely composed of two monoterpenes, geraniol and citral, both of which are end-products of, and therefore block, mevalonate metabolism.

Peppermint oil and irritable bowel syndrome

Peppermint oil is the treatment of choice for irritable bowel syndrome (IBS), the standard dose being 0.2ml three times daily by mouth before food. Rees *et al.* (1979) and Dew, Evans and Rhodes (1984) both report improvements in IBS, though Nash *et al.* (1986) failed to demonstrate superiority of peppermint oil over placebo. See also Lech *et al.* (1988). It has been hypothesized that the action of peppermint oil in IBS is due to the action of menthol, the oil's major constituent, which has been shown to inhibit calcium ion influx in smooth muscle (p. 158). The oil has also been used to reduce colonic spasm during endoscopy (Leicester and Hunt, 1982), an application which could hardly be further from traditional aromatherapy massage.

'Gouttes aux essences' for respiratory tract infections

Ferley *et al.* (1989) failed to show a clear effect of internal aromatherapy in preventing supervening infections in patients with chronic bronchitis. A total of 182 elderly subjects with chronic bronchitis were randomized to 20 drops three times daily of 'gouttes aux essences' or placebo over a 5-month period. Gouttes aux essences contains 1.5% peppermint oil and 0.5% each of lavender, cinnamon, thyme and clove oil. The mean number of bronchial infections was similar in both groups, as was the number of patients who remained symptom-free, the duration of infections, the severity of fever and general physician assessment. Patients receiving true aromatherapy used fewer antibiotics (81% v. 89%) but this difference did not reach statistical signif-icance. A subgroup analysis suggested that aromatherapy may have had some beneficial effect for those patients who normally suffered a large number of infections, but a further trial would be required to substantiate this claim.

In summary, essential oils and essential oil constituents are found in pharmacological preparations for irritable bowel syndrome, ureteral stones and gall stones. There is reasonable evidence that these prepa-rations are of benefit. However, there has been no research on individualized essential oil prescription.

TOPICALLY ADMINISTERED ESSENTIAL OILS

A number of trials have investigated localized topical application of essential oils to treat conditions confined to a particular area of the body surface. Many mouthrinses contain essential oils components and these have been shown to have effects on plaque and gingivitis. Tea-tree oil has been found to be of benefit for a number of different skin conditions. However, in one of the largest and most rigorous aromatherapy studies ever conducted, lavender was not found to improve the rate of perineal healing in women after childbirth.

Mouthrinses

Possibly the most widespread application of essential oils for medici-nal purposes is the use of mouthrinses for the prevention and treatment of tooth and gum disease. Listerine is a trademarked prod-uct of the Warner-Lambert Co. It contains menthol, eucalyptol and thymol obtained from natural sources. Fornell, Sundin and Lindhe (1975), Lamster et al. (1983) and Gordon, Lamster and Seiger (1985) have demonstrated statistically significant reductions in both plaque and gingivitis after rinsing with Listerine. This effect is ascribed to the antimicrobial properties of the essential oils. However, Finkelstein, Yost and Grossman (1990) report findings which suggest that, though antimicrobial mouthrinses (including those containing essential oils) do reduce plaque on visible surfaces, they do not penetrate sufficiently between teeth to affect interdental plaque and inflammation. McKenzie et al. (1992) failed to demonstrate a clinically significant benefit of Listerine on plaque for institutionalized adults with learn-ing disabilities, a group which suffers a higher than average incidence of periodontal disease. Listerine did significantly reduce gingivitis, though gingival scores were still indicative of disease after 12 months.

Only one trial of an essential oil mouthrinse other than Listerine has been reported. Moran, Addy and Roberts (1992) compared a mouthrinse containing eugenol, thymol, camomile and myrrh with a variety of other products. The essential oil mouthrinse was found to be significantly superior to placebo and second only to chlorhexidine in controlling plaque regrowth. However, it did cause 'mucosal erosions in a significant number of subjects', suggesting that high doses of essential oils can cause adverse reactions.

Tea-tree oil

In the early part of this century, essential oil of tea-tree was widely used as a germicidal agent in Australia. Peña (1962) described the use of this agent for vaginal infections. Treatment consisted of tampons saturated in 40% tea-tree oil and regular douches of a 0.4% solution. Patients reportedly commented on the pleasant odour and soothing effect of the treatment and efficacy was claimed to be comparable to standard anti-trichomonal therapy. Peña also reports on a series of successful treatment of furunculosis using undiluted oil directly on the boil.

The efficacy of tea-tree oil has recently been assessed using more rigorous methodology. Bassett, Pannowitz and Barnetson (1990) compared topical application of 5% tea-tree oil gel with that of 5% benzoyl peroxide (a standard anti-acne agent) in a randomized trial of 124 subjects with mild or moderate acne. Both preparations significantly reduced counts of inflamed and non-inflamed lesions. After 3 months, mean numbers of inflamed and non-inflamed lesions for subjects in the tea-tree oil group had fallen by 50% ($p < 0.001$) and 30% ($p < 0.05$) respectively.

Benzoyl peroxide was significantly superior to tea-tree oil for the main outcome measure – reduction of lesions – and for skin oiliness. This difference was attributed to the slower onset of the essential oil preparation. However, benzoyl peroxide scored significantly worse for scaling, pruritus and dryness, and caused a greater number of adverse effects (79%) than tea-tree oil (44%). The authors claim that 5% tea-tree oil gel is therefore an effective topical treatment for acne. However, the lack of a group receiving an inactive preparation entails that a placebo explanation for the effects of tea-tree cannot be excluded. It would be worthwhile to repeat the study using a placebo gel and possibly also a higher-concentration tea-tree gel.

Tong, Altman and Barnetson (1992) conducted a randomized trial of tea-tree oil gel in the treatment of tinea pedis ('athlete's foot'). In this trial, 104 patients were randomized to receive 10% tea-tree oil in sorbolene gel, 1% tolnaftate cream (a standard antifungal preparation) or a placebo cream. Though only tolnaftate showed a significantly higher rate of mycological cure than placebo, tea-tree oil gel demonstrated significantly superior clinical outcome versus placebo at $p = 0.022$. Two-thirds of the tea-tree group experienced improvements in symptoms (such as itching) compared to 41% and 58% in the placebo and tolnaftate groups respectively. The authors concluded that symptomatic improvement, without mycological cure, was the basis for the popular use of tea-tree oil for athlete's foot.

The poor mycological response to tea-tree oil is perhaps surprising given its in vitro activity against two of the organisms most commonly implicated in tinea pedis (Beylier, 1979). Tong, Altman and Barnetson comment that this may have been due to the relatively low concentration used in the trial. However, they point out that tea-tree oil is difficult to make up into a topical cream and that a 10% formulation is possibly the highest concentration that retains physical stability.

The tinea pedis trial is of relatively high quality – possibly the only serious reservation is that the active preparations may have been distinguishable from the placebo gel – and it is therefore worth drawing some tentative conclusions. Firstly, tea-tree oil does appear to have activity over and above that of placebo. Secondly, the action of tea-tree oil may be multifactorial, that is, it may have an effect on inflammation or itching which is independent from any anti-mycological action. This would support aromatherapists' claims that individual oils have a variety of different, overlapping properties. However, the trial appears to warn against any simple extrapolation from in vitro to clinical properties of essential oils. In the laboratory, tea-tree oil is effective against organisms pathogenic for tinea pedis; in practice, it does not effect a mycological cure in infected patients.

A third trial of topical tea-tree oil for fungal infections has recently been published. In a double-blind study, Buck, Nidorf and Addino (1994) randomized 117 patients with onychomycosis (a fungal infection of the nails) to 100% tea-tree oil or clotrimazole, a standard anti-fungal agent. Baseline assessments were similar in both groups. At the end of the 6-month treatment period, 18% of subjects in the tea-tree group had a negative culture as opposed to 11% of those using clotrimazole. Disease was recorded by physicians as fully or partially resolved in about 60% of all patients at termination of therapy. Subjective reports of cure at 3-month follow-up were approximately 55% in both groups. There were no statistically significant differences between treatments. Though clotrimazole is a standard anti-fungal agent, it has not been assessed against placebo in onychomycosis. So though tea-tree oil is of equivalent, moderate benefit, it may be that this is a function of the natural course of the disease or of a placebo effect.

Lavender for perineal healing

A trial worth discussing in particular detail is that of Dale and Cornwell (1994), who examined the role of lavender in relieving perineal discomfort following childbirth. This trial is particularly interesting for two reasons. Firstly, it is one of the few trials which investigates an important claim made by aromatherapy authors. Price (1993: 235) specifically states that lavender will hasten the healing of 'birthwounds'. Tisserand (1977) and Davis (1988) claim that lavender has analgesic and anti-inflammatory properties. They also ascribe specific obstetrical and gynaecological actions to lavender – for example, reduction of menstrual and labour pain. Valnet (1980) states that lavender is indicated for wounds of all kinds. All four authors also claim that lavender has antimicrobial properties. Reed and Norfolk (1993) report that at an orthodox midwifery service, lavender oil is used for perineal wounds to 'promote healing, help prevent infection and provide pain relief'. If these statements are correct, lavender should reduce perineal discomfort.

The second reason why the Dale trial is of particular interest is that it was based upon an uncontrolled pilot study. In this study, mothers were given lavender oil as a bath additive after childbirth and 85% claimed that it reduced perineal discomfort. This is exactly the sort of anecdotal data upon which much aromatherapy is based and the study therefore gives us an insight as to the reliability of such knowledge.

In the trial, 635 women were recruited from a postnatal ward in a district general hospital. They were randomized to receive a 52 ml bottle of either lavender oil, an indistinguishable synthetic lavender oil or an inert aromatic compound. The women were instructed to add six drops a day to their bath water. Outcome measures included visual analogue scales of pain and mood, medication use, presence of infection and the day by which the perineum was healed. With the exception of a slightly lower rate of instrumental delivery in controls, the groups were similar at baseline.

Lavender oil was not found to be an effective treatment for perineal healing. Scores were similar for all groups, with no statistically significant difference recorded for any comparison on any outcome variable. Data 'dredging' reveals that pain scores for those receiving lavender were slightly lower than those in the control group in the first half of the trial, especially on day 5. However, this result does not reach statistical significance and may be explained by the higher use of medication in this group. Moreover, the rate of infection in the true lavender group was over twice that of controls. In fact, this is the only outcome variable which approaches statistical significance ($p = 0.08$).

In short, the trial does not provide any evidence to support the claim that lavender has analgesic and anti-inflammatory properties and that it is of benefit for wounds. In particular, no support is provided for any clinically significant antibiotic properties of lavender. Price (personal communication) has complained that 'no Latin name was specified for the lavender used; this can indicate that an inferior or adulterated oil may have been used'. But George Dodd (personal communication), a leading aromatherapist, prepared the oils for the trial and has vouched for their good quality. It is possible that insufficient dosage was used, although both Price (1993) and Davis (1988) do recommend six drops per bath. It is also possible that it is bathing, rather than lavender, which is ineffective and that another means of administration, such as a compress, would be of benefit. However, what the trial does demonstrate is that anecdotal reports of the properties of essential oils are not always reliable. When merely asked, in the pilot study, women reported that lavender oil was of benefit for perineal discomfort. But when data was collected in a more systematic fashion, including comparisons with control groups, no effect was found. Given that aromatherapy knowledge is primarily based on anecdotal reports, the negative result of this trial surely presents a serious challenge to aromatherapists.

Other trials of topical essential oil application

A few other trials of topical essential oil application are worth reporting in brief. Maiche, Grohn and Maki Hokkonen (1991) found that an ointment containing essential oil of camomile was no more effective than a placebo ointment in preventing acute radiation skin reaction during radiotherapy. However, there was some trend towards fewer cases of dark erythema (reddening of the skin) in the camomile oil group. Korting et al. (1993) found that a distillate of witch hazel suppressed experimentally induced erythema when made up with an ointment containing phosphatidylcholine, which aids skin penetration. Camomile cream was found to have no effect.

Ginsberg and Farnaey (1987) found that a proprietary topical application – Rado-Salil ointment – was of benefit for low back pain. A total of 40 patients were randomized to receive either Rado-Salil or an indistinguishable placebo ointment. Highly significant improvements were found in pain, muscular contracture, functional assessment and medication usage in the experimental group, but not in controls. Rado-Salil contains a number of compounds commonly found in essential oils, including menthol and methyl salicylate. The effects of Deep Heat, another topical application containing these two compounds, have been assessed in a laboratory setting (p. 148).

In summary, a number of commercial mouthwashes contain essential oils or fractions thereof and most trials show at least some effect of such mouthwashes on gingivitis and plaque regrowth. This may be attributed to the antibacterial action of essential oils. There is good-quality evidence that topical tea-tree oil appears to be effective in the treatment of certain skin infections. However, in a large, randomized study of perineal healing, lavender oil was found to be no more effective than placebo. This trial is of particular interest not only because of its quality, but because it is one of the few trials directly to examine a claim made by aromatherapists.

INHALATION OF ESSENTIAL OILS FOR RESPIRATORY CONDITIONS

Inhalation of essential oils added to boiling water, and aromatic ointments rubbed on the chest, are traditional treatments for respiratory conditions which developed independently from professional aromatherapy. There is some evidence that these treatments are of value. Most research has investigated patented products consisting of essential oil compounds rather than whole essential oils. An exception is Saller *et al.* (1990), who found that steam inhalation of camomile extract relieved the symptoms of the common cold in 15 patients. Improvement was dose-dependent – in other words, higher doses of camomile extract gave greater relief – and statistically significant compared to placebo. That said, the study was reported only briefly and this precludes any critical appraisal of its value.

A study of higher methodological quality is reported by Cohen (1982). In this, 24 non-smoking adults with common colds were randomized to inhale hot water vapour (control) or a mixture of 9% eucalyptus oil, 56% menthol and 35% camphor. Moderate improvements in respiratory function were recorded on a number of tests. On some measures, for example, forced vital capacity and forced expiratory volume, there were statistically significant differences between treated subjects and controls. The authors conclude that the aromatic inhalation attenuated the changes in airways dynamics occurring during the common cold. The study therefore provides some support to this traditional treatment practice. It would be worth repeating this experiment to include subjective outcome measures to assess whether inhalation of essential oils provides symptomatic relief in the common cold.

Berger and colleagues have undertaken a series of studies examining the effects of Vicks VapoRub on the symptoms of acute bronchitis in children. In the first trial (Berger, Jarosh and Madreiter, 1978a), 60 children were randomized to topical application of VapoRub or plain Vaseline. Statistically significant improvements in frequency and amplitude of breathing were recorded. Effects were maximal shortly after the initiation of treatment but persisted at a reduced level until the 70-minute follow-up, which constituted the end of the experiment. This diminution of effect could possibly be explained in terms of evaporation of the active constituents of the treatment. A second report (Berger, Jarosh and Madreiter, 1978b) involved a reanalysis of the same data to determine restlessness. It was found that treatment increased 'quiet periods' by up to 200% in the treated group but not in controls. This effect was maintained over the 70-minute follow-up period and would seem to support the traditional use of VapoRub in children before bedtime. In a separate study Berger *et al.* (1978) found that treatment with VapoRub, but not Vaseline, increased skin temperature by 1°C ($p < 0.05$). Because rectal temperature was unaffected, this effect was attributed to dilation of blood vessels in the treated area. A similar effect was noted in healthy children. However, the time course was shorter, suggesting that bronchitis changes the response to VapoRub treatment.

VapoRub is a patented product consisting of eucalyptus oil, menthol, camphor and turpentine oil. Although Berger's results seem to suggest a role for VapoRub in the alleviation of symptoms in bronchitis, it should be mentioned that many experimental details were missing from the published reports. It would therefore be premature to draw firm conclusions about this product.

In a double-blind, randomized controlled trial, 100 male patients with chronic obstructive pulmonary disease received either Pinimenthol, a patented preparation containing camphor, eucalyptus, menthol and essential oils of two pine species (*Pinus silvestris* and *Pinus pumila*) in Vaseline (Linsenmann and Swoboda, 1986). Patients applied the preparations to the chest and back three times daily. Outcome measures, including lung function and assessments of cough, dyspnoea (laboured breathing) and wheezing, were taken at 1, 7 and 14 days after commencement of treatment. Moderate improvements in lung function found in patients receiving Pinimenthol were statistically superior to those of the placebo group. Symptoms of dyspnoea and cough, and presence of wheezing, also improved significantly more in the treatment group than in controls. For example, 30% of those receiving Pinimenthol, as against 14% of controls, reported an improvement in dyspnoea. For more on the effects of essential oils on respiratory conditions, see the basic research described on page 156.

In sum, the clinical data provide some support for traditional ointments and inhalations containing essential oils and/or essential fractions for the alleviation of respiratory infections. Aromatherapy treatment of respiratory conditions has not been evaluated.

HERB STUDIES

Aromatherapists have a somewhat uneasy relationship to herbal medicine. For example, while Davis (1988: 100) claims that an 'aromatherapist can find [in Culpeper] useful indications on the properties and uses of many oils', Price (1993: 120) states that the 'effects of a plant are not always the same as those of its essential oil' and cautions against use of the traditional herbal manuals. Despite this warning, many indications and properties of essential oils are similar to those given by herbalists.

Valerian is a particularly interesting case in point. Aqueous extracts of this herb have been shown to improve sleep (Lindahl and Lindwall, 1989; Schulz, Stolz and Muller, 1994). It is possibly on these grounds that Price (1993: 278), Tisserand (1988: 136), Lawless (1994b: 201) and many others would feel justified in ascribing sedative properties to valerian oil and give insomnia as an indication. However, Houghton (1994) reports that 'insufficient volatile oil is present in standard extracts of valerian used pharmaceutically to account for the sedative effects'. Rather, the sedative properties of valerian are ascribed to a class of compounds called valepotriates. These are found in alcoholic tinctures (used by herbalists) but not in essential oils. Interestingly, experiments measuring psychophysiological effects of essential oils in animal models (p. 151) do not find a sedative action of valerian, possibly confirming Houghton's hypothesis. It is beyond the scope of this book to investigate the presumed mode of action of all herbs that have similar properties and indications to essential oils; the valerian story, however, is a suitable warning against simple extrapolation from herbal data.

MISCELLANEOUS STUDIES

Some studies go somewhat beyond the bounds of traditional aromatherapy practice. Rose and Behm (1994) found that vapour of black pepper essential oil could be of benefit for smoking cessation; 48 cigarette smokers participated in a 3-hour session conducted after overnight deprivation from smoking. Subjects puffed at will on a special cigarette-like device which delivered the vapour of an essential oil. They were randomly assigned to black pepper oil, mint/menthol or control. Reported craving for cigarettes was significantly reduced in the pepper condition relative to each of the two control conditions. In addition, subjects inhaling black pepper oil had significantly fewer psychological and somatic symptoms of anxiety. The intensity of reported chest sensations was also significantly higher for the pepper condition. The authors concluded that respiratory tract sensations are important in alleviating smoking withdrawal symptoms and that cigarette substitutes delivering pepper constituents may prove useful in smoking cessation treatment.

In southern India, the traditional treatment to suppress puerperal lactation in mothers of stillborn infants involves direct application of jasmine flowers to the breasts. Shrivastav *et al*. (1988) randomized 60 women to application of jasmine flowers or bromocriptine (standard therapy). Jasmine flowers were found to reduce both serum prolactin and clinical signs of lactation. This confirms an earlier study in a rat model (Abraham, Sarada Devi and Sheela, 1979). It is interesting to speculate on the mechanism of this effect. Though an olfactory route cannot be ruled out, Abraham and colleagues found that jasmine flowers were most effective if applied directly to the breasts. This suggests that passage of some substance from the flowers into the breast is important. Essential oils, or constituents thereof, might be a suitable candidate.

BASIC RESEARCH ON AROMATHERAPY

Plants contain pharmacologically active substances and have been subject to pharmacological research. Many tens of thousands of papers have been written on plant pharmacology. Research has included chemical analyses of plant material and investigations of substances derived from plants using human, animal and in vitro models. A large proportion of this research is relevant for aromatherapy, so much, in fact, that it is impractical to conduct a complete review in a text of this nature. An overview of the most important and representative studies is given below.

RESEARCH ON THE ADMINISTRATION OF ESSENTIAL OILS (1): BIOAVAILABILITY

One of the most fundamental claims in aromatherapy is that the therapy is something more than just massage plus smell. Though essential oils certainly do have pharmacological properties (see, for example, p. 133) the oils must enter the bloodstream for these properties to be of value. Most aromatherapy practice in the UK and US consists of topical application of essential oils in baths and massage and inhalation of vapour. It is therefore vital that aromatherapists demonstrate passage of essential oils into the bloodstream after topical application and inhalation. Indeed, aromatherapists have long claimed that this does occur because essential oils are fat-soluble and hence pass through the skin. There is now some good evidence that this claim holds.

Bioavailability of essential oils after topical application

Jäger *et al.* (1992a) demonstrated that lavender oil can penetrate the skin: 1.5 g of a 2% solution of lavender oil in peanut oil was gently massaged into the stomach of a male volunteer for 10 minutes. Blood samples were taken at the end of the massage and at regular intervals thereafter. Gas chromatography revealed traces of linalool and linalyl acetate, the two major constituents of lavender oil, 5 minutes after the end of the massage. Maximal concentration was reached at 20-minute follow-up with levels of 121 ng/ml and 100 ng/ml respectively. Levels returned almost to baseline after 90 minutes indicating elimination of the lavender oil from the bloodstream. Similarly, Bronough (1990) demonstrated the passage of a number of aromatic compounds (mainly benzyl derivatives) through the skin in humans and Rhesus monkeys. Collins *et al.* (1984) detected methyl salicylate (the major component of wintergreen oil) in venous blood after topical application by means of an aerosol spray. Villar *et al.* (1994) have reported symptoms of poisoning, such as uncoordination and muscle tremors, in cats and dogs following dermal applications of tea tree oil. This provides further evidence for the passage of essential oil components into the bloodstream through the skin. Cornwell and Barry (1994) have gone so far as to investigate the possibility of using substances derived from essential oils as skin penetration enhancers. Diliberto, Usha and Birnbaum (1988) studied the pattern of distribution and elimination of citral (the major constituent of lemongrass oil) after oral, intravenous and dermal administration in rats. Citral was readily absorbed and rapidly metabolized, elimination occurring in urine, faeces and expired air. This supports the claim that essential oils may have widespread actions on a variety of body systems after topical application, and might explain aromatherapists' otherwise somewhat surprising assertion that massage with some essential oils is of benefit for digestive complaints. Schäfer and Schäfer (1981) report on two studies in which radioactive camphor was topically applied to the shaved thorax of rats. At 15 minutes, 60% of the camphor remained on the skin; at 60 minutes, this had fallen to 38%. Only 0.3% of the camphor was eliminated in expired air, the rest having evaporated or been distributed throughout the rest of the body.

Bioavailability of essential oils after inhalation

There is evidence that essential oil constituents enter the bloodstream after inhalation. Kovar *et al.* (1987) reported increases in locomotor activity in mice after inhalation of rosemary oil. A major constituent of rosemary – 1,8-cineole – was detected in blood drawn from the mice for about 2 hours after exposure. Serum levels of 1,8-cineole correlated with initial dose of rosemary vapour and increases in locomotor activity. Similar results were reported for oral administration of rosemary oil, suggesting that changes in behaviour following inhalation of rosemary oil are likely to involve a pharmacological mechanism.

This work was expanded upon by Buchbauer *et al.* (1993). The study is reported in more detail below. What is of interest here is that aromatic compounds were detected in mice serum after inhalation of essential oils and constituent compounds. For example, after inhalation of neroli oil, measurable quantities of geraniol, a constituent compound, were detected in serum samples. Aromatic compounds were also found to be present in blood after inhalation of sandalwood oil, rose oil, orange flower oil, lavender oil and anise oil. In similar experiments, Jäger *et al.* (1992b) identified fractions of neroli oil, primarily linalool, in blood samples after inhalation and Jirovetz *et al.* (1992) identified santalol and santalene in serum samples after inhalation of sandalwood oil.

Absorption of inhaled aromatic compounds has also been demonstrated in humans by Falk-Filipsson. These studies involved volunteers breathing from a controlled source while undergoing light exercise on a stationary bicycle. Both alpha-pinene (Falk *et al.*, 1990) – a component of many oils, particularly juniper – and d-limonene (Falk-Filipsson, 1993) – a constituent of lemon oil – were detected in capillary blood after inhalation. Approximately 60% of the compound was absorbed in each case. Almost all of this was metabolized, with only 0.001% of absorbed substance recovered from subjects' urine at the conclusion of the study. Elimination rates were rapid: serum levels fell towards baseline levels within 6 hours.

Such research demonstrates that at least some substances in essential oils are absorbed into the bloodstream via inhalation or through the skin. This is not perhaps surprising, given that a number of drugs are now administered in the form of nasal sprays (Chien, 1985) or skin patches and provides a partial research basis for the aromatherapeutic practices of massage and vaporization. However, essential oils reach the bloodstream in low doses and are eliminated relatively rapidly. The current research data does not suggest a mechanism for any long-lasting effect of treatment with essential oils.

RESEARCH ON THE ADMINISTRATION OF ESSENTIAL OILS
(2): SKIN SENSITIZATION

One of the most interesting claims of aromatherapy is that the toxic effects of one substance found in an essential oil can be reduced or 'buffered' by the effects of another. It is said, for example, that the presence of an essential oil constituent which is, say, a skin irritant, is offset by the presence of other components which negate this effect. There are two studies which indicate that this claim may well hold. Opdyke (1976) reports that buffering actions of essential oil constituents were noticed accidentally while undertaking a series of experiments to assess skin sensitization (an allergic process; see page 256). It was found that, whereas certain essential oil constituents could cause sensitization when applied to the skin in their pure form, whole essential oils did not often do so. For example, whereas a 1% solution of citral resulted in a sensitization reaction in some individuals, a 4% solution of lemongrass oil (which is 85% citral) was well tolerated. Opdyke went on to demonstrate a similar effect when 4% citral was tested with 1% solutions of d-limonene, alpha-pinene or mixed citrus terpenes (constituents found with citral in a variety of essential oils). Similarly, though cinnamic aldehyde was found to cause skin sensitization in some subjects, cinnamon leaf oil did not. Moreover, no irritation was observed when cinnamic aldehyde was tested in a 1:1 mixture with eugenol or d-limonene, despite being present in a much greater concentration than that which caused sensitization when tested in a pure form. Opdyke described this effect as 'quenching'.

Hanau et al. (1983) also found that d-limonene influenced delayed skin sensitivity induced by citral. Guinea pigs were sensitized to citral alone or to citral and limonene. No differences were found in erythema (reddening of the skin), but significant improvements on histological examination were found in the citral plus limonene group. This indicates that the adverse effects of one essential oil component can be offset by the presence of another. This supports Opdyke's (1976) observations and provides at least some evidence for the claim that the presence of many compounds in an essential oil buffers at least some potential adverse effects.

ANTIMICROBIAL ACTIVITY OF ESSENTIAL OILS

Many essential oils are active against bacterial and fungal pathogens. This should not be seen as surprising: plants need to avoid infection and production of anti-microbial compounds provides an important defence mechanism.

It is probable that more research has been conducted on the anti-microbial activity of essential oils than on all other properties combined. Janssen, Scheffer and Svendsen (1987) give a useful overview of significant research from the 1970s and early 1980s. The review confirms that many essential oils have antimicrobial activity but concludes that this is often difficult to quantify because of variations in the test methods and insufficient description of the essential oils and microorganisms in different studies. Of particular interest is the finding that the time of day, stage of development and location from which the plant is harvested, as well as the isolation technique used, can all influence an oil's antimicrobial activity. For example, it is reported that antimicrobial activity of essential oil of *Thymus pulegoides* varied depending on the region of Poland where the plant was collected. It is also reported that different chemotypes (p. 30) of *Thymus vulgaris* have varying antimicrobial activity. The strongest antifungal chemotype, for instance, had eight times the activity of the weakest against *Candida albicans*. Marotti *et al.* (1994) studied variations in the antimicrobial activity of fennel oil. Up to four-fold differences in activity were found across two varieties harvested at three different stages. For example, the essential oil from Florence fennel showed a 30% decrease in activity against the bacterium *Clostridium sporogenes* when harvested at the 'late waxy seed' stage compared to the 'early waxy seed' stage. Oil from plants harvested at the 'ripe seed' stage showed a further 15% fall in activity.

A particularly interesting paper is that by Remmal *et al.* (1993a, b) who criticize the method typically used in assays of antimicrobial activity. Remmal *et al.* point out that solvents and detergents are normally used to help disperse the essential oil. By comparing the results of a novel technique, which involves dispersion of the oils directly into the culture medium, with those commonly found in the literature, Remmal *et al.* claim that conventional methods underestimate the antimicrobial potency of essential oils. This is ascribed to the action of the detergents and solvents.

The essential oils featuring in the majority of studies on antimicrobial activity are not commonly used by aromatherapists. As an example of a representative study, Hammerschmidt *et al.* (1993) found that essential oil of *Jasonia candicans* had anti-bacterial properties against *Pseudomonas aeruginosa* and *Bacillus subtilis* as well as activity against *Candida albicans* and a number of other fungi. *Jasonia candicans* is a herb used in Egyptian folk medicine, but the use of its essential oil has not appeared in the aromatherapy literature.

However, some oils commonly used by aromatherapists have demonstrated antimicrobial properties *in vitro*. Papers of particular interest include that of Zani *et al.* (1991), who reported anti-bacterial activity of a number of oils including roman camomile, sage, savory, thyme and bergamot, and Panizzi *et al.* (1993) ,who studied thyme, savory and rosemary. Perrucci *et al.* (1994) found that thyme and savory had particularly strong activity against various fungi isolated from animals, even those resistant to synthetic anti-mycotics. Rosemary and lavender were found to have a less marked effect. De

Blasi *et al.* (1990) found that, in addition to activity against bacteria and fungi, some essential oils are effective against pathogenic amoebae *in vitro*. Knoblock *et al.* (1989) correlated antibacterial and antifungal properties of a variety of essential oil fractions with physical characteristics such as solubility in water. See also Beylier (1979), Ogunlana *et al.* (1987), Gabbrielli *et al.* (1988), Dube, Upadhyay and Tripath (1989), Deans and Svoboda (1990), Carson and Riley (1993, 1994), Onawunmi and Ogunlana (1986), Onawunmi, Yisak and Ogunlana (1984) and Juven *et al.* (1994).

The constituents of essential oils have also been demonstrated to have antimicrobial properties. Moleyar and Narasimham (1992) studied the antibacterial activity of 15 essential oil components towards a variety of pathogens including *Staphylococcus* and *Enterobacter*. Citral, geraniol, eugenol and menthol were all found to have high antibacterial activity. Hammerschmidt (1993) reported activity of 1,8-cineole, camphor and borneol against *Candida albicans*, though these compounds were not effective against several other fungi. See also Onawunmi (1989).

The clinical implications of these studies are not entirely clear. An essential oil demonstrating an *in vitro* effect on a certain strain of bacteria may not have a useful clinical effect on an infection caused by that strain. This is because, to be effective, the oil needs to be delivered to the site of infection consistently, in an appropriate dose and unmodified by possible interactions with other substances in the body. It remains for clinical trials to assess the value of aromatherapy in the treatment of infection. With a few notable exceptions, these have yet to be undertaken.

TOPICAL PREPARATIONS IN HUMAN VOLUNTEERS

Deep Heat is an over-the-counter preparation containing eucalyptus oil, menthol (the major constituent of peppermint oil) and methyl salicylate (the major constituent of wintergreen oil). It is said to be a rubefacient, that is, it increases local blood flow. Collins *et al.* (1984) applied Deep Heat by means of an aerosol to the forearms of healthy volunteers. The preparation caused erythema and increased local skin temperature, suggesting increased local blood flow and thus confirming a rubefacient action. Other findings of interest include increased oxygen levels and decreased platelet aggregation in venous blood. These effects were ascribed to the passage of pharmacologically active substances into the bloodstream.

Göbel, Schmidt and Soyka (1994) investigated the effects of topical peppermint and eucalyptus oil on experimentally induced headache in 32 healthy volunteers. In a double-blind, randomized, cross-over design, subjects received one of four applications to the forehead: 10% peppermint oil (P), 5% eucalyptus oil (E), both (E+P) or only trace amounts of both (placebo). In each case, the preparation was made up to 10 g with ethanol. Both the P and E+P preparations led to a relaxation of the temporal muscles during the headache and to decreased emotional irritation as measured by a standard psychological test. The E+P preparation reduced CNV amplitude (p. 164, indicating either a sedative or distraction effect, both a positive response in headache. Interestingly, only the P preparation reduced pain ratings, suggesting that the analgesic actions of peppermint are antagonized by eucalyptus oil. Placebo and eucalyptus oil alone had no effect. Göbel, Schmidt and Soyka claim that the analgesic effects of essential oils derive from the activation of nerves sensitive to cold and cites unpublished data to support this contention. In conclusion, Collins *et al.* (1984) and Göbel, Schmidt and Soyka (1994) provide some support for the traditional use of pain-relieving ointments and other topical applications.

PSYCHOPHYSIOLOGICAL ACTION OF ESSENTIAL OILS IN ANIMAL MODELS

Kovar *et al.*'s (1987) report on the stimulation of locomotor activity in mice following inhalation of rosemary oil has already been reported (p. 144). A similar experiment which raises a number of interesting questions is that of Ortiz de Urbina *et al.* (1989). Intraperitoneal injection of essential oil of *Calamintha sylvatica* was found to exert sedating effects on rats. The three major fractions of the oils – pulegone, menthone, 1,8-cineole – were then examined independently. It was found that the whole essential oil had a more persistent sedative effect than the component fractions and that, in addition, a much lower dose was required. This lends support to aromatherapists' claims that the various constituent compounds in essential oils work synergistically. What is also of interest is that 1,8-cineole was found to have a sedating effect, the opposite result to that of Kovar *et al.* (1987). There are three possible explanations for this discrepancy, each important for the interpretation of animal studies on essential oils. Firstly, Kovar *et al.* may have been wrong in assuming that a positive correlation between serum 1,8-cineole and locomotor activity indicated a causal relationship. It is quite possible that the stimulating effects of rosemary oil were due to a component other than 1,8-cineole. Also possible, though perhaps less likely, is that the route of administration mediates the effects of an essential oil. It may be that injection of an oil intraperitoneally, in other words, directly into the body cavity, has a different effect to oral administration or inhalation. Finally, the psychomotor effects of essential oils may be hormetic (Sagan, 1989), that is, they may have opposite properties either side of a dosage threshold (Figure 5.1.) It is possible that 1,8-cineole has stimulating properties in low doses (Kovar *et al.*, 1987) and sedating properties at high doses (Ortiz de Urbina *et al.*, 1989).

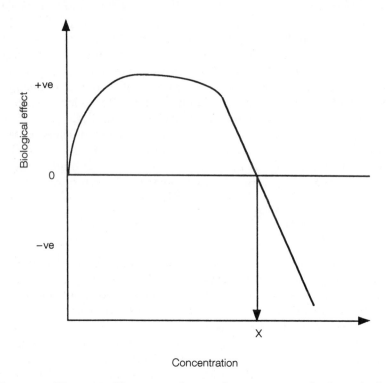

Concentration

Figure 5.1 Hormesis. The same substance has an opposite biological effect on either side of the threshold concentration x. A typical example might be growth rate of bacteria against concentration of sugar.

Using a similar experimental design to that of Kovar and Ortiz de Urbina, Rossi *et al.* (1988) found that high doses of essential oil of *Anthemis nobile* (camomile) caused sedation in rats. The rats were given intraperitoneal injections of 350 mg/kg essential oil and spontaneous motility was subsequently measured. Treatment caused reductions in motility of between 55% and 80%, depending on the variety of plant from which the oil was extracted. This effect lasted for about one hour. Moran *et al.* (1989) found that high doses (707 mg/kg) of essential oil of *Artemisia caerulescens* (wormwood) injected intraperitoneally in rats led to a decrease in motor activity and muscle tone, respiratory depression, central nervous system depression, hypothermia and hyperglycaemia. In support of horme-sis, two constituents of wormwood oil, camphor and alpha-thujone, were found to be sedative at low doses and convulsant at high doses.

Perhaps the most extensive research on the action of essential oils in animal models has been undertaken by Buchbauer, Jirovetz and Jäger of the Institute of Pharmaceutical Chemistry at the University of Vienna. Jäger *et al.* (1992b) have shown that neroli oil and two of its major constituents, citronellal and phenylethyl acetate, cause sedation in mice. Inhalation of these substances led to significant falls in motility compared to controls. In a more comprehensive experiment (Buchbauer *et al.*, 1993), mice were exposed to a 1-hour inhalation period of an essential oil or fragrance compound. Motility was assessed by measuring the number of footfalls on a sensitive electronic grid. Sandalwood, rose, neroli and lavender oil were found to have sedative effects after inhalation. Valerian oil, as well as several oils not widely used by aromatherapists, had no significant effect on motility. Numerous important constituent compounds of essential oils were also found to have sedative effects on inhalation. These include: anethole, bornyl salicylate, coumarin and, in particu-lar, 2-phenylethyl acetate, benzaldehyde, citronellal and geranyl acetate. Compounds with stimulant effects after inhalation include: geraniol, isoborneol, isoeugenol, nerol, methyl salicylate, alpha-pinene and thymol.

A second experiment was conducted in which mice were pretreated by injection of caffeine solution directly into the body cavity. Although in general this moderated the sedative effects of essential oils and fragrance compounds, some, including lavender and sandalwood, still reduced motility. In Buchbauer *et al.*'s words these substances 'were able to compensate caffeine-induced over-agitation'. What is of partic-ular interest is that some compounds, including eugenol, which had neutral or stimulant properties in untreated mice, had sedative effects in caffeine-pretreated animals. For other compounds, such as geraniol, stimulant activity was abolished by caffeine pretreatment. A further result of interest is that lavender oil sedated caffeine-pretreated animals more than untreated controls.

Guillemain, Rousseau and Delaveau (1989) also claim that inhala-tion of lavender oil leads to sedation in mice, though this is not supported by the data presented. Ten mice were given essential oil of lavender in olive oil by mouth at a dose of about 0.008 ml per animal. A control group received plain olive oil. The mice then completed a number of tests (e.g. mazes) and, though the results of the mice receiv-ing lavender oil suggested a sedative effect, the difference between groups did not reach statistical significance. There was, however, a significant effect on barbiturate-induced sleeping times: mice slept longer after receiving lavender oil and barbiturate than after receiving barbiturate alone.

Implications of the animal psychophysiological studies

It is illuminating to look at the composition of essential oils in the light of Buchbauer *et al.*'s data. Lavender oil was a more effective sedative than either of its major two constituents (linalool and linalyl acetate) in isolation, especially in caffeine-pretreated animals. This supports the contention of aromatherapists that constituent compounds in essential oils work synergistically.

The claims of aromatherapists could be examined further. Clary sage oil is claimed to be a muscle relaxant useful in stress and tension (Davis, 1988: 89). Like lavender, it contains a high proportion (85–90%) of linalool and linalyl acetate. Buchbauer *et al.*'s reporting of sedative activity in both these compounds might be thought to provide experimental evidence for Davis's claim. It is interesting that clary sage also contains small proportions (0.05–0.25%) of alpha-pinene, nerol and geraniol, all stimulants according to Buchbauer *et al.* It would perhaps be tempting to ascribe the alleged 'euphoric' qualities of essential oils to these minor constituents. However, coriander also contains a high proportion of linalool and a lower percentage of the stimulants found in clary sage. Yet, Price (1993: 267), Lawless (1994b: 139) and Valnet (1980: 118) all describe coriander as stimulating. As another example, juniper oil contains a large proportion of alpha-pinene. So perhaps Price (1993: 267), Lawless (1994b: 157) and Davis (1988: 192) are correct in claiming nervous exhaustion as an indication for this oil. On the other hand, aniseed is given stimulating properties by Price (1993: 267) and Valnet (1980: 95) though its major constituent, anethole, is given as a sedative by Buchbauer *et al.*

In short, a single essential oil contains a mixture of compounds, some of which stimulate and some of which sedate in their pure form. Some of the traditional properties ascribed by aromatherapists to essential oils accord well with the sedative or stimulant actions of the oil's major constituents: others do not appear to do so.

That said, it is as well to be extremely cautious in interpreting Buchbauer's data. Firstly, a replication with statistical evaluation of the results is necessary. For example, the paradoxical results of some oils in caffeine-treated mice may be due to chance variation. Moreover, there are always dangers associated with extrapolating animal experiments to humans. In particular, it is not known whether a substance which causes a mouse to increase locomotor activity acts as a stimulant in humans. The doses used in animal experiments are usually extremely high: Jäger *et al.* (1992b), for example, used inhalation of 1.3 g of oil for four mice. The equivalent dose for a human can only be guessed at but, say, a quarter of a litre would not be an exaggeration. Perhaps most importantly, the effects of psychotropic substances in humans are psychosocially mediated (p. 58). In other words, it may not be possible to make simple generalisations about the psychological effects of essential oils based upon animal models simply because human psychology is different.

PHARMACOLOGICAL EFFECTS OF ESSENTIAL OILS IN ANIMAL AND ISOLATED TISSUE MODELS

A number of workers have administered essential oils to animals or isolated tissue in the hope of determining their pharmacological properties. Particular essential oils or essential oil fractions have been shown to increase the metabolism of sedative drugs, reduce pain and inflammation, treat convulsions, increase both the production of bile and its passage into the gut, suppress the insulin response to a glucose tolerance test, inhibit contraction of smooth muscle and a number of other properties. The doses used in these experiments were high and the clinical implications are not clear.

Essential oils and drug metabolism

A number of aromatherapists and other clinicians have expressed concerns over possible interactions between essential oils and conventional medications. In an important study, Jori *et al.* (1969) investigated the effects of essential oils on drug metabolism. Pentobarbital-induced sleeping in rats was used as the study model. Pentobarbital is a sedative drug which causes rats to fall asleep; substances which interfere with its metabolism alter the duration of this effect. Though alpha- and beta-pinene, menthol, guaiacol and whole oil of *Pinus pumila* were found to have no effect, 1,8-cineole did significantly interfere with pentobarbital. Sleeping times and brain levels of the drug were reduced by about 50% for both subcutaneous injection and aerosol inhalation. Relatively high doses were used: 250 mg/kg for injections or 30 minutes of inhalation with the oil nebulized at 50 mg/minute. The effects were persistent, with sleeping times reduced even if administration of 1,8-cineole occurred 36 hours before that of pentobarbital. Activity of liver enzymes was found to be increased by both subcutaneous and aerosol routes and this may provide a mechanism for 1,8-cineole's mediating effect on the drug. In an extension of this work involving human volunteers (Jori *et al.*, 1970), 10 minutes' inhalation of 1,8-cineole for 10 days increased metabolism of aminopyrine. A similar pretreatment regime in rats reduced plasma and/or brain levels of a variety of drugs, including pentobarbital and amphetamine. Other workers reporting induction of liver enzymes and/or increased metabolism and excretion of drugs following pretreatment with essential oil fractions include Seto and Keup (1969), Roffey, Walker and Gibson (1990), Rompelberg, Verhagen and van Bladeren (1993) and Chadha and Madyastha (1984). Gershbein (1977) investigated the effect of subcutaneous injections of high doses (up to 3000 mg/kg) of essential oils and fractions on liver regeneration in partially hepatectomized rats (those with livers partially removed). Most substances had no effect but essential oils of anise, fennel, tarragon, nutmeg, mace and cumin, as well as several aromatic compounds, did lead to increased liver regeneration. Given the extremely high doses, and the route of administration, the implications for practice are unclear.

Similar results have been reported for whole essential oils by Wade *et al.* (1968), who found that inhalation of cedarwood oil resulted in induction of hepatic enzymes, with a consequent 75% fall in hexobarbital sleeping times. Cedarwood oil also enhanced the disappearance of dicumarol (a sedative) from the bloodstream. Inhalation of pine oil, from pine shavings, had a similar, if milder, effect on sleeping times and again this is attributed to increased hexobarbital metabolism. Wade *et al.*'s work is a replication and extension of that of Ferguson (1966), who found that cedar-chip bedding caused a reduction in hexobarbital- and pentobarbital-induced sleeping times in rats.

Analgesic and anti-inflammatory properties of essential oils

Though some essential oils are said to have analgesic properties, relatively little research has been undertaken. Lorenzetti *et al.* (1991) demonstrated that an infusion of lemongrass leaves (a popular remedy in many South American countries) produces a dose-dependent analgesia in rats. Because the tea was active against hyperalgesia (increased sensitivity to pain) induced by subplantar injections of carrageenin and prostaglandin E_2, but not against that induced by dibutryl cyclic AMP, it was concluded that lemongrass analgesia involves a peripheral site of action, rather than having an effect on the central nervous system. Oral administration of the essential oil produced similar results. The analgesic effect of the oil was attributed to myrcene, a minor constituent present in proportions of about 0.5%. Neral and geranial, the major constituents of lemongrass oil, had analgesic activity a little under half of that of myrcene. The activity of the whole oil was about 85% of that of myrcene, suggesting some synergistic activity. Interestingly, repeated administration of myrcene did not produce drug tolerance in the same manner as, for example, morphine. Myrcene is found in a high proportion of essential oils, including coriander, petitgrain, rosemary, lavender and juniper.

Rossi *et al.* (1988) used artificially induced inflammation in a rat model to investigate the anti-inflammatory effects of the essential oil of *Anthemis nobile* (camomile). Intraperitoneal injection of 350 mg/kg was found to inhibit inflammation by approximately 30%. The oil was also reported to have anti-diuretic properties in this paper. Tubaro *et al.* (1984) found that a hydroalcoholic extract of *Chamomila recuitta* reduced croton-induced oedema in mice in a dose-dependent manner. Ocete *et al.* (1989) found dose-dependent anti-inflammatory activity of *Bupleurum gibraltaricum* after both oral and intraperitoneal administration. Delta-3-carene was reported to be responsible for this effect. The compound inhibited oxytocin- but not acetylcholine-induced contractions of isolated rat uteri. The author argues that this rules out a non-specific relaxant action and indicates a prostaglandin-related mechanism for the oil's anti-inflammatory properties. Though *Bupleurum gibraltaricum* is not commonly used in clinical practice, delta-3-carene is found in low concentration in a number of oils used by aromatherapists.

Essential oil treatment of induced convulsions

In an experiment of particular interest, Yamada, Mimaki and Sashida (1994) found that lavender oil had an anticonvulsive effect in a laboratory model. Convulsions were induced in mice by intraperitoneal injection of pentetrazol, nicotine and strychnine or by electroconvulsive shock. The animals were pretreated by 15 minutes inhalation of various doses (0.3–1 ml) of lavender oil. Compared to controls, lavender oil reduced convulsions and death resulting from low-dose pentetrazol and from nicotine, for which there was a dose-dependent effect. Furthermore, lavender oil reduced tonic extension, clonic convulsion and death resulting from electroconvulsive shock, though tonic flexion was unaffected. These data reconfirm the sedative properties of lavender (see above) and suggest that the oil may have significant neuropharmacological properties. In a further study on seizures, Nwaiwu and Akah(1986) found that the volatile oil of *Tetrapleura tetraptera* (not commonly used by aromatherapists) protected against leptazinol-induced convulsions in mice.

Essential oils and bile

There is also some experimental support for an effect of essential oils on both the production of bile and its passage into the gut. Mörsdorf

(1966) suggested that cyclic terpenes, such as those found in many essential oils, increase bile flow. Hoefler *et al.* (1987) showed that ethanolic extracts of rosemary have choleretic properties in rats. The extracts were also shown to protect against carbon tetrachloride poisoning of the liver. Extracts of young sprouts had a stronger action that those of grown plants. Lallement-Guilbert and Bezanger-Beauesne (1970), on the other hand, found that though some constituents of rosemary increased biliary flow in rats, the essential oil did not. The picture is perhaps further confused by Mongold *et al.* (1991), who found that an aqueous alcoholic extract of rosemary (similar but not identical to the essential oil) had both a choleretic and cholagogic effect (stimulates flow of bile into the intestine). Kodama *et al.* (1976) found that d-limonene, found in numerous oils, including rosemary, lowered the ratio of bile acids and phospholipids to cholesterol in rats. Clegg *et al.* (1980) showed that menthol, cineol, borneol and menthone inhibited H MG-CoA reductase, an enzyme which is important in the biochemical pathway for the production of cholesterol in the liver.

Rangelov *et al.* (1988) studied the effects of topical application of 0.01 g/kg essential oils on bile in guinea pigs. Cholagogic effects were ascribed to rose, German camomile and fennel oil. Oils said to be choleretic included thyme, fennel, rose and caraway. There was no effect of peppermint, coriander or dill. Diliberto, Usha and Birnbaum (1988) found that a major constituent of lemongrass oil had a cholagogic effect in rats (see above for experimental details). However, these papers lack experimental detail and are poorly presented. Similarly, extra caution is warranted in interpreting Nikolaevskii *et al.*'s (1990) claim that inhalation of lavender oil is angioprotective. Though the oil had no effect on cholesterol levels, the authors report that lavender 'reduced affectation of the aorta by the atherosclerotic plaques'.

Expectorant action of essential oils

Boyd and Sheppard (1966) found that steam inhalation of Friars' Balsam, a traditional expectorant remedy, had no effect on the output and composition of respiratory tract fluid in rabbits. Neither eucalyptus (Boyd and Pearson, 1946) nor anise (Boyd and Hicks, 1955) had an effect on respiratory tract fluid when given intragastrically. These results were confirmed in a further experiment using steam inhalation with rabbits (Boyd and Sheppard, 1968). Only cedar leaf oil affected respiratory tract fluid, leading Boyd to conclude that, though this particular oil merited further investigation, other essential oils do not have a specific expectorant action: though they add a pleasant aroma to steam inhalation, it is the warm, moist air which is of benefit. But in a later trial, Boyd and Sheppard (1970) found that citral and geraniol, constituents of lemongrass oil, exhibited significant expectorant properties. Both compounds increased the volume and soluble mucus content and decreased the specific gravity of respiratory tract fluid in the rabbit model. Low doses (5 mg/kg) were more effective than high doses.

In a further animal study on essential oils for respiratory conditions, Schäfer and Schäfer (1981) examined the effects of Pinimenthol, a patented topical application, on respiratory tract fluid in rabbits and acetylcholine-induced bronchospasm in guinea pigs. The remedy consists of eucalyptus oil, menthol, camphor and essential oils of two pine species (*Pinus silvestris* and *Pinus pumila*) in Vaseline. Schäfer administered the remedy by tracheal tube or by topical application to the thorax. Tracheal administration led to immediate falls in bronchospasm compared to controls. This effect was maximal at 25 minutes, with a 50% improvement in respiratory function. Topical application lead to only minor reductions in bronchospasm and these did not reach statistical significance. The volume of respiratory tract fluid secretions was increased by about 50% for both tracheal and topical application; viscosity of the respiratory tract fluid was reduced. The authors conclude that Pinimenthol has a marked expectorant action. However, its bronchodilatory properties are dose-dependent, an effect on bronchospasm occurring only when Pinimenthol was delivered directly to the bronchi. Interestingly, Linsenmann and Swoboda (1986) found that topical application of Pinimenthol was of benefit for patients with chronic obstructive pulmonary disease (p. 141), further highlighting the difficulties of interpreting the results of animal research. Other clinical trials on aromatic inhalations for respiratory conditions are discussed on page 140.

Synergy and essential oils: nutmeg oil and platelet aggregation

One of the most important claims of aromatherapists is that the effects of whole essential oils cannot always be deduced from the actions of their constituents in isolation. The constituents of an oil are said to act synergistically and it is claimed that seeking particular active principles is likely to lead to decreased efficacy and increased side-effects. Though there is some evidence that synergism does occur in some instances (see, for example, p. 152), this has not always been found to be the case.

Janssens *et al.* (1990) reported that inhibition of platelet aggregation by nutmeg oil could be largely explained by the presence of two constituents: eugenol and isoeugenol. In this study, the effects of whole nutmeg oil on platelet aggregation in rabbit blood were compared with theoretical values calculated by assuming that the oil consisted of eugenol, isoeugenol and a pharmacologically inert fraction. The former values were lower, suggesting decreased efficacy of the whole oil. Moreover, artificial combination of fractions found to have a minor effect on platelet aggregation did not reveal any potentiating effects of one compound upon another. In other words, the effects of nutmeg oil on platelet aggregation are best explained in terms of a small number of active compounds, rather than the synergistic effects of different constituents.

Essential oils and cancer

There are reports of anticancer activity of certain oils. Shwaireb (1993) claims that topical application of caraway oil inhibited experimentally induced skin tumours in mice. Likewise Fang *et al.* (1989) reported that some constituents of geranium oil exhibit 'marginal' antitumour activity. These findings should be interpreted with caution. A large number of substances have been found to either cause or cure cancer in the laboratory and there is no simple relationship between such findings and a substance's potential for therapeutic use. The results of the studies reported here do not, on their own, suggest efficacy of essential oils against cancer.

Essential oils and smooth muscle: calcium channel activity

Peppermint oil is the treatment of choice for irritable bowel syndrome and there is some good evidence that it is an effective treatment for this condition (p. 134). Rosemary is also a traditional treatment for indigestion and bowel disorders. A number of experiments have been conducted to determine the mechanism of action of these two essential oils. Hills and Aaronson (1991) found that peppermint oil reduced contractions in guinea pig taenia coli (fibrous bands of tissue surrounding the large intestine) induced by a variety of substances including acetylcholine, histamine and carbachol. Peppermint oil also inhibited spontaneous contractile activity of guinea pig colon and rabbit jejunum. Electrophysiological measurements in the latter case showed that peppermint oil inhibited calcium influx in a dose-dependent manner. This reduces muscle contraction because contraction of smooth muscle is dependent on free calcium within the muscle cell.

Taylor, Luscombe and Duthie (1983) found that peppermint oil inhibited gastrointestinal smooth muscle. In a further experiment (Taylor, Luscombe and Duthie, 1984), using human taenia coli, peppermint oil was found to exhibit specific calcium antagonist activity. Menthol, the major constituent of peppermint oil, was found to be primarily responsible for this property. A further replication (Taylor *et al.*, 1985), using human bowel tissue in calcium-free solution, suggests that menthol inhibits gastrointestinal smooth muscle by decreasing influx of extracellular calcium while having no effects on its intracellular mobilization. Hawthorn *et al.* (1988) also found that peppermint oil blocked calcium-channel activity in guinea pig intestine and heart muscle. Menthol was found to be as effective as peppermint oil and was therefore considered to be its active constituent. Further evidence of the effect of peppermint oil on heart muscle comes from a report of two cases of atrial fibrillation following excess intake of peppermint (Thomas, 1962).

Giachetti, Taddei and Taddei (1988) assessed the spasmolytic activity of essential oils on smooth muscle in a guinea pig model. The Oddi's sphincter (the muscle controlling flow of bile into the gut) was contracted by an injection of morphine. Various doses of essential oils were then injected to see which would reverse this effect. Peppermint had the greatest activity, followed by sage and then rosemary oil. In a reversal of this effect, high doses of peppermint were found to induce spasm. For an overview of pharmacological studies on peppermint, see Balacs (1992).

Aqel (1991) reported that rosemary oil inhibits acetylcholine-, histamine- and potassium-induced contractions of rabbit and guinea pig tracheal smooth muscle. This paper also reports the results of unpublished data suggesting that rosemary oil also inhibits both spontaneous movement and acetylcholine-induced contractions of rabbit and guinea pig intestines. In an interesting additional experiment, rosemary oil was shown to reduce histamine-induced contractions of tracheal smooth muscle in a calcium-free solution. This suggests that rosemary oil may interfere with release of calcium from intracellular sources in addition to any action on extracellular calcium influx. Aqel (1992) found that rosemary oil inhibition of potassium- or noradrenaline-induced contractions in rabbit aorta was not abolished by the presence of increased calcium or by the use of calcium-free solution. This confirms that rosemary inhibits both the entry and intracellular mobilization of calcium. Antispasmodic action has also been ascribed to essential oils of clove, sage, thyme and melissa in an animal model (Debelmas and Rochat, 1967).

Blocking of calcium channels is an important pharmacological property and may explain why some essential oils increase local blood flow (see, for example, the research on Deep Heat). The mechanism of this calcium-channel blocking has been investigated by Melzig and Teuscher (1991), who found that a variety of essential oils – including fennel, peppermint, and anise – and essential oil constituents – including menthol, anethole, eugenol and thymol – inhibited adenosine uptake in aortic endothelial tissue. Inhibition of adenosine uptake causes accumulation of adenosine nucleotides and it is this which causes blocking of calcium channels.

Miscellaneous studies

Aromatherapists claim that certain oils can be of benefit for menstrual disorders. There is at least some theoretical support for this notion from animal studies. Albert-Puleo (1980) has reviewed the evidence that fennel and anise oil have oestrogenic properties. Gomez and Turner (1939), for example, showed that anol, which is present in both oils, promotes the development of the mammary glands in adult virgin and immature female rabbits and rats.

Ortiz de Urbina *et al.* (1989) found that intraperitoneal injection of *Calamintha sylvatica* oil in rats reduced pyrexia (fever) induced by subcutaneous injection of beer yeast. The three major components – pulegone, 1,8-cineole and menthone – were tested individually and it was the pulegone which was found to be primarily responsible for the oil's antipyretic activity.

A study of interest with respect to safety is that of al-Hader, Hasan and Aqel (1994), who showed that 25 mg/kg of rosemary oil administered intramuscularly suppressed insulin response to a glucose tolerance test in rabbits. Plasma glucose levels were 55% higher than controls after 120 minutes ($p < 0.001$). Rosemary oil treatment also caused hyperglycaemia in rabbits with alloxan-induced diabetes. The authors suggest that the effect of rosemary oil on insulin secretion was due to its properties as a calcium antagonist (see above). It would be worth considering whether this study should be taken as the basis for contraindicating rosemary, and possibly other calcium antagonist oils such as peppermint and sage, in diabetes.

IMPLICATIONS OF THE PHARMACOLOGICAL RESEARCH ON AROMATHERAPY

Certain essential oils have been shown to have pharmacological effects in animal and isolated tissue models. This is perhaps not surprising given that essential oils contain a cocktail of organic substances. Practitioners have sometimes used the evidence discussed above as a vindication of aromatherapy practice. There are two problems with doing so. Firstly, the clinical value of a treatment cannot necessarily be assessed from its effects on animals or tissue models. Many of the animal studies have used large doses of essential oil administered by injection for maximum bioavailability. Rossi *et al.* (1988), for example, used a dose of 350 mg/kg administered intraperitoneally to examine the effects of camomile on inflammation. A quick calculation shows that this dose is many times higher than that used in traditional aromatherapy practice. In the case of isolated tissue models, the effects depend on a certain dose of essential oil being present for a certain length of time, conditions which cannot be guaranteed in the living body.

The second reason why the pharmacological research cannot be taken as validation of aromatherapy practice is because the number of claims made by practitioners vastly exceeds those which have been studied. For example, in just one of six tables of properties and indications for essential oils (Price, 1993: 278), 30 essential oils are tabulated with 40 properties; 251 individual claims for the properties of essential oils are made on this table alone. While there is evidence that some essential oils do have some pharmacological properties, this is swamped by the vast number of claims made by aromatherapists.

RESEARCH ON OLFACTION

Aromatherapists are often at pains to emphasize that the odour of an essential oil may of itself exert a beneficial effect on health. Though this sometimes shades into the somewhat overly romanticized – 'Why have we let the flowers die in the garden of our soul? Even the dried up petals have been blown away!' (Lawless, 1994b: 38) – the point is a good one: perhaps, like touch, the effects of odour on our mood are so widely recognized that they do not need scientific confirmation. That said, there is surely a role for research in identifying both the nature and the scope of the health effects of odour.

There is extensive observational evidence that smell can indeed have psychological and physiological effects. The existence of pheromones, volatile chemicals, as a means of communication in the insect world is well-known. What is perhaps not as widely recognized is the importance of odour cues in higher animals. For example, the presence of an unfamiliar male rat can cause a pregnant female to abort (Kaba and Keverne, 1988). This has be prevented in the laboratory by drug treatment of the olfactory bulb of the brain suggesting that the phenomenon is related to odour and that an olfactory bond is formed between mating pairs. Menstrual synchrony (similar timing of menstruation) in human females is another example of a physiological change in mammals thought to be mediated by odour (Weller and Weller, 1993). For a more detailed discussion, see Schwartz and Natyncuk (1990).

Experiments on the effects of odour in humans can roughly be divided into two categories: those which investigate the effect of an ambient odour on mood and cognitive functioning, and those which directly measure nervous system responses to the presentation of an odour. As might be imagined, the literature on olfaction is extensive. The following brief overview will cover some of the more representative studies, particularly those using essential oils as the odour stimulus. All the studies detailed below involved healthy volunteers, rather than a clinical population.

PSYCHOLOGICAL EFFECTS OF AMBIENT ODOUR

In a typical trial (Warm, Dember and Parasuraman, 1990), subjects watched two parallel lines on a VDU screen and were required to press a button when the lines moved slightly apart. Presence of peppermint odour increased detection, indicating greater vigilance and arousal. A similar result is given by Lorig (1992), who reports on an unpublished experiment in which subjects were asked to indicate when they though 60 seconds had passed from a given signal. Average scores in the control condition were somewhat greater than 60 but were reduced towards a correct answer by the presence of peppermint, once more suggesting that this odour leads to arousal. A third study indicating a stimulating effect of peppermint is that of Bordia *et al.* (1990). Subjects were given the task of awakening and pressing a switch at a particular cue. Both awakening and switch-pressing were enhanced by the presentation of peppermint odour, though only the latter achieved statistical significance. See also Warm, Dember and Parasuraman (1991).

Miyake *et al.* (1991) report in short an experiment measuring the effects of essential oil odours on sleep latency in subjects having undergone a stressful arithmetic task. Bitter orange oil was found to decrease sleep latency (time taken to fall asleep) significantly whereas marjoram, linden, valerian, sweet fennel and spike lavender had (apparently) no effect. This suggests that, while some oils traditionally claimed to be effective for insomnia do not appear to be of value, bitter orange oil can promote sleep even in conditions of mental stress. Other studies published only in abstract form include those of Nagai *et al.* (1991), who suggest that the odour of sweet fennel oil can reduce mental stress and fatigue caused by an arithmetic task, and Karamat *et al.* (1992), who found that lavender oil increased reaction times on a vigilance task. Jasmine oil had the opposite effect. This suggests that the former oil is a sedative and the latter a stimulant. Karamat *et al.* also report a separate experiment in which lavender oil was found to influence decision times, but not motor action, suggesting that the oil's action on the nervous system is central rather than peripheral.

However, although of interest, the lack of experimental detail presented in these papers makes them unsuitable as a basis for generalizations about the psychological effects of essential oils. Moreover, the result of most ambient odour experiments are much more complex. Warrenburg and Schwartz (1990) did not find differences in muscle tone, skin resistance and skin temperature response to three different odorants (neroli, apple spice and galbanum) in two different conditions (relaxation or mental arithmetic task). Subjects were divided into those who liked the smell of neroli and those who did not. The former had a better response across odour conditions, suggesting that liking neroli predisposed subjects to be generally more relaxed and attentive. In this case, rather than neroli improving psychological characteristics, liking the smell of neroli was associated with a particular personality type.

Knasko (1992) undertook a sophisticated experiment in which the presence or absence of the scent of lavender, lemon or DMS (a mildly unpleasant smell) was found to be correlated with subject performance in tests assessing creativity, personality, mood and health symptoms. Each subject took the tests twice and a different odour was presented on each occasion. Mood was found primarily to be affected, not by the presence of an odour as such, but by the order in which subjects were presented with the odour. For example, subjects who received the smell of a scent the first time they undertook the psychological tests were in a significantly less pleasant mood when they experienced a no odour condition the second time around. Highly complex interactions were also found between personality traits and the effects of odour on task performance and mood. For example, lavender improved mood, but only in subjects with an external locus of control, that is, those who believe that their health is affected primarily by external factors such as 'catching a bug' rather than by factors over which they have control, such as diet or lifestyle. In a further trial, Knasko (1993) reported that, compared to a no-odour control condition, the presence of pleasant (lemon or ylang ylang) or unpleasant odours had no effect on the performance of reasoning tasks, health symptoms or mood in college students. However, subjects exposed to odour, particularly those in the malodour group, believed that it had affected their performance. So again, the effects of an ambient odour are not any inherent effect but appear to be dependent upon belief.

Ludvigson and Rottman (1989) similarly reported that psychological reactions to an odour were mediated by a number of factors. Subjects were exposed to lavender, cloves or no odour while undertaking cognitive tests. Subjects attended twice, being exposed to odour at one session only. Mood was assessed using a variety of scales. Lavender was found to reduce arithmetical reasoning compared to no odour, suggesting a sedative action. Those in the lavender group also enjoyed the experiment more. However, sub-jects who were exposed to no odour at their first session reported unfavourable reactions when lavender was presented during their second session. One possible explanation could be that individuals experiencing lavender the first time they undertook the tests expe-rienced lowered levels of apprehension. Those who experienced it on the second test found it either an annoying distraction, if they had previously experienced no odour, or simply a pleasant change from cloves. The authors conclude that 'the effects of ambient odour will not submit to a simple generalization such as that lavender is relaxing'.

EFFECTS OF ODOUR ON THE NERVOUS SYSTEM

Other workers have attempted to look at the psychological effects of odour by more direct means. In possibly the most widely reported experiment of this sort, Torri et al. (1991) measured the electrical response of the brain to odours. The experiment utilized a phenom-enon known as contingent negative variation (CNV), which is a slight change in electrical activity that occurs when a subject expects an event to take place. Subjects were presented with the odour of an essential oil, shortly after which a buzzer sounded. This was fol-lowed 2 seconds later by a light which subjects had to turn off by flicking a switch. CNV was found to be reduced by a number of essential oils traditionally thought to be sedative (e.g. lavender) and increased by oils thought to be stimulant (e.g. basil). However, there were some anomalies. Neroli, thought by aromatherapists to be a sedative, was found to increase CNV, suggesting a stimulant effect. Rose oil also decreased CNV, whereas valerian had no effect. Oils were found not to have an effect on reaction time, heart rate or galvanic skin resistance. This suggests that any stimulant or seda-tive actions of essential oils do not operate through conventionally understood mechanisms. Kikuchi et al. (1991) have published a short report of a similar experiment in which heart rate variations to an expected stimulus were recorded. Lemon odour increased the anticipation response whereas rose had the opposite effect, con-firming the traditional view of lemon as stimulating and rose as sedating.

Once again, considerable caution is warranted in the interpretation of such results. Teece, Savignas-Brown and Meinbresse (1976) have pointed out that highly arousing stimuli may be distracting and thus reduce CNV amplitude. Kanamura et al. (1988) measured skin poten-tial at the same time as CNV. Compared to the no-odour control condition, skin potential was higher for jasmine and lavender and lower for camomile. In other words, the result for lavender was in the opposite direction to that predicted by CNV data.

COGNITIVE MEDIATION OF THE EFFECTS OF ODOUR

Lorig and Roberts (1990) have cast doubt on whether CNV changes really indicate a direct psychological response, suggesting that they might be cognitively mediated. Three odours (jasmine, lavender, galbanum) were presented individually. A mixture of all three was then presented along with the suggestion that it consisted of only one of the three previously presented odours. The CNV data and subjective ratings of pleasantness mirrored the odour the subject *thought* was being presented. In other words, the same odour (the mixture) elicited a different CNV response depending on what subjects thought they were smelling. This replicates the result of an earlier study (Lorig and Schwartz, 1989), which measured brain wave responses to odour presentation without using CNV methodology. Food odours were found to reduce high-frequency brain waves. These are associated with arousal, suggesting that food odours are a relaxing stimulus. However, imagery of food affected brain-wave patterns in a similar way. In a later review, Lorig (1992) suggests that odours are suggestive of experiences and that it is the imagery that causes psychophysiological changes, rather than a direct odour effect. For example, lavender may be associated with, say, a walk in the country on a summer day. The odour of lavender may therefore suggest – consciously or unconsciously – summer walks and induce relaxation because the recalled experience is relaxing. This is no more than classical Pavlovian conditioning: a stimulus (a ringing bell/the smell of lavender) is paired with an event (feeding/a walk in the country) which produces a response (salivation/relaxation). On repetition, the stimulus alone will causes the response.

There is direct evidence that classical conditioning can indeed occur with odour presentation. Kirk-Smith (1983) had subjects undertake a stressful cognitive task while exposed to extremely low concentrations of an odour known as TUA. It was found that subsequent exposure to the odour alone induced a stress response. Interestingly, when subjects were presented with detectable levels of TUA, they denied ever having experienced it. There are two important conclusions to be drawn from this study. Firstly, odours may have effects even if they are not consciously perceived. Secondly, odours may cause particular psychological changes if they have previously been paired with stimuli causing those changes. Moreover, this conditioning process can take place very rapidly, after only one experience of the pairing of stimuli.

Ehrlichman and Halpern (1988) have demonstrated that odours can affect memory recall. College students recalled memories cued by neutral words (such as 'light switch') during presentation of a neutral, unpleasant or pleasant odour. These memories were later rated by the subjects as happy or unhappy. Overall, the pleasant odour elicited happy memories whereas the unpleasant odour produced the opposite effect. The trend was strengthened in those who found the odours either particularly pleasant or unpleasant. Odour may therefore affect mood by recall of positive experiences, further strengthening the classical conditioning hypothesis. King (1991) reports using the phenomenon of odour conditioning in a clinical setting. Relaxation was induced in stressed and anxious patients while they were exposed to artificially produced seaside odours. The odours could be later be used outside the clinic to bring about relaxation.

Knasko, Gilbert and Sabini (1990) provide further evidence that the psychological effects of odour may be indirect. Subjects were told that they were being subjected to either a pleasant, unpleasant or neutral odour but were informed that they might not be able to detect the scents being used. In fact no odours were presented. Nonetheless, the mere suggestion of a positive odour improved self-reports of pleasantness, mood and physical symptoms. In other words, a feigned odour caused a measurable psychological change.

In summarizing the effects of odour exposure, Lorig (1992) therefore concludes:

> The data ... do not support the implicit claims associated with aromatherapy which suggest that odours have direct effects on well-being ... aromatherapy's effect may be due more to the expectation of health benefit than to any specific characteristic of odours *per se*.

An aromatherapist might well point out that it need not matter how the odour of an essential oil elicits a particular change in a patient, the important question is whether or not it does so. However, while one is tempted to support such an emphasis on clinical data, it must surely be accepted that the psychological effects of odour appear somewhat more complex than aromatherapists' repeated claims that particular oils are sedative, uplifting or stimulating. It should also be pointed out that there is very little clinical data on the therapeutic value of odour: clinical trials assessing the effects of odour on patients have apparently yet to be conducted.

In summary, odours can affect mood, cognitive functioning and simple behaviours in certain situations, whether or not they are perceived consciously. However, the effects of odour are mediated both by prior experience and expectation and by the degree to which the odour is liked or disliked by the subject. As such, the effects of odour are influenced by learning (and are therefore culture specific) and vary from individual to individual.

Readers interested in olfaction research are referred to Jellinek's (1994) review of 'aroma-chology'. Aromatherapists may be particularly interested in Jellinek's claim that, with respect to the psychological effects of odour, 'there is no fundamental difference between ... single essential oils, single aroma chemicals (natural or synthetic) and blends of natural and synthetic materials (fragrance compositions)'.

RESEARCH ON AROMATHERAPY AND ESSENTIAL OILS: A SUMMARY OF THE MAIN FINDINGS

Research on aromatherapy can be divided into two main categories: clinical research, in which the effects of aromatherapy or essential oils are assessed using clinical endpoints (for example, symptoms) in a patient population, and basic research, in which the effects of essential oils are assessed by examining healthy volunteers, animals or isolated tissue models. Studies on olfaction are also of interest.

CLINICAL RESEARCH

- Aromatherapy treatment often involves massage. The research literature on massage is therefore a useful resource for the evaluation of aromatherapy.
- There is a dearth of good quality clinical research investigating aromatherapy as typically used by practitioners.
- There is only limited evidence that essential oils have sedative actions in institutional populations. Most trials have been of extremely low quality and a significant number have either never been published or are reported with insufficient methodological detail.
- Though some trials show that the use of essential oils in massage increases its sedative effect, a larger number do not.
- Certain pharmacological preparations contain essential oils or essential oil constituents. Preliminary trials suggest that peppermint oil is of benefit for irritable bowel syndrome and that a mixture of essential fractions is of benefit for ureteral stones and gall stones.
- One orally administered essential oil product was found to have no preventative effect on infections in elderly patients with chronic bronchitis.
- A number of commercial mouthwashes contain essential oils or fractions thereof. Most trials show at least some effect of such mouthwashes on gingivitis and plaque regrowth.

- There is good-quality evidence that topical tea-tree oil is effective in the treatment of certain skin infections.
- In a large, randomized study of perineal healing, lavender oil was found to be no more effective than placebo.
- There is some evidence that topically applied and inhaled essential oils ease breathing in respiratory tract infections.
- Research on herbs does not always apply to essential oils: valerian is known to be a sedative but the active ingredient is not present in the essential oil.

In sum, the clinical research on aromatherapy is extremely disappointing. There are few good-quality clinical trials and the vast majority of claims made by aromatherapists (for example, the treatment of arthritis, sinusitis or period pain) remain unevaluated. Most trials examine traditional essential oil products (e.g. Vicks VapoRub for respiratory infections) and are only indirectly related to aromatherapy. Even where there is evidence of effect, such as tea-tree oil for acne, the practices of aromatherapists (oils used, dosages, frequency and duration of treatment) may not reflect those used in the trial.

BASIC RESEARCH

- At least some substances in essential oils are absorbed into the bloodstream by inhalation and topical application. However, blood levels are extremely low and elimination is relatively rapid.
- There is some evidence that the irritant effects of whole essential oils are lower than those of constituent fractions.
- Many essential oils demonstrate marked in vitro antimicrobial activity.
- There is some evidence that essential oils traditionally used in ointments for pain relief (eucalyptus, peppermint, wintergreen) have desirable effects on blood flow, muscle tension and pain.
- Certain essential oils have been found to have sedative effects in animal models. In one study, inhalation of lavender was found to reduce artificially induced convulsions in mice.
- Certain essential oils may speed the metabolism and excretion of drugs.
- Anti-inflammatory effects of some essential oils and essential oil fractions have been demonstrated in animal models.
- Essential oils have been shown to have effects both on the production of bile and its passage into the gut.
- A number of essential oils, peppermint and rosemary oil in particular, have been found to inhibit smooth muscle contraction in

isolated tissue models. This is thought to result from an effect on calcium-channel activity.

- In some studies, effects of whole essential oils were greater than those of constituent fractions, suggesting that individual compounds in essential oils may act synergistically. However, in other trials, the action of a whole oil could be largely explained in terms of one or two active ingredients.
- Few studies have compared the effects of mixtures of oils to those of single oils. One study found that peppermint oil reduced the pain of artificially induced headache but that a mixture of peppermint and eucalyptus oil had no effect. This suggests that individual oils in mixtures can have antagonistic actions on one another.

In sum, essential oils do appear to be both pharmacologically active and bioavailable. However, it does not follow that because essential oils have effects in the laboratory they are necessarily of clinical value. In animal experiments, for example, extremely large doses of essential oils are used. It is unclear whether the much lower doses used in aromatherapy have similar effects. The overwhelming majority of claims made by aromatherapists remain unevaluated.

OLFACTION

- Chemical signals are used as a form of communication in the animal world.
- Studies on olfaction have either examined the effects of an ambient odour on mood or have attempted to measure the effects of an odour on the nervous system directly by using electroencephalography. All studies have used healthy volunteers, rather than a clinical population.
- A number of simple studies, reported in brief, purport to show psychological effects (e.g. arousal) due to the presence of an odour.
- Most of the ambient odour experiments reported in detail do not find a simple relationship between odours and changes in psychological state.
- Research on the effects of essential oils on the nervous system has found that changes in brain electrical activity (stimulation or sedation) often correlate with the traditional properties ascribed by practitioners. There are, however, some notable exceptions.
- There is evidence that these changes are the result of expectation and may not be due to an inherent effect of odour on the nervous system.
- The effects of an odour are mediated by expectation and classical conditioning. It may not be possible to make simple statements about the effects of an odour on psychological state.

PART TWO
Practice

The therapeutic use of massage and aromatherapy: an overview

6

The next three chapters will discuss the use of massage and aromatherapy in a variety of conventional health-care settings. The aim is to give the reader a general introduction to the scope, effects and management of massage and aromatherapy. The settings and client groups described are intended to be representative rather than comprehensive, to give some insight into the use of massage and aromatherapy in conventional settings rather than to be a complete description of practice.

The methodological problems of gathering information about practice have been discussed in the Preface. To recap briefly: it would be impossible to give a definitive description of practice in a book of this nature. The following chapters aim to sketch out a rough 'first draft' as a means of providing useful information. They are based on impressions gained from discussions with patients, carers, practitioners and other health-care staff. The discussions reflect the author's personal understanding and are not intended as knowledge claims.

Some practitioners may find that the description of massage and aromatherapy given in the following chapters does not fully correspond with their own personal notions of practice. In particular, they may find that the practices described tend to be primarily non-specific in nature. For example, the use of massage to aid relaxation and help with sleep problems is discussed; the treatment of migraine is not. Similarly, no mention is made of the aromatherapeutic treatment of hypertension, though the self-help remedy of sedative oils in a warm bath is discussed. Practitioners are often quick to point out, for example, that 'real' aromatherapy involves treating the 'whole' person, for whatever symptoms they present, and that oils are chosen on an individualized basis.

But however well or poorly the descriptions of practice given below chime with practitioners' own views, they do reflect how massage and aromatherapy have generally been used in health-service settings. Practitioners have been given certain roles within multidisciplinary health-care teams and this has often limited the nature of their practice. This issue is dealt with further in a special section starting on page 231, which discusses massage and aromatherapy when practised by autonomous clinicians, and Chapter 10, which discusses how to organize massage and aromatherapy in conventional health settings.

DO THE EFFECTS OF MASSAGE AND AROMATHERAPY DEPEND ON THE CLIENT GROUP?

Many of the effects of massage and aromatherapy are non-specific and, as such, will be similar across client groups. For example, an aromatherapy massage is generally a relaxing experience regardless of an individual's particular condition or symptoms. There are some condition-specific issues: the use of massage to improve growth in premature infants would be a good example. But there are number of consistent 'themes' in different client groups' experience of and response to massage and aromatherapy. Some of these themes are discussed below, with advice on where to locate fuller discussions.

- *Muscle tension.* It is claimed that massage and aromatherapy treatment can relieve muscle tension. This can sometimes lead to short-term improvements in mobility. Muscle tension and mobility is said to be a particular issue in physical disability, AIDS and primary care.
- *Blood circulation.* Certain forms of massage are said to improve blood circulation. Aromatherapists say that essential oils can also stimulate local blood flow. This is reportedly of value in physical disability, cancer care and where patients spend significant periods of time in bed or in a wheelchair (e.g. ICU, AIDS in some cases).
- *Pain.* Massage and aromatherapy are reported to have short-term effects on pain. This is of particular importance in physical disability, cancer care, hospice care, primary care and AIDS.
- *Fatigue.* Invigorating massage techniques can be used in an attempt to relieve fatigue. Certain essential oils are said to be stimulant. Massage and aromatherapy treatment of fatigue is reportedly of

benefit in cancer, AIDS, mental health and primary care in particular.

- *Infection.* Essential oils are known to be antimicrobial. More controversially, both massage and aromatherapy are claimed to stimulate the immune system. Complementary treatment of infection is an issue of particular interest in the treatment of disabled children and people with AIDS.
- *Relaxation.* Massage and aromatherapy treatment can be a relaxing experience. Patients may also undertake self-help with essential oils as inhalations or in the bath. Relaxation is generally beneficial, particularly where patients are anxious, such as in cancer care, disabled children, hospice care, mental health, HIV and AIDS and ICU. Massage and aromatherapy can also give patients a concrete experience of relaxation as a prelude to the use of self-regulation techniques such as meditation. This is an important issue in cardiovascular rehabilitation, primary care and mental health.
- *Counselling.* Massage is said to aid the counselling process in some cases. This has been found to be of particular value in hospice care, mental health, primary care and HIV and AIDS.
- *Self-image.* Some patients have reported that touch received during massage treatment has improved their self-image. This is an issue of particular importance in physical disability, cardiovascular rehabilitation, mental health, primary care and HIV and AIDS.
- *Relationships.* Certain types of massage have been said to foster relationships and communication. This is of particular interest in the treatment of disabled children, profound and severe learning disability, cardiovascular rehabilitation, intensive care and midwifery. Interestingly, the way in which massage has fostered relationships is different in each of these client groups.
- *One-to-one care.* The quality of one-to-one care and attention associated with a massage or aromatherapy treatment is not common in health care. This has been found to be important in physical disability, primary care, mental health, HIV and AIDS, hospice care and cancer care.
- *Support for staff and carers.* Massage and aromatherapy can be an important means of providing support to staff and carers. Though an important issue in all settings, such support is said to be of particular relevance in hospice care and for carers of disabled children.

Some issues appear to be important for almost all client groups discussed in this book.

- *Sleep*. Massage and aromatherapy are reported to improve sleep.
- *Pleasure*. A good aromatherapy or massage treatment can be a very pleasurable experience.
- *General well-being*. Most people report feeling generally better in themselves after massage or aromatherapy treatment.

Disability

7

PHYSICAL DISABILITY

INTRODUCTION AND OVERVIEW OF PRACTICE

This section will focus on the use of massage and aromatherapy by adults and older children with physical disabilities. Typical conditions include arthritis, stroke, multiple sclerosis, spinal injury and cerebral palsy. Older people who have problems with self-care will also be included in this section.

Physical disability may arise from a number of different causes. Moreover, physical disability does not equate with physical ill-health. As a result, adults with physical disabilities, unlike many of the client groups discussed in this book, do not share a specific subset of health-care settings. Certain units, such as spinal injuries units or rheumatology departments, are primarily used by disabled people. However, large numbers of disabled people live in the community and do not use specialist medical services.

Consequently, massage and aromatherapy with physically disabled adults and older children has predominantly consisted of consultation with individual private practitioners working in the community. The financial burden that this imposes has restricted practice, particularly as disabled people often have limited economic resources. That said, day care facilities maintained by local government have made increasing use of massage and aromatherapy in recent years. Practitioners may make weekly visits to such centres, sometimes on an unpaid basis, to give short massages to a number of individuals. Due to time constraints, physical impairment and, often, unsuitable rooms, these massages tend to take place through clothes with the client sitting upright in a chair. At some centres, massage has taken the form of a class in which relaxation exercises and self-massage may be taught.

HEALTH ISSUES

Physical symptoms

The classic effects of massage – improved circulation, relief of muscular tension, alleviation of pain – are of particular relevance in physical disability. Many of these symptoms are common in disabled people, not necessarily as a result of the primary complaint, but from associated behaviours or processes. For example, poor gait, resulting from neurological impairment, may lead to increased muscle tension in the upper back and neck. Similarly, the use of a wheelchair may compromise blood circulation and result in oedema (swelling) of the feet and ankles.

As discussed on page 18, the use of massage as a specific treatment for musculoskeletal conditions is not the prime focus of this book. Nonetheless, physically disabled adults who have experienced non-specific massage or aromatherapy do frequently report improvements in muscle tone and circulation.

> Massage relieves all the pain and stiffness in my neck and shoulders. It also gets the circulation going a bit: my feet are now warm and there is more feeling there.

Though such benefits are primarily a matter of increased comfort and quality of life, short-term improvements in mobility are not uncommon. One elderly woman with arthritis has claimed that, since receiving massage:

> My hands are now much more supple. Before, I couldn't really do things like making tea or taking a bath without help. Now I can do more things for myself.

Pain relief has also been widely reported. Though this often stems from relief of muscular aches, pain may be a primary symptom of a disability – in rheumatoid arthritis, for example – and massage has been used by some individuals primarily as a means of pain relief. It must be stressed that improvements in circulation, muscular tension and pain resulting from massage treatment are generally short-term. Typical comments include:

> I feel marvellous after a massage, really supple. I can turn my head right round. But by next morning I'm just as stiff as normal.

I can't believe the [pain] relief I get! But it normally lasts only half the week and by the time my next session comes around, I'm back where I started.

This is not an unusual feature of the health care of people with disabilities. Many health problems associated with disability result from an effectively permanent condition or process. Such health problems are therefore managed, rather than cured, and this often depends on continuing treatment. Practitioners of massage therefore do not see the relative brevity of action of massage as precluding a useful role in the health care of disabled people.

Essential oils are often used in the treatment of physically disabled people to enhance the effects of massage. For example, a number of essential oils are said to be rubefacient, that is, they are thought to promote local blood flow. These are typically used by aromatherapists to treat rheumatic or arthritic pain and to improve circulation. Other oils may be used for pain relief or muscular tension.

Sleep is often compromised by physical disability. Pain, low levels of activity and physical impairment may all contribute to poor sleep patterns. Massage is popularly seen as a soporific and people with physical disabilities have said that massage has improved both the quantity and quality of their sleep.

Many essential oils appear to have sedative properties and aromatherapists believe that they can treat sleep problems associated with disability. Oils are typically used as a home remedy, in the bath or a vaporizer before bed-time. Classical conditioning (p. 165) no doubt has an important function in this respect, the repeated association of sleep with a particular odour resulting in sleep being elicited by that odour. It is not known whether the use of essential oils in the long term as an aid to sleep leads to adverse side-effects, tolerance or addiction. Aromatherapists say that this is unlikely, on the grounds that the sedative action of oils is relatively mild.

One intriguing possibility is that massage may aid body-awareness in people who are physically disabled. This rests on the idea that imprecisions or distortions in an individual's mental picture of his or her body can interfere with efficient functioning. There have been reports of improvements in physical functioning following increased body-awareness after massage treatment. However, whether massage has any specific or generally applicable role in this regard is open to speculation. Physiotherapists may point to massage practitioners' relative lack of knowledge of neurology and rehabilitation. On the other hand, massage practitioners do emphasise the importance of body-awareness (p. 42).

Self-image

A significant number of disabled people see themselves as ugly or deformed. Moreover, particularly where disability has been acquired, by accident or disease, they may experience frustration and anger at the body, often expressed as 'my body has let me down'. A counsellor for disabled people has reported that 'a large proportion of the clients I see positively hate their own body'. Though such perceptions may be socially and politically engendered – and though they are amenable to social and political intervention – massage may also have a role in the re-establishing a positive self-image in those with physical disabilities.

Touch has been linked to self-esteem in a number of observational studies (p. 111). Given that these studies often use complex psychology to come to relatively obvious conclusions, the more intuitive approach of massage practitioners is sometimes refreshing:

> To be the recipient of a good massage is to receive care in the most direct and human way: through touch. It is to have someone say: you are worthwhile, I sympathize with you. A caring touch can communicate trust, empathy and respect. All this may be especially important for elderly or disabled people who may be rarely touched other than to be moved around.

It is interesting to compare these comments with those of Forsythe (1988), a doctor who has multiple sclerosis, who relates an experience of receiving massage from a friend:

> My own angry feelings about myself and my intense dislike of my body made it almost impossible for me to let her near enough to touch me: I was frighteningly vulnerable. Her work ... began to lessen the loathing I felt for my body.

Those with congenital disabilities have also commented on improvements in body image and awareness after massage:

> When I was being massaged, it felt like a stroke up my back was traversing three countries. Massage made me aware of the splits and divisions in me. I certainly gain self-acceptance through touch.

The experiences of pleasure and well-being resulting from massage can also play an important role. For someone who has found their body a source of frustration, and perhaps of pain, the realization that it can also be a source of pleasure and relaxation can be profoundly important.

Particular emphasis has been placed on the importance of touch in work with elderly people, particularly those who are socially isolated. Practitioners commonly use the phrase: 'touching the untouched' to describe massage with this client group.

PROFESSIONAL ISSUES

There are a number of complex non-medical issues involved in disability work. Practitioners wishing to 'help the disabled' have often been surprised to find that many disabled people tend to play down the medical aspects of disability. The reasons for this are plain: disabled people are often treated as a function of their condition and endure extreme prejudice as a result. For example, those with physical disabilities are often deemed incapable of intellectual effort, even to the point of making trivial decisions ('Does he take sugar?'). Disabled people also point out that popular fiction often associates moral weakness with physical stigmata (Dr Strangelove, Captain Hook) and that the media rarely portrays disabled people outside the role of 'heroes' or 'cabbages'. Disabled people are excluded from many things that able-bodied people take for granted: public transport is almost always inaccessible for people in wheelchairs; likewise, physical barriers such as steps and narrow doors often prevent those with disabilities from using shops, cinemas, libraries, restaurants and hotels. Employment opportunities are often restricted, by inaccessible buildings and by the prejudice of employers. In sum, whereas able-bodied health professionals see disability as a problem of individual health, disabled people themselves tend to see disability as a social problem.

Another aim of the disability movement has been to ensure that disabled people are allowed to participate in the decisions which affect their lives. Many disabled people feel disempowered, particularly in medical contexts, and it is important for a practitioner to ensure that clients are given the maximum possible choice over treatment decisions. For example, some practitioners who work in day centres have asked potential clients direct to their faces if they wanted treatment. It would be embarrassing and difficult for most people to refuse in such a situation, even more so for someone used to being at the mercy of other people's decisions. It is preferable to allow the individual concerned to make up their mind in another room and relay their decision through a third party if necessary.

A number of different professionals may liaise on the care of a person with a disability. These may include a social worker, a physiotherapist, an occupational therapist, a consultant, a GP, 'key workers' and workers at day centres and other units. It is important for complementary practitioners to maintain effective relations with these individuals, though this often presents considerable logistical problems.

Finally, the role of carers should not be overlooked. Caring for a disabled person can be a stressful, exhausting and seemingly endless experience. Some practitioners have made efforts to include therapy for carers in their treatment programmes.

SUMMARY

The role of massage and aromatherapy for adults with physical disabilities appears to be:

• the treatment of general aches and pains and poor blood circulation;
• aiding sleep;
• improving general well-being, body awareness and self-image.

CHILDREN WITH DISABILITIES

INTRODUCTION AND OVERVIEW OF PRACTICE

This section will discuss the use of massage and aromatherapy with children who have physical or learning disabilities. Typical conditions include Down's syndrome, cerebral palsy and autism. 'Children' will be taken as referring to those aged 12 or below.

Other sections in this chapter discuss the specifics of physical and learning disability in more detail. This section examines issues particular to childhood. Compared to older children and adults with disabilities, disabled children are characterized by a relatively greater degree of medical intervention, lack of autonomy and the possibility that treatment may have long-term effects.

Non-conventional therapies have traditionally been used on a wide scale by parents of disabled children. It is not unusual, for example, for parents to travel abroad to obtain unorthodox treatments or to spend many hours a day putting their child through unproven exercise regimes.

The use of massage and aromatherapy with disabled children exhibits a somewhat unusual pattern of practice. This is a function, at least in part, of a wide variety in both professional services and healthcare settings. A disabled child may receive health services from parents, general practitioners, hospital consultants, physiotherapists, occupational therapists, speech therapists, social workers and clinical psychologists; health settings may be as varied as hospitals, home, community health centres, schools, residential institutions and voluntary organizations. Many of these individuals and settings provide an opportunity for massage and aromatherapy. Typically, simple techniques are used by carers or professionals with only limited training. For example, massage may be used be a mother to help her child fall asleep or by a teacher to help build communication skills in a child with profound disabilities.

HEALTH ISSUES

Neurological impairment

Many physically disabled children have neurological impairments that lead to abnormalities of muscle tone. Though this may manifest as hypotonia (muscle flaccidity), increases in muscle tone, such as spasm or spasticity, are more usual. Massage is reported to bring about short-term improvements in such conditions. There are a number of reasons given to explain this effect.

One of the more obvious points is that high muscle tone is promoted by stress and anxiety. Similarly, pain may lead to increases in muscle tone. Massage is said to be of short-term benefit for pain and this may therefore be an important factor in reducing abnormally high muscle tone in children with neurological impairments. Specific physical manipulations such as stretches form an important element in physiotherapy for disabled children. However, the relevance of this to massage as practised by nurses and complementary practitioners is unclear. Such practitioners do not always have the skills required to assess and implement the specialist techniques used by physiotherapists.

The experiences of disabled children who have received massage and aromatherapy are most often reported indirectly through the observations of parents. The role of bias and expectation in distorting observations is therefore possibly at its highest. Nonetheless, parents do seem to be in agreement that massage can lead to short-term improvements in muscle tone. Typical comments are that massage has helped to calm 'jerky muscle spasms' or that a child's hands have 'opened out' after massage.

Another common observation is that of improved circulation following a massage. For example, one mother commented that 'Anne's hands and feet are normally ice cold, but they feel soft and warm after a treatment session'.

Blood circulation is often a specific problem in children with neurological impairments because tense muscles may impinge on blood vessels.

It is uncertain what specific role, if any, essential oils play in treating the primary physical symptoms of neurological impairment in children. Numerous oils are said to reduce spasm. However, though it has been shown that essential oils can reduce spasm in smooth muscle (p. 158) it is not known whether they have any effect on spasm in skeletal muscle. Other oils are said to improve blood circulation and may be used where this is thought to be appropriate.

RECURRENT SECONDARY SYMPTOMS

In practice, the main role of massage and aromatherapy with disabled children appears to be the treatment of emotional and behaviour problems (see below) and the treatment of recurrent secondary symptoms.

A number of recurrent health problems are associated with disability, especially in children. This is because aspects of a disabled person's physical condition, or lifestyle, may promote specific conditions. Perhaps the most well-known secondary symptom associated with disability is the pressure sore, caused by constant sitting and/or bed rest. In disabled children, the two secondary conditions of greatest interest for massage and aromatherapy are constipation and recurrent upper respiratory tract infection.

Recurrent constipation results from an interplay of different factors in a disabled child. Increased tone of the muscles of the abdominal wall is certainly an important factor, as is low intake of fibre and fluid in some children with feeding difficulties. Moreover, the passage of food through the gut is promoted by movements such as walking and bending which may be reduced in the disabled child. Massage of the abdomen is being used increasingly as a specific therapy for constipation, and constipation-related incontinence, in a number of different institutional settings. Though there are many anecdotal claims of success, there is, as yet, little support from the research literature. As was discussed on page 91, a German trial has indicated that massage is not an effective treatment for constipation. However, the particular aetiology of constipation in children with disabilities may make it difficult to extrapolate from this study. A beneficial effect of massage on bowel function may be attributed not so much to direct stimulation of the colon (the hypothesis under test in the German research) as to decreased abdominal muscle tone, relief from pain and improvements in anxiety. Support for this view comes from the fact that massage has been reported to be of benefit in painful conditions of the digestive tract other than constipation: for example, indigestion and 'colic' have been treated with some success in disabled children.

Recurrent respiratory tract infections are also a common feature of childhood disability. The reason for this is not completely understood but may be due to breathing difficulties, low levels of exercise and possibly lowered immune function. In children with Down's syndrome, recurrent colds and flu may be due to constriction of the nasal sinus passages associated with the altered cranial bone structure found in this condition.

Aromatherapists claim to have considerable success in treating recurrent respiratory infections in disabled children and these claims appear to be supported by the experiences of their clients. For example, the coordinator of a voluntary group which sponsors aromatherapy has commented: 'A number of the mothers at the centre have commented that, since the aromatherapist started work here, the number of respiratory infections that the children get has reduced to a more normal level.'

Aromatherapists give three reasons why essential oils are of benefit in recurrent infection. Firstly, essential oils are said to have anti-infective properties. This is at least partly supported by the scientific evidence (p. 147). However, though it is known that many oils have *in vitro* antibiotic activity, it is not known whether these oils demonstrate similar properties *in vivo*; moreover, many of the oils said to be of benefit in respiratory infections (e.g. lavender) are yet to be tested for antibiotic activity. Similarly, the claim that certain oils are anti-viral has never been thoroughly investigated.

The second reason often given for the benefit of aromatherapy in recurrent infection is that certain oils are said to palliate the symptoms of infection. For example, eucalyptus is a well-known decongestant and has traditionally been used in steam inhalations. It is a constituent of over-the-counter remedies such as Olbas Oil and Vicks VapoRub. See page 140 for a description of clinical research on this subject.

Thirdly, and perhaps most controversially, aromatherapists have claimed that essential oils act to strengthen the immune system. It may be possible to use a psychoneuroimmunological perspective to explain this effect: stress and anxiety are thought to suppress immune response, therefore a therapy that reduces stress and anxiety may have a positive effect on immune function. A further discussion of massage and aromatherapy in the treatment and prevention of infection is given in the section on AIDS on page 199.

Emotional and behavioural problems

Though emotional and behavioural problems are common in disabled children, many parents have fought for recognition that such problems are not always organic or even pathological. For example, a child with severe physical disabilities may exhibit what an ablebodied person could perceive as problem behaviours. These might, however, be perfectly appropriate attempts to communicate pain or frustration.

One of the commonest behavioural problems is poor sleep patterns and it seems that practitioners of massage and aromatherapy can often provide a useful service. Certain massage strokes can be very soporific; moreover, a number of essential oils are said to have sedative properties. Many parents have found that their children have fallen asleep during a massage session and/or that they have slept well the night following the massage. Given that it is impractical for a parent to take a child to a practitioner every day, many parents use simple techniques with their children before bedtime. Some have learnt simple calming massage strokes, often with the help and advice of an experienced practitioner. Others have used essential oils either in the bath or in a vaporizer. In addition to any direct sedative effect, the smell of the oils can create an appropriate 'mood' for bedtime and may induce relaxation by classical conditioning (p. 165).

Similar techniques can be used during the day to calm irritable and distracted children. Often even a gentle hand or foot rub can be effective in helping to calm a child and diffuse tension. This is one of the reasons why a large number of those who work with disabled children are learning simple massage techniques to use on an *ad hoc* basis. For example, teachers working in special schools have taken basic classes in massage to use in the classroom.

> Denise has inexplicable outbursts of temper and violence towards objects. She can be very excitable, but through massage becomes much quieter and calmer. There is benefit for her in just keeping still in a relaxed way.

Other uses of massage with disabled children overlap with those for people with learning disability. For example, self-harm may be found in adults or children with disabilities: massage has been found to be an effective treatment in at least some instances. For this and other aspects of massage in work with children who have learning disabilities, see the section on page 188.

Other health issues

One mother described massage treatment as a 'special time emotionally' for her child. It is clear that many children do enjoy massage enormously: it is relaxing and physically pleasurable. The reason why this is an issue of particular importance is that disabled children often have to undergo numerous sessions of medical treatment. Much of this therapy may simply be boring, but it can also be unpleasant or painful. For example, physiotherapy techniques aimed at preventing or treating contractures may cause pain to a child. A number of practitioners have pointed out the importance of the massage session as an occasion when therapy 'feels good'. An additional issue is that, through massage, a child can learn that his or her body can be a source of pleasure and relaxation, as well as pain and frustration. The role of massage in promoting improved self-concept is discussed further on page 180; what may be worthy of particular consideration here is the role of a therapy thought to improve self-concept at a time when that self-concept is first forming.

PROFESSIONAL ISSUES

The major professional issue for massage and aromatherapy with disabled children is the use of simple techniques by non-practitioners. Parents, teachers and other care workers may learn a few basic massage strokes for calming children or for use before bedtime and this may be supplemented by knowledge of a few oils.

This is not a development which should be discouraged. It is clearly impossible for a specialist practitioner to be available at all times when massage might be appropriate for a disabled child. Moreover, massage can be a useful way for parents to become involved in the health care of their children and for teachers and other care workers to foster relationships (see also p. 190).

However, it is important for practitioners to help define the scope and limits of non-professional practice. For example, it would be clearly inappropriate for a parent or teacher to treat a specific health problem, such as a recurrent urinary tract infection, or to use massage to attempt bring about changes in muscle tone.

'Caring for the carers' is mentioned several times throughout this book. Parenting a disabled child can be stressful and exhausting, the inherent difficulties of bringing up a child being compounded by the additional problems connected with disability and the necessity of having to deal with (and often fight) health professionals and social services. Some voluntary groups have demonstrated an enlightened attitude in this respect. One centre which provides an aromatherapy service has a regular 'Mothers' day' on which it is the parents, rather than the children, who enjoy the benefit of a relaxing massage.

SUMMARY

The role of massage and aromatherapy for children with disabilities appears to be:

- short-term relief from spasm, muscle pain and poor blood circulation;
- treatment of constipation;
- treatment of recurrent respiratory tract infections;
- calming irritable or distracted children;
- providing support to carers.

SEVERE LEARNING DISABILITY AND PROFOUND DISABILITY

INTRODUCTION AND OVERVIEW OF PRACTICE

This section discusses the use of massage and aromatherapy with older children and adults who have severe learning disabilities or profound disabilities. Learning disability is defined as where lowered ability to learn new skills and concepts significantly interferes with an individual's ability to lead a normal life. Though the terms 'learning difficulties', 'mental handicap' and 'mental retardation' are also used to refer to this client group, the latter two are now thought to be inaccurate and pejorative. Profound disability is where individuals have sensory impairments in addition to learning disabilities.

There are a number of different conditions or syndromes associated with people who have learning disabilities. These include Down's syndrome, cerebral palsy and fragile X syndrome. However, decreasing reference is made to specific syndromes as this reinforces a medical rather than a social model of disability.

Historically, people with learning and profound disabilities were confined to large institutions. This was as much due to the perceived need to 'protect' society from what were seen as evil and sick individuals as it was to the provision of an appropriate environment for people with learning disabilities. Recent models of care have emphasized a more client-centred and community-based approach and what is known as normalization, or more recently, social role valorization. Larger institutions have closed and people with learning disabilities have been rehoused in small group homes in the community. Simple hand and foot massage has been used by some support workers in this setting.

Aromatherapy and massage have also been used within a day-centre setting either to aid relaxation, as a leisure activity, or as part of the educational curriculum. The popularity of the therapies stems primarily from the realization that touch and smell can be an important means of communicating with people who have profound disabilities. Current interest has grown to the extent that institutions such as the Royal National Institute for the Blind now offer formal training in massage and aromatherapy to care workers.

HEALTH ISSUES

Many of the health issues pertinent to profound and severe learning disability have already been discussed in the chapters referring to adults with physical disabilities and disabled children. For example, body awareness (p. 179) can be a problem in some people with profound disabilities. This chapter will focus on the use of massage and aromatherapy for communication and intellectual development.

Sensory stimulation

For people with profound disabilities – those who have impaired hearing and/or vision in addition to learning disabilities – touch and smell may become the most significant means of obtaining sensory information about the world. They may also be an effective means of conveying that the outside world is of interest, and worth interacting with. This is important because people with profound disabilities often need help to explore their environment.

'Multisensory massage' (Sanderson and Harrison, 1991) is a term used to describe the use of a variety of massage tools plus oils or creams perfumed with essential oils to provide experiences of touch, smell, texture and vibration. Some massage tools are simple, cheap wooden items such as the handle roller, 'footsie', or twin or six-ball massager, all of which are widely available from health stores. More sophisticated massage tools, such as hand-held electrical massagers with interchangeable heads, can also be used. Electrical massage tools can be attached to large, sensitive switches so that they can be switched on or off by the person receiving the treatment. This can help people with profound or severe learning disabilities to understand that they can affect the world around them and that they can make choices.

The use of essential oils provides an additional means of developing the ability to exercise control. A multisensory massage session often starts by helping the individual to choose an essential oil to use for the day. Uplifting and refreshing oils are usually used because the session focuses on learning and experiencing rather than relaxation. Most people with profound disabilities cannot speak, but experienced workers are generally able to determine an individual's preference by their physical reactions when they smell an oil.

Essential oils can be used as a form of sensory stimulation without massage. A 'smell bank' is an area of the classroom which is reserved for helping pupils to understand about smells. It consists of a series of containers with different smells and often includes a small selection of essential oils.

Interactive massage

Many people with profound and severe learning disabilities have a degree of what is termed 'tactile defensiveness'. They may associate touch with an unwanted functional activity: touch can come to signify change and invasion of personal space.

Gentle massage can be used to overcome tactile defensiveness. This is important in two respects. Firstly, it is an aid to teaching self-care. For example, in order to teach someone with a visual impairment how to reach out to grasp a cup, the teacher must guide and hold the pupil's hand. This will be much easier if the pupil has been accustomed to touch by massage.

In addition, massage can help build relationships in a more general sense. Recent innovations in work with people who have learning disabilities have placed the forming of interpersonal bonds at the centre of education and made the development of relationships the most important goal of any therapy. A number of workers have reported that interactive massage has been the key to developing relationships with some pupils.

Massage also allows therapists and care staff to convey warmth in an appropriate manner.

> People with profound disabilities often become isolated from any special, caring touch. It's inappropriate for staff to go around hugging and cuddling pupils, but we can use hand and foot massage.

For many people with profound or severe learning disabilities touch and massage need to be introduced slowly and carefully. There is a sequence that most people with profound disabilities progress through when they are introduced to any new activity (resists, tolerates, cooperates passively, enjoys, responds cooperatively, leads, imitates, initiates). When this sequence is applied to massage it is known as 'interactive massage' (Sanderson and Harrison, 1991) and can help therapists and support staff to identify how well someone is learning to accept touch.

Challenging behaviour

Some people with profound or severe learning disabilities exhibit challenging behaviours such as self-harm or regurgitation. A number of workers have hypothesized that such self-stimulatory behaviours are caused by a lack of external stimulation. Massage provides a form of stimulation and is therefore seen as an appropriate treatment. Others have pointed out that any pleasurable and relaxing activity is likely to be a calming influence on those exhibiting excitable and disrupted behaviour.

> Jean was continually thrashing backwards and forwards, punching her head with her fists, slapping her head and face …. The aromatherapist spent two hours with her using a massage oil made up with relaxing essential oils. At first any contact with Jean was met with total rejection … [but] during the last half-hour … Jean appeared relaxed and was lying back in the bean bag, with her hands behind her head, smiling and sometimes laughing.
>
> *Sanderson and Harrison, 1991: 65–66*

Even more dramatic cases have been reported in the literature, one involving complete cessation of self-harm after 10 years of unsuccessful treatment (p. 123). That said, the role of massage and aromatherapy should not be overestimated: they certainly do not provide a panacea for the profound problems that challenging behaviour may present.

Location smells

Some units have used essential oils to provide environmental cues. Different essential oils are vaporized in a number of specific locations to create an association between an odour and a place. An example given by Sanderson and Harrison (1991) is the smell of pine, familiar in bathrooms through the use of perfumed cleaning agents. This effect can be reinforced by regularly vaporizing the essential oil. When the person with profound disabilities is taken to the bathroom, the odour acts both as cue to their location and to the forthcoming activity: 'I can smell a familiar smell (pine), I must be in the bathroom, therefore I am going to have a bath'. Location smells can be particularly valuable for helping an individual identify his or her own property. Essential oils can be used on handkerchiefs in clothes drawers and vaporized in bedrooms to give the person a sense of knowing what is theirs. This creates a reassuring familiarity and identification with surroundings.

Essential oils can also be used to help identify people. In one school for children with severe learning disabilities, every member of staff wears a fabric bracelet scented with a different essential oil. This is found to help the children to differentiate between staff.

PROFESSIONAL ISSUES

Massage and aromatherapy for people with profound or severe learning disabilities has generally involved the use of simple techniques by care staff rather than specialist practitioners. This is partly because the role of massage and aromatherapy has been largely an everyday activity to aid general teaching and care tasks (e.g. the development of relationships) rather than a special session of therapy to treat specific symptoms. However, some specialist practitioners have volunteered to work with people with profound disabilities. Though it was anticipated that practitioners might experience problems working with this client group, this has not turned out to be the case.

That said, it is worth re-emphasising that massage and aromatherapy practice need to be placed in the context of conventional approaches to learning disability. For example, one common guiding concept is that of 'the five accomplishments' (O'Brien, 1986). These are choice, community participation, respect, relationships and competence. For example, when considering the area of choice, people with disabilities may have had the majority of choices made for them. It is therefore important to give people as much choice as possible when introducing them to massage and aromatherapy. This includes choice of oils, choice of which part of the body to massage and choice of when and where to receive the massage.

SUMMARY

Massage and aromatherapy for people with severe learning disability or profound disability are normally used by parents and care staff, rather than specialist practitioners. The role of massage and aromatherapy for this client group appears to be:

- sensory stimulation;
- aiding the development of relationships;
- treatment of self-harm and other challenging behaviours;
- essential oils can be used to identify people and places.

Disease

8

CANCER CARE
Caroline Stevensen, MacMillan Clinical Nurse Specialist in
Complementary Therapies, Royal London Homoeopathic NHS Trust,
London, and Andrew Vickers

INTRODUCTION AND OVERVIEW OF PRACTICE

This section will discuss the use of massage and aromatherapy with people who are living with cancer. For hospice care see page 222.

Cancer will affect approximately one person in three. As a result of recent advances in therapy, significant numbers of people survive an initial cancer episode and live with the disease, often for many years. This has allowed increased recognition of the importance of the psychological and spiritual aspects of cancer care, a development which has also been fuelled by patient advocacy groups. Organizations representing women's health issues in particular have been effective at articulating and lobbying for patient-centred models of care, especially those that acknowledge that cancer is not purely a medical experience for the patient but raises profound psychological and spiritual issues.

Programmes of psychological and spiritual support in cancer were initially developed in specialist centres, such as the Bristol Cancer Help Centre in the UK, and by patient self-advocacy organizations. In recent years, such programmes have become more mainstream: the provision of counselling, self-help groups, relaxation techniques and complementary therapies is now reasonably commonplace in general and specialist secondary centres alike. In 1994, the National Health Service went so far as to make research into the alleviation of psychological distress in cancer a priority area.

Massage and aromatherapy have found a place in a number of cancer care programmes. The overall rationale for their use has been to comfort patients and to improve quality of life.

HEALTH ISSUES

Psychological distress

People living with cancer may be affected by a number of psychological and emotional difficulties. These include fear of harsh treatment regimes, pain, disease recurrence and death; anxiety, related to an unknown life expectancy, the possible loss of income and the effect on loved ones; depression due to fatigue, pain, uncertainty and the loss of social role; loneliness and bitterness. The use of massage and aromatherapy in cancer care has developed, at least in part, from a recognition of its value in reducing anxiety and for its particular appropriateness for some of the psychological problems listed above. For example, the use of touch can be a useful way of overcoming loneliness in a patient.

> They're too busy, the nurses. They're rushing round the wards ... with massage, as soon as the hands go on, you know she's there, she's calm, she's touching you, she has time for you.
>
> *Patient quoted by Turton (1989)*

Other patients have reported a deep sense of relaxation and release of muscular tension following treatment, often commenting that massage has helped them to break the anxiety–muscle tension–anxiety cycle. This can be an important prelude to the use of self-regulation techniques such as relaxation therapy or meditation. Stress and anxiety can lead to sleeping difficulties and massage and aromatherapy have been reported to lead to improved sleep in some cancer patients. It is not uncommon for patients to report 'the best night's sleep I can remember' after an aromatherapy massage given before bedtime.

Massage and aromatherapy have also been claimed to be a useful treatment for depression in some patients. Sensitive use of touch is a form of social support and can be particularly useful where depression leads to social withdrawal. Certain essential oils are said to have psychological actions (pp 58 and 164) and aromatherapists may use appropriate mood-altering oils in massage with depressed patients. Treatment has been said to be especially useful for patients who find words inadequate or feelings difficult to express. The trust built up through the use of touch may provide the atmosphere necessary for further emotional expression. Massage has also helped certain patients become more aware of their physical tension, with the result that they recognize more readily their emotional needs. See also page 219.

Altered body-image can be a problem for many cancer patients. Many feel that they have suddenly become the site of their tumour and that a small lump is suddenly 'all that matters'. Others may feel 'split in two', that the diseased part of their body is somehow not part of them. As with other conditions, massage has been reported to improve cancer patients' perceptions of their own body. In the words of one nurse: 'massage leads to an acknowledgement and acceptance of the changes that occur with cancer'.

Many of the issues of body-image in cancer are similar to those in physical disability; see page 180 for a further discussion.

It may be worth briefly discussing the links between psychology and cancer. It has been said that stress, and even personality, can contribute to the cause of cancer and that various psychological factors, such as attitude or social support, can affect its outcome. There is evidence, for example, that psychosocial support improves survival in patients with metastatic breast cancer (Speigel *et al.*, 1989). It is tempting to speculate as to whether massage and aromatherapy could improve outcome in cancer by relieving stress and improving social support. However, there is no reliable evidence that they do indeed have this effect and it would be wise to be cautious in making any claims for the value of massage or aromatherapy in cancer beyond that of improving quality of life.

Physical problems

Physical problems experienced by people with cancer can include pain, constipation, impaired mobility, nausea, fatigue, skin problems and recurrent infections. Massage and aromatherapy are said to offer short-term relief in some cases.

Pain in cancer can be due to a number of different causes: surgery, tumour growth or lymphoedema, to name but a few. Massage and aromatherapy have been reported to be a useful adjunct to conventional pain management strategies in some patients. Though reduction of anxiety is likely to play an important role, massage may also be an effective treatment for the physical causes of pain, of which lymphoedema deserves special consideration. Lymphoedema is the accumulation of fluid in the limbs, particularly the arms, resulting from poor functioning of the lymphatic system. This can be caused by cancerous invasion of the lymph nodes, surgical removal of lymph vessels or damage due to radiotherapy. The standard treatment for lymphoedema consists of massage, bandaging and exercise. However, a specialized form of massage is used and this requires a specific training. Practitioners of massage and aromatherapy may not be sufficiently conversant with the effects of cancer on the lymphatic system to offer a useful service in the treatment of lymphoedema. Nonspecific massage does seem to be of benefit for general muscular aches and pain and for oedema resulting from prolonged bed rest.

One particularly intriguing possibility is the use of massage and aromatherapy to alleviate the fatigue and lethargy common at some stages of cancer. Massage can be invigorating, as well as relaxing, and certain essential oils are also said to stimulate. One practitioner has described how 'patients often come in dragging their feet as a result of fatigue from radiotherapy. After treatment they seem to spring off the table and trip down the corridor.'

Aromatherapists claim that they may be able to help some of the skin problems common in cancer. Eczema or psoriasis occur in some patients, possibly as a result of stress, and radiotherapy and chemotherapy can cause dry and fragile skin. Many essential oils are said to be of benefit for the skin. Camomile, for example, is a traditional aromatherapy treatment for eczema.

PROFESSIONAL ISSUES

The possibility of interactions between essential oils and chemotherapy agents has worried some practitioners working in cancer care. Those with experience of the field point out that essential oils are relatively mild and enter the bloodstream in low doses and are therefore unlikely to affect the extremely potent drugs used in cancer treatment. That said, adverse effects from massage and aromatherapy are perhaps more probable in cancer care than in most other settings, simply because both the disease and its treatment can weaken a number of body systems. For example, certain forms of chemotherapy can cause the skin to bruise easily, entailing that massage must be conducted with particular care. Chemotherapy-related nausea is also an important consideration: exposure to the odour of an essential oil while experiencing nausea can lead to a conditioned association so that the odour can provoke nausea at a later stage. See Chapter 11 for more on adverse effects and contraindications of massage and aromatherapy.

Working with cancer patients can also raise a number of complex psychological issues for a practitioner. These are discussed in the section on hospice care in Chapter 9.

SUMMARY

The role of massage and aromatherapy for people with cancer appears to be:

- alleviation of stress and anxiety associated with living with cancer;
- emotional support for problems such as loneliness;
- treatment of pain and fatigue in some patients.

HIV AND AIDS

INTRODUCTION AND OVERVIEW OF PRACTICE

This section will discuss the use of massage and aromatherapy with people who are infected with the human immunodeficiency virus (HIV). Some have symptoms characteristic of acquired immuno-deficiency syndrome (AIDS). Others, while not necessarily suffering symptoms of AIDS, live with the possibility of a disabling and potentially fatal disease. There are a number of similarities between the problems faced by people with HIV and AIDS and those faced by people with physical disabilities, so the reader is advised to read the section starting on page 177.

People with HIV and AIDS have not always been content with conventional treatments. Therapeutic options in HIV and AIDS are limited and the recent demonstration that zidovudine is not an effective prophylactic treatment for asymptomatic HIV (the Concorde trial) has further weakened faith in conventional medical approaches. Many individuals are also unhappy about the medical model of AIDS and the process of medical treatment. Some, for example, have complained that the medical profession has ignored the real needs of individuals in their quest to eliminate HIV. Others claim that their treatment has reflected the homophobic attitudes of many doctors.

As a result, a number of specialist centres have been established to deal with the health needs of people with HIV and AIDS. Such centres are community-based and are often funded partly or wholly by charitable donations. They are generally run by users of the service. Most emphasize information, self-help and peer support. Though these centres do tend to involve conventional health professionals, a variety of complementary therapies are commonly practised. Massage and aromatherapy are particularly widespread and popular. The majority of massage and aromatherapy practice with people with HIV and AIDS takes place in these specialist centres.

HEALTH ISSUES

Physical symptoms

A number of physical symptoms are common in people with AIDS. Perhaps most important are infections and tumours, both of which can be fatal. People with AIDS may also suffer a variety of minor symptoms, some of which can seriously interfere with quality of life. These include: neuropathies, poor mobility, stiff and aching muscles, breathing difficulties, headache, digestion and bowel problems, fatigue and insomnia. Some of these problems are also common in people with HIV and this has been attributed to the stress of an HIV diagnosis. Massage and aromatherapy have been reported to be of benefit for many of the symptoms listed above. One doctor has claimed that 'massage and aromatherapy seem to lead to pain relief and improved mobility in many of our users. That said, the effect is moderate and seems to depend on continuing treatment.'

Short-term improvements in pain, mobility, sleep and digestion may result primarily from relaxation. These symptoms are discussed further in the section on Physical Disability (p. 177). Massage and aromatherapy also seem to lead to a perceived increase in levels of general well-being in many cases. People with HIV and AIDS have claimed that treatment led to an 'overall improvement in health' or that 'the problems are still there but they don't bother me so much'.

Breathlessness occurs in some people with AIDS as a result of infection or due to the presence of Kaposi's sarcoma in the lungs. Massage and aromatherapy are said to be of benefit for a variety of reasons. Breathing difficulties are often exacerbated by anxiety and this can cause a downward spiral in which breathing difficulties lead to anxiety which impairs breathing. The spiral can be broken by relaxation and some practitioners have reported that patients have breathed more slowly and deeply and with less effort after a treatment. Massage treatment may also be of benefit by reducing physical tension in the chest and abdomen. This is an interesting claim (it mirrors that of osteopaths and chiropractors who say that they are able to help asthma by physical manipulation) and is worthy of further research.

Practitioners also say that they are able to ameliorate fatigue in some patients. Though this may be a function of improved sleep and general mood, and decreased pain, practitioners may also use specific techniques to increase energy levels. These include reflexology, acupressure and hands-on healing. Certain essential oils are said to be stimulating, uplifting or 'fortifying' and may be used in particular cases.

Infections and immune function

Immune function is the key issue in HIV and AIDS: it is the weakening of the immune system in AIDS which causes the infections and cancers which lead to death. Many practitioners say that treatment can stimulate the immune system and/or fight infection and some give this as the main rationale for their work. This claim is an important one and requires further examination. Because there is no clinical research on the effects of massage and aromatherapy on immunity in AIDS and HIV, and because anecdotal reports are unlikely to give an insight into the effects of treatment on the immune system, this section will consist of a discussion of the background theoretical issues.

Essential oils have been shown to have antimicrobial properties in the laboratory (p. 147). However, this does not necessarily imply that the oils are of clinical value. At the current time of writing there is no rigorous, clinical evidence that essential oils are effective for the sort of infections important in AIDS. Moreover, though trials of tea tree oil have demonstrated that it is of benefit for a number of different skin infections, this may not be through any direct action on the pathogenic organism (p. 136).

The more general claim that massage and aromatherapy boost the immune system is even more problematic. A number of essential oils are said to be immune stimulants. This is not as unusual a claim as it sounds: several herbs, most notably *echinacea*, have been shown to stimulate the immune system (Bräunig, Dorn and Knick, 1992; Tomoda *et al.*, 1994). However, there is no evidence that any essential oil has this effect. On the other hand, some practitioners have taken a psychoneuroimmunological perspective: stress is known to lower the immune system; massage and aromatherapy are therefore of benefit because they relieve stress. Unfortunately, it is not entirely clear whether this is a valid argument and reliable evidence is hard to come by. Perhaps the only relevant study found that relaxation therapy does not affect immune function in men with HIV (Coates *et al.*, 1989), so the psychoneuroimmunological argument is not necessarily valid in HIV.

There is, however, some evidence for a direct effect of massage on the immune system. Both Groër *et al.* (1994) and Green and Green (1987) found that a back rub raises levels of salivary immunoglobulin A (s-IgA). Though this is associated with resistance to respiratory tract infections, the duration of s-IgA enhancement remains unknown and so its clinical significance is unclear. Specific massage techniques, for example, manual lymph drainage, have been said to be of benefit for immune functioning and are used for people with HIV and AIDS by some practitioners. These techniques have not been evaluated at the current time of writing.

In summary, practitioners of massage and aromatherapy claim to be able to boost the immune system of people with HIV and AIDS. Though there is no clinical evidence to support this claim, there are at least some theoretical reasons why massage and aromatherapy may be of benefit. Good quality research is clearly required.

Psychosocial issues

Psychosocial support is generally the main reason given for the use of massage and aromatherapy with people who have HIV or AIDS. Treatment is said to relieve 'stress' generally, but also to ameliorate specific psychosocial problems. Anxiety and depression are a common consequence of a diagnosis of serious disease. This can be exacerbated by job and housing difficulties and by bereavement: many people with HIV and AIDS have friends who have died of the disease. A number of workers have also pointed out that worrying 'Have I got AIDS?' at the sign of a cold or other minor health problem is a major stress for people with HIV.

Massage and aromatherapy can be deeply relaxing and some individuals have reported this to be of particular benefit. A number of practitioners have used massage as part of an educative process, a concrete experience of relaxation as prelude to the use of self-regulation techniques. This principle is discussed on pages 203 and 220. The general feelings of well-being resulting from treatment can also be important. The comment of one patient following a massage was 'I feel so much lighter' and this seems a good description of the improvement in mood often experienced after treatment. See the section on cancer (pp. 194–195) for a fuller discussion of massage and aromatherapy for the treatment of the emotional problems associated with serious disease.

Treatment may also have a role in facilitating the psychotherapeutic process in people with HIV and AIDS. This is claimed to occur for a variety of reasons. The trust built up with a practitioner has been said to be important, as has relaxation, on the grounds that individuals generally find it easier to disclose personal information when they are relaxed. Some practitioners have claimed that emotions can become 'locked into muscle tissue' and that soft-tissue work can lead to emotional release. For more on the links between counselling and massage, see pages 24, 207 and 219.

Touch may have a particular role for people with HIV and AIDS because of a cluster of issues concerning stigmatization, isolation and social rejection. One practitioner commented that when she started work in the early 1980s, people with AIDS were considered 'society's pariahs'. Though attitudes have no doubt improved, people with HIV and AIDS still suffer a degree of stigmatization and rejection. This can be compounded by homophobia, especially where an individual has decided to 'come out' to friends and family as a result of an HIV diagnosis. Fears of infection can further isolate people with HIV and AIDS. Physical contact can be an important means of ameliorating feelings of rejection and isolation. One user commented: 'It was wonderful to be touched by someone who wasn't wearing gloves.'

Massage has also been said to be an important source of touch. It is often thought that in countries such as the US and the UK, most instances of touch occur between sexual partners, if not necessarily during sex itself. Many people with AIDS and HIV do not have active sex lives and may go without touch. Massage can provide an appropriate means of touch gratification.

It is so nice to be touched after all these years.

The experiences of physical pleasure resulting from massage can be particularly important. The realization that the body can be a source of pleasure and relaxation may be of benefit to anyone whose body has been a source of suffering, perhaps particularly where that suffering has been itself been caused by pleasure. See page 180 for more on massage and self-esteem.

Some people with HIV and AIDS, however, have reacted against this concept of massage as a means of overcoming isolation and stigmatization.

If I want to be massaged, I ask my friends. I certainly don't need a professional to lay her hands on and 'accept' me. I feel great about myself.

PROFESSIONAL ISSUES

Practitioners working in specialist HIV and AIDS units need to be aware of the special issues and perceptions of the gay community. Certainly not all practitioners have been completely free of common social prejudices about gay people. Practitioners should also be aware that HIV and AIDS is a social, as well as a medical issue. The most pressing problems for a person newly diagnosed as HIV-positive may have little to do with health: rather it is mortgages, insurance policies and workplace discrimination that are likely to be of most immediate concern.

Though some workers have voiced concerns about the possibility of HIV transmission during massage, the risk of infection is probably negligible. Simple, common-sense procedures to avoid contact with bodily fluids are probably the only necessary safety precautions.

Kaposi's sarcoma is thought by some to be a contraindication for massage. A recent consensus appears to be that, though direct pressure on tumours should be avoided, massage is no more likely to cause the spread of tumour than everyday activities such as walking, sitting or lying down.

Some of the specialist HIV and AIDS centres have not developed effective systems of interdisciplinary health care. Users are usually offered a 'smorgasbord' of different therapies to chose from as they wish, with individual practitioners often working independently, in relative isolation from one another. This situation is particularly common where complementary practitioners volunteer to give free treatment. The problems associated with this approach are discussed on page 246.

SUMMARY

The role of massage and aromatherapy for people with HIV and AIDS appears to be:

- relief from general aches and pains;
- improvements in sleep, digestion, breathing and fatigue in some patients;
- alleviation of stress and anxiety associated with living with HIV;
- providing touch;
- some practitioners claim to be able to treat infections and improve immune function: it is not clear whether this is indeed the case.

CARDIOVASCULAR REHABILITATION

INTRODUCTION AND OVERVIEW OF PRACTICE

This section will discuss the use of massage and aromatherapy in cardiovascular rehabilitation. Cardiovascular disease is one of the commonest causes of death and disability in the Western world and occurs in various forms. Some diseases, such as angina pectoris, have a relatively gradual onset and cause long-term disability. Cardiovascular disease may also present suddenly, as a 'heart attack' in which muscle tissue dies due to a lack of oxygen caused by compromised blood supply. A heart attack is technically known as a myocardial infarction (MI).

Medical care of cardiovascular disease may involve intensive care (p. 277) and hospice care (p. 222). This section will concentrate on rehabilitation following discharge after hospitalization for MI or for surgery, such as coronary bypass, to prevent MI. The overall aim of cardiovascular rehabilitation is to reduce disability and to lower the probability of further cardiovascular events. In the last few years, a limited number of centres have developed structured rehabilitation programmes which include advice and education on diet, lifestyle, exercise and smoking. These complement drug therapy and regular diagnostic screening. Rehabilitation has also sometimes included pro- grammes of stress reduction. Where massage and aromatherapy have found a place in cardiac rehabilitation, they have typically done so as a part of such programmes.

HEALTH ISSUES

Stress reduction

Stress and anxiety have long been acknowledged to place strain on the cardiovascular system. As everyone knows, one sign of stress is a rapidly beating heart. High levels of arousal are also associated with increased and sometimes inappropriate activity and this can of itself place undue strain on the heart. Massage and aromatherapy can be seen simply as therapies to reduce stress and anxiety. A massage treatment is relaxing and is seen to reduce stress; use of appropriate relaxing odours in aromatherapy is said to add to this effect.

Practitioners who work in cardiovascular rehabilitation say that it is misleading to see a massage or aromatherapy consultation simply as a unidirectional therapy for stress. Though massage and aromather- apy can be used to treat, for example, acute anxiety in a hospital set- ting, their use in rehabilitation is more concerned with eliciting long- term changes in a patient. In this view, massage is seen not so much as a treatment but as an educative process. A common idea is that mas- sage teaches relaxation as a prelude to using self-regulatory tech- niques, such as meditation, on a daily basis.

Massage is a concrete experience of relaxation that a patient can tap into.

In other words, massage can teach a patient what a relaxed state feels like. This helps them to incorporate periods of relaxation in their daily life. Practitioners also point out that massage aids body aware- ness, thereby enabling patients to feel areas of tension and tightness. Patients who have experienced massage are said to recognize stress more readily and therefore cope with it effectively.

Massage and aromatherapy can also be incorporated into lifestyle changes. The massage sections of some rehabilitation programmes can be as short as a single, 2-hour session involving one practitioner and a dozen patients with their spouses or partners. Practitioners have treated such sessions as an opportunity to teach a few simple massage techniques, such as a neck and shoulder rub, which patients can exchange with their spouses or partners on a regular basis. Practitioners may also recommend the use of essential oils in the bath as an aid to relaxation.

That said, a number of practitioners do see massage and aromatherapy treatment as having direct therapeutic value. Some (Freeman, 1987) claim to be able to reduce blood pressure in hypertensives, though there is little rigorous evidence that massage can indeed have this effect (p. 101) . Others make the more general point that, because tension can be held in muscle tissue, chronically tense and anxious patients are unlikely to benefit from self-regulatory techniques, such as daily relaxation sessions, simply because of the degree of physical tension held in their body. For example, relaxed, diaphragmatic breathing can be difficult if the abdomen is tense or the shoulders raised. Massage and aromatherapy treatment to decrease muscle tension is said to be an important prerequisite for self-directed relaxation in such patients.

Psychological and interpersonal issues

MI is often a sudden, catastrophic event which can radically affect an individual's perception of their own body. Patients may feel vulnerable or 'damaged', and the knowledge that the future may bring another, perhaps fatal MI can further compromise a patient's self-image. Massage can play an important role in restoring a positive body image in cardiovascular rehabilitation. Simply to receive caring touch can improve a patient's self-esteem. The feelings of pleasure and relaxation resulting from a massage can also be of benefit: for someone who has found their body a source of frustration, and perhaps of pain, the realization that it can also be a source of pleasure and relaxation can be profoundly important. See page 180 for a full discussion of the role of massage in restoring a positive self-image.

An issue of particular interest in cardiac rehabilitation is a patient's relationship with their partner or spouse. Relationships are likely to be altered by MI due to the fear of illness, disability and death and the resulting psychological imbalance between partners. The misconception that sex can precipitate MI can also complicate relationships. Some practitioners have taught massage specifically as a means of re-establishing relationships and of increasing confidence between a couple. Partners are shown simple massage techniques to practise on one another during the class and it is suggested that these are used on a regular basis at home. In addition to aiding relationships, massage may also allow a patient to reverse care roles by giving care to his or her partner. This not only involves 'care for the carers' but may aid a patient's self-esteem.

PROFESSIONAL ISSUES

Massage has been said to be contraindicated after MI because changes in blood flow resulting from massage may put undue strain on a weak heart. As it happens, there is evidence that gentle massage does not cause significant physiological changes in coronary patients (see p. 264 for a full discussion). That said, it would be wise for a practitioner to avoid vigorous massage and to liaise with a patient's doctor if massage was thought to constitute a risk.

There are various reasons why massage and aromatherapy may not always have a receptive patient audience in cardiovascular rehabilitation. As part of a rehabilitation package, massage may not have been specifically sought out by patients. Moreover, patients may not wish to see themselves as in need of 'hands-on' care once they have left hospital.

Massage and aromatherapy is yet to become common in cardiovascular rehabilitation. One consequence is that there is often medical resistance to, or at least neglect of, the inclusion of massage and aromatherapy in cardiovascular rehabilitation programmes. The field was established relatively recently and it is likely that new insights will develop over the next few years.

SUMMARY

The role of massage and aromatherapy in cardiovascular rehabilitation appears to be:

- reduction of stress by providing a concrete experience of relaxation;
- aiding relationships, particularly between patients and their partners;
- improving self-image.

Special health care settings

9

INTRODUCTION AND OVERVIEW OF PRACTICE

This section will discuss the use of massage and aromatherapy in primary care. Known as general practice in the UK, and as family practice in the US, primary care is normally the first point of contact between patients and the health service and often one of the few settings to which patients can self-refer. As such, a majority of the population come into regular contact with primary care.

Traditionally, primary care acted as a kind of filter. General practitioners (GPs) provided certain simple medical services but referred cases requiring specialist attention to secondary-care centres such as hospitals. Recently, there has been a move away from hospital care towards the provision of more services in the community. Primary-care centres have begun to provide an increasing range of interventions, including physiotherapy, health promotion, counselling and even minor surgery. In the UK, the expansion and diversification of general practice has been fuelled by the advent of fundholding, which gives GPs more freedom to purchase services as they see fit.

The increasing use of massage and aromatherapy in primary care has resulted from both local political changes, such as fundholding, and from long-term trends such as the move away from hospital care. Though it is sometimes a practice nurse who provides treatment, it is more often the case that a specialist practitioner is hired in for one or two sessions a week. Some primary-care centres have offered massage and aromatherapy as part of multidisciplinary stress reduction clinics.

HEALTH ISSUES

Stress-related illness in primary care

It is widely acknowledged that patients with persistent non-specific illness or minor psychological distress constitute a significant proportion of any GP's caseload. This is problematic because conventional treatment options for such patients are limited. It is unclear, for example, what a GP can do for a patient who returns repeatedly to complain of headaches, fatigue and mild depression, despite an absence of organic findings.

Massage and aromatherapy treatment are said to provide a useful service to such patients. There are several issues of note. At its most basic level, massage and aromatherapy treatment provides care to those who might not otherwise receive medical services, despite feeling in need. Hands-on therapy is a particularly effective means of helping patients to feel cared for.

When I go for the massage I feel accepted, unjudged.

Massage was an oasis at a time when I was in a very low state and it was a bridge that supported me.

It also appears that treatment can be of benefit because many cases of non-specific illness or minor psychological distress are related to psychosocial stress: fatigue, headaches, mild depression or gastro-intestinal disturbances are good examples. Practitioners have found that relaxation following treatment has led to relatively rapid improvements in a significant number of patients and they attribute this to relief from the effects of stress.

But for some patients referred to practitioners of massage and aromatherapy in primary care, stress itself may be the presenting complaint. Such patients include those experiencing bereavements or other major life changes and those in stressful jobs. Massage and aromatherapy are said to be particularly appropriate treatments for such patients simply because they provide deep relaxation. However, the importance of counselling and a positive therapeutic relationship should not be underestimated. Hands-on treatment can help build up trust and rapport and this can aid discussion of personal problems (see also p. 219). As one practitioner put it:

I can give a patient attention, unconditional attention. Through touch, I can communicate my care, support and acceptance. Patients often tell me personal matters and then remark that they don't feel able to say such things to anyone else.

Patients are also more likely to feel comfortable enough to discuss difficult issues when they are relaxed. Some practitioners have described massage as a 'way in' for people who are resistant to counselling. Moreover, there is the point that patients are normally asked to talk and explain their problems. During a massage, no talking is necessary. Paradoxically, this may help the counselling process (see also the section on mental health, p. 216). One practitioner reports that:

> A patient came in full of words. When I said 'You don't have to talk' she said 'Phew!' and relaxed on the couch.

The following remark from a patient is also of interest:

> I was very surprised after the first massage that I had been able to bring into the open all these fears and feelings. I most certainly would have been far less forthcoming and far less frank in a situation of psychotherapy, i.e. sitting, fully-dressed, face to face with a counsellor.

The issue of counselling brings up a more general point, which is that massage and aromatherapy are said by some practitioners to be most effective as part of an multimodal programme of stress management. This can include attention to diet and lifestyle, and the teaching of techniques such as breathing exercises or sequential muscle relaxation. One nurse working in primary care works out a treatment plan with each patient. She says that many of the patients she sees have diet or lifestyle problems that exacerbate stress. A typical case might go without breakfast, take no break at lunch and drink 15 cups of coffee a day. The use of alcohol and television to relax can further exacerbate stress-related problems. A course of treatment might involve six massages spread out over 2 months, a relaxation tape to use daily at home, aromatherapy oils to use in the bath and some simple diet and lifestyle guidance.

Although such interventions do appear to be of benefit, simply raising the issue of stress, and pointing out that symptoms may be stress-related can be of great importance. One practitioner sends each patient a 'stress questionnaire' before commencing treatment, primarily as a means of orienting patients to the importance of stress.

'Low-touch' patients

A significant proportion of primary-care patients lead isolated lives and experience a lack of caring touch. Elderly people are widely acknowledged to be touch-deprived. Single parents, those living alone and those caring for disabled relatives may also come into the category of what one practitioner has described as 'the untouched'.

> Touch had never been common in my family. Massage has been complementary in giving me a structured experience of touch. The main benefit though was relearning to be at ease with my

body, relax my mind, without being overcome with weeping or anxieties.

Such individuals may present with physical symptoms, such as headache or muscular pain, but often need little more than contact and emotional support. The role of massage and aromatherapy treatment for this group of patients is similar to that for those with non-specific illness: it is a means of providing appropriate care for those who feel in need, yet for whom conventional options are limited.

Massage has also been reported to be of benefit for those with altered body image, such as those with physical disabilities, anorexia or chronic disease. See pages 180 and 204 for more on the links between touch, massage and self-image.

Chronic musculoskeletal pain

Patients with persistent musculoskeletal pain, particularly elderly people, have been referred to practitioners of massage and aroma-therapy in some primary-care centres. Practitioners say that they can sometimes address the immediate cause of pain, for example, muscle spasm. This is especially true of practitioners who use specific soft-tissue techniques such as those described on page 25. Similarly, some aromatherapists claim to be able to treat conditions such as arthritis or back pain by the use of essential oils (p. 253).

Pain relief from non-specific aromatherapy and massage is said to be only short-term, but patients commonly report that 'the pains are not getting worse any more'. Some patients also experience short-term improvements in mobility and posture. In many cases, however, the role of massage and aromatherapy treatment moves away from the treatment of the immediate cause of musculoskeletal pain. One prac-titioner has emphasized the importance of individual diagnosis and treatment. Some patients simply need emotional support: they want to lie down on the massage couch, relax completely and have someone touch them. One patient described this as 'having something for me'. But other patients demand more directly therapeutic intervention from practitioners, seeking relief from particular symptoms. That said, pain is an affective state and it is often difficult to make clear distinc-tions between physical and psychological interventions .

Massage and aromatherapy have also been of benefit by improving sleep in some chronic pain patients. Patients reportedly sleep deeply during and for a few nights after a treatment. Home use of essential oils has also been said to improve sleep. Though this may reflect an inherent sedative effect, essential oils can provide a 'cue' to sleep, particularly where a certain odour has been linked to relaxation by a prior use during a massage. See page 165 for more on classical conditioning and odour.

PROFESSIONAL ISSUES

Complementary practitioners working in primary care are likely to meet a very different client population from that found in private practice. It is now almost a truism that whereas complementary practitioners tend to work with middle-aged people on higher incomes, poor people from the extreme ends of the age spectrum tend to constitute the majority of a GP's case load. The range of ethnic origin and social background is also likely to be far greater in primary care. One practitioner has reported working with a patient from East Africa who had idiosyncratic beliefs about the cause of his ill-health. This caused a number of communication difficulties. Needless to say, such patients rarely form part of complementary practitioner's private clientele.

An associated issue is that complementary practitioners may be unused to working with patients who have not chosen to receive massage or aromatherapy treatment. This can sometimes lead to problems, especially where treatment is given as part of a stress-reduction package involving dietary advice and relaxation exercises. Some patients fail to cooperate with these self-help measures and it can be difficult for practitioners to know how to change such behaviour.

Full interdisciplinary collaboration is especially important in primary care. This is partly due to the importance of ensuring appropriate referrals and partly because GPs continue to be responsible for a patient's care after the conclusion of treatment and so require feedback as to progress. Some primary-care centres have established sophisticated methods of audit and feedback to improve communication. Others have found that practice meetings are sufficient to ensure adequate dialogue between GPs and complementary practitioners. However, interdisciplinary collaboration is difficult and rarely achieved. It is all too common for a masseur or aromatherapist to work in almost complete isolation, attending the surgery one half-day per week, having referrals arranged by the receptionist and experiencing virtually no contact with medical staff. See Chapter 10 for a full discussion of appropriate management practices.

One problem sometimes encountered in primary care, as well as several other settings, is dependence on treatment. This is not only because massage is an extremely enjoyable experience, but because its effects are often short-term. Practitioners may need to emphasize from the beginning that patients will receive only a certain number of appointments. One further means of avoiding dependence is to encourage patients, or their partners, to learn simple techniques to use at home.

SUMMARY

The role of massage and aromatherapy in primary care appears to be:

- treatment of non-specific or stress-related illness, such as fatigue or mild depression;
- aiding counselling;
- provision of touch for isolated individuals, particularly those who feel in need of care;
- emotional support for people with chronic pain.

MIDWIFERY: PREGNANCY AND THE FIRST MONTHS OF LIFE

INTRODUCTION AND OVERVIEW OF PRACTICE

Pregnancy and childbirth is one of the few areas in medicine in which a natural process becomes the focus of health care. The aims of such care are two-fold: the prevention of morbidity associated with pregnancy and childbirth, and the control of symptoms, such as pain during labour, which are a common or inevitable part of giving birth.

The course of the last 20 years has seen increasing dissatisfaction with what is seen as the overmedicalization of pregnancy and labour. Birth is perceived to have been appropriated by the medical profession and turned into a technical problem. Moves towards 'natural childbirth' have been prompted by the desire to meet the psychological and spiritual needs of mother, father and baby. These needs are felt to have been neglected in the focus on the physical and medical aspects of birth.

The increasing use of massage and aromatherapy in midwifery is, at least in part, a function of the revival of interest in natural childbirth and the reaction against unnecessary medical intervention. In the wake of the thalidomide disaster, the fear of drug-taking during pregnancy has also been a stimulus for interest in safer means of treating pregnancy-related symptoms.

In addition, increasing attention has recently been paid to traditional health practices. The inclination to educate and eliminate 'superstitious' health beliefs has been replaced by a more curious and open-minded attitude. In this respect, baby massage, which is ubiquitous in many parts of Africa, Asia and the Pacific, has become the focus of considerable interest.

Health care during pregnancy and the first months of life takes place in many different settings, some of them informal. Pregnant women may receive care by way of general practice, specialist antenatal units and general hospital services. Birth may take place at home or in hospital units of varying degrees of specialization. Of particular interest is the role of the midwife, a specialist health professional for pregnancy and childbirth, and the health visitor, who monitors development in the early months of a child's life. Both midwives and health visitors appear to have shown an increasing interest in massage and aromatherapy in recent years.

HEALTH ISSUES

Pregnancy

Massage is widely used as a relaxation therapy and for the relief of aches and pains in pregnant women. The vast majority of this practice is informal, with massages given by friends and family. However, health professionals have sometimes chosen to treat, for example, more marked cases of anxiety, with massage treatment. A number of pregnancy-related symptoms have been said to respond to aromatherapy. Some of these, such as constipation, insomnia, oedema and mild backache, might seem to be relatively obvious indications. Others, such as morning sickness, stretch marks, varicose veins, hypertension and fainting, constitute perhaps somewhat stronger claims. It is worth mentioning that there is excellent evidence (p. 89) that a simple form of acupressure is of benefit for morning sickness.

Labour

Back rubs and massages from friends and relatives are a traditional form of support during labour. Research has shown (p. 121) that this form of touch is generally perceived positively: it is seen to convey concern, caring and reassurance. Massage is perhaps at its most informal during labour and is possibly no more deserving of academic attention than soothing words or cool drinks.

What is interesting, and worthy of attention, is the claim that essential oils are useful analgesics and can affect the course of labour. Davis (1988: 199) has claimed, for example, that 'during labour, lavender will both reduce pain and strengthen contractions'. Tisserand (1977: 247) states that '[lavender] makes for a speedy delivery without increasing the severity of contractions'. Practitioners also say that essential oils have also been of benefit for pain, nausea and general mood. A significant number of midwives have been using essential oils for this purpose and say that the results have been positive.

> Women using lavender baths progress well into their labour and appear to be more relaxed. As yet we do not have the hard evidence, but it could be that lavender oil may have accelerated some labours.

It would not be unusual if essential oils improved the overall birth experience of some women, if only because they provide a pleasant atmosphere by virtue of their smell. The claim that essential oils have pharmacological effects on pain and duration of labour, however, is important and should be researched, especially if the use of oils for this purpose is as widespread as it appears to be.

Postnatal care

Aromatherapy oils have been prescribed by midwives as a bath additive for the treatment of perineal discomfort. A large trial of lavender for perineal healing is discussed on page 138. The negative result of this trial suggests that it would be wise to be cautious before attributing specific actions to essential oils. Claims for the actions of essential oils in postnatal care include: treatment of mastitis, regulation of the flow of breast milk, and promoting expulsion of the placenta.

A number of midwives have reportedly used massage and aromatherapy for the treatment of a form of postnatal depression which they described as 'third-day blues'. One commented that, though she refers more severe cases, she was confident in her ability to treat 'low-level depression, feeling under the weather and being listless'. Essential oils are said to have an important mood-modifying function in such cases.

Massage of premature and low-birth-weight neonates

The use of massage as a treatment for premature neonates has been extensively researched (p. 80). Almost all studies show increased weight gain and/or maturation following the massage intervention. A typical treatment consists of 5 minutes of gentle stroking of the whole body of the baby, 5 minutes of kinaesthetic stimulation by extension and flexion of the limbs and 5 more minutes of stroking. This is repeated three times a day. The massage may be given by nursing staff, parents or, in some cases, volunteers. Though this type of tactile stimulation appears to have a broad range of application, a number of workers have stressed the need for care in the choice of subjects to receive touch interventions. Treatment should always be decided on a case-by-case basis and in some instances, for example, medically unstable infants, touch stimulation can be counterproductive (p. 82).

The RISS programme is a special form of massage treatment which focuses more specifically on mother–child interaction. Mothers are encouraged to engage in four types of stimulation: massage (tactile), talking (auditory), eye contact (visual) and rocking (vestibular). There is evidence that RISS aids weight gain and mother–child interactions (p. 83).

Given the extent of the research demonstrating improvements in medical outcomes attributable to infant massage, it is perhaps easy to forget the more subtle benefits claimed for this technique. The technological nature of the neonatal intensive care unit (NICU) can be a cause of anxiety to parents and they can find comfort in the use of a conspicuously gentle and human technique. Moreover, giving a massage to a premature infant may help overcome the sense of being a 'helpless bystander'. Many parents have appreciated being able to participate in the care of their child in this way. One physiotherapist who has taught parents to massage babies in intensive care has commented that:

> The mothers in NICU are 'all-at-sea'. They feel afraid, vulnerable and guilty. Getting them to massage the baby helps to calm them down and makes them feel involved. It is also important for new mothers whose handling skills have not developed: some of the mothers have never held a baby before.

However, this worker tries not to stress the 'bonding' aspect of neonatal massage. Some parents are said to want to wait to get home before they will consider a baby theirs. This is a reasonable strategy for coping with the stress of a premature child. Attempts to force the strategy's abandonment, by encouraging a parent to bond with a child, are likely to be counterproductive.

Baby massage

Massage is a routine nurturing practice in some cultures. It is traditionally thought to improve coordination, increase weight gain and aid development of the skeleton. Some health professionals have attempted to encourage similar practices in the West by establishing baby massage groups for new mothers. These are generally run on an informal 'drop-in' basis at a set time each week and cater for about a dozen mother and baby pairs at a time. A typical session might involve 20–30 minutes of baby massage followed by a guided relaxation, postnatal exercises or a health education class for the mothers. During the group, the mothers massage their own child by following a demonstration given by the professional leading the session. The mothers are encouraged to practise massage with their babies every day. Emphasis is given to the overall feel and skills of massage, rather than to specific strokes and techniques.

One of the most important functions of baby massage groups is that of basic social support for mothers. The groups allow young mothers to meet each other, compare experiences and exchange general baby-care advice. This may help to overcome the feelings of isolation experienced by many mothers, particularly those in inner-city areas. Contact, friendship and solidarity with other mothers have rated highly on evaluations of baby massage groups by mothers. Mothers of disabled children have appreciated the mutual integration and support from mothers of the able-bodied.

The massage groups also ensure continued contact between mothers and health professionals. Mothers find the groups highly enjoyable and there is often a special attempt to provide a welcoming environment by choosing a pleasant room with music and essential oils. This provides an impetus for mothers to visit the massage group and allows health professionals an opportunity to assess the health of both mother and child.

A number of health professionals have reported that the baby massage groups can increase confidence and help develop basic mothering skills in certain cases. Some mothers are uncomfortable handling their babies and massage is said to provide a useful mechanism for addressing this difficulty. Continuing massage at home can cement the relationship between mother and child, especially as mothers are encouraged to maintain eye-contact and talk during the massage. One mother commented that 'massage is a special time for us. It's a time for me to relax with the baby. I even take the phone off the hook.'

The effects of massage on normally developing babies are not known. Some health visitors have reported that, in their clinical impression, massaged babies are less prone to infections and reach developmental milestones, such as unaided sitting, more rapidly. These claims may well hold, especially given that the effects of massage on development may be mediated by improved mother–child bonding and that massage has been shown to be of benefit for preterm neonates. Good-quality research is clearly required.

PROFESSIONAL ISSUES

The practice of massage and aromatherapy in pregnancy and the first months of life is not generally the domain of specialist practitioners. The majority of practice appears to consist of simple self-help remedies suggested by midwives or of massage given by friends and relatives. Specialist practitioners may play a role in the treatment of specific pregnancy related disorders, but this has been rare in ortho- dox maternity settings.

Some concern has been expressed over possible adverse effects of essential oils during pregnancy. The danger most widely discussed in the aromatherapy literature is miscarriage in early pregnancy. Oils said to be emmenagogue (i.e. those that increase menstrual flow) are therefore contraindicated for pregnant women. Similarly, oils consid- ered to have strong effects are not recommended for use with pregnant women or babies. Practitioners generally restrict the oils used in pregnancy and the first months of life to a limited number of those perceived to be safer and gentler. See Chapter 11 for more on safety issues.

SUMMARY

The role of massage and aromatherapy in pregnancy and the first few weeks of life appears to be:

- relaxation, and treatment of general aches and pains in pregnancy and labour;
- massage of premature infants improves weight gain and can help parents feel involved in the care of a child;
- baby-massage groups provide social support and help mothers to develop confidence and basic mothering skills;
- aromatherapists claim that essential oils aid pregnancy and childbirth in specific ways, such as treating morning sickness, strengthening contractions during labour and helping the expul- sion of the placenta. These claims are unsubstantiated.

MENTAL HEALTH

INTRODUCTION AND OVERVIEW OF PRACTICE

This section will focus on the use of massage and aromatherapy with people who have mental health difficulties. Though this has been traditionally defined in terms of a diagnosis of a discrete psychiatric condition, for example, manic depression or schizophrenia, such disease labels are the subject of considerable controversy and will be avoided here.

Some of the arguments against labelling have been theoretical and have been put forward by conventional health professionals. For example, some authorities have pointed out that the existence of characteristic psychological symptoms does not necessarily imply the existence of an underlying disease entity, that is, a disordered brain. Doubt has also been case on the clinical value of labels. It has been claimed, for example, that different psychiatrists often given radically different diagnoses to the same individual. However, the recent shift in understanding and care of mental health has also resulted from the grassroots activism of users of mental health services. Often describing themselves as 'survivors' of the psychiatric system, users have seen disease labels as a potent symbol of a medical model of treatment which they see as fundamentally flawed. They have advocated alternative models of care which place greater emphasis on the participation of the individual. It is argued that users of mental health services should be able to make choices about their treatment and that information should be provided to help them make those choices. Respect for the individual, and in particular, recognizing that users are individuals, rather than diseases, has also been emphasized.

The move away from the medical model has been one of the main factors in the growth of massage and aromatherapy in mental health care. Certainly, the general health beliefs of many users and user-advocacy organizations do reflect many of those of complementary practitioners. Also important has been the move away from large institutions, dominated by the psychiatric profession, to smaller, inter-disciplinary projects based in the community. Such projects are often run partly or wholly by voluntary organizations and have generally had a large degree of freedom over the services provided to users. Practitioners of massage and aromatherapy have often worked as volunteers at such units. Nurses and other support staff based at community projects have sometimes learnt simple self-help techniques for use in particular cases.

HEALTH ISSUES

Stress and mental health

'Stress' is a widely used concept in mental health care. It is usually taken to refer to adverse psychosocial events that cause or exacerbate mental health problems. An associated concept is that of a 'crisis', an acute episode of distress when the individual finds it particularly difficult to cope. Massage and aromatherapy have been brought into mental health services primarily because it was thought that they might have a role in alleviating stress and in coping with crises.

One mental health worker who runs a 'drop-in' centre for people with long-term mental health problems has undertaken training in massage. She has found that short neck and shoulder rubs can be of particular benefit if a user becomes upset.

> Massage is good for calming people down so that they can talk. It helps 'ground' clients: when they're upset they may be crying, moving their head about, clenching their fists; after a massage they are generally calmer. Often they talk, and you find out that they're upset because of something simple, like an estranged child's birthday.

A number of people have pointed out that users of traditional psychiatric services would normally have been held down, injected with sedatives and put in isolation during a crisis. The importance of sensitive, one-to-one attention is perhaps therefore hard to overestimate. As one user pointed out:

> Where in normal mental health services do you get such good-quality time and attention? All you normally get is a jab up the backside.

Some see massage and aromatherapy as having a more preventative role. In this view, by inducing relaxation and aiding sleep, treatment can prevent stress building up to the point at which it precipitates a crisis.

> Aromatherapy helps me deal with stress. It's stopped me following the health problem I am supposed to have. I am off the medication and I need something to deal with whatever it was which necessitated lithium in the first place. Aromatherapy supports me.

> Massage showed me that I can let go and nothing terrible will happen.

Practitioners of aromatherapy say that essential oils can be of benefit for reducing general levels of stress. Particular oils are said to be soothing, calming or sedative and have sometimes been promoted as an alternative to traditional psychotropic medication. However, this is not necessarily a good thing. Some users have complained that essential oils made them feel as though they were 'on drugs'. Because they did not like this feeling, the individuals concerned asked practitioners to use milder oils or lower doses.

Psychosocial development

Talking therapies are an important part of many mental health services. It is thought that counselling, psychotherapy and group work can help individuals understand the reasons behind their mental health problems and develop coping strategies for the future. Some aspects of this work may be indirect. For example, therapy may aim to develop self-confidence and trust in the value of relationships on the grounds that insecurity and poor relationships can exacerbate mental health difficulties.

Some units have used massage and aromatherapy specifically to aid this therapeutic process. Touch, it is thought, can aid talk. One centre, for example, develops programmes of care for its users and massage typically comes early in this programme, with counselling starting only after a number of sessions of massage treatment.

Massage is a 'safe' therapy simply because you don't have to talk. Users are normally asked to talk about their problems, dig into childhood memories and so on. But unless someone feels nurtured, cared for, they simply aren't going to open up.

In this view, massage helps develop trust and confidence, and this in turn aids the psychotherapeutic process. Massage is also thought to help in the general sense of 'relaxed body, relaxed mind': users are said to be ready to talk or more open to change if they are relaxed. Practitioners frequently report that individuals will, without prompting, discuss personal and emotional issues during or just after massage treatment.

Some practitioners claim that massage can have a more directly psychotherapeutic role. Massage is said to be able to release emotions which have been 'locked into' the body. A simple example might be hunched shoulders. In the short term, hunched shoulders are an expression of anxiety or fear. Some practitioners believe that chronic anxiety or fear causes persisting changes in muscle tone so that the shoulders become permanently hunched. This is said to cause a positive feedback cycle in which negative emotions cause changes in muscle tone and certain patterns of muscle tension re-elicit negative emotions. Though this theoretical model is intuitively plausible – tension does cause us to hunch our shoulders and hunching our shoulders does seem to induce tension – it remains unevaluated at the current time of writing. Nonetheless, many practitioners do believe that work on soft tissue can directly address psychological problems and explain the elicitation of emotions by massage in terms of this effect (see p. 24).

Massage has also had a rehabilitative role in mental health care. One practitioner who teaches massage to groups with tranquillizer dependency has described his classes as 'an apprenticeship into contact with people: enabling intimacy and trust'. Furthermore, the feelings of worth and self-esteem that often result from a course of massage treatment can also be important in helping individuals to re-establish themselves after a crisis or a period in care.

Substance dependence and abuse

Substance dependence and abuse can be either a cause or a consequence of mental health care. People who are addicted to alcohol or recreational drugs often seek mental health services. On the other hand, some people become dependent on medication used to treat mental health problems. Dependence on tranquillizers, for example, is particularly widespread.

Massage and aromatherapy have been used in the treatment of substance dependence. Some practitioners say that treatment aids the elimination of 'toxins' from the body. Others have pointed out that massage and aromatherapy can be an effective treatment for some of the symptoms associated with withdrawal, for example, physical pain. However, many workers stress a more general psychotherapeutic role. There is often an underlying psychological reason why people abuse alcohol and recreational drugs and massage and aromatherapy are said to aid the psychotherapeutic process in some cases (see above).

According to some workers, massage and aromatherapy may also be of benefit by providing a suitable surrogate for experiences associated with substance use. For example, treatment, like recreational drugs, is pleasurable:

> Massage can give people the experience of feeling good without recourse to drugs.

> Using aromatherapy oils in the bath is a way of spoiling myself in a way that doesn't harm me and isn't a form of self-abuse.

Similarly, in tranquillizer addiction, the therapies can provide an alternative means of dealing with anxiety. This is not so much a case that an individual will deal with a specific crisis by having a massage, or sniffing an oil, instead of taking medication. Rather, massage and aromatherapy are said to help individuals to generate the confidence that they can deal with anxiety other than by the use of tranquillizers. As one mental health worker put it: 'Massage can help people to relax by giving them a concrete experience of relaxation.'

Physical abuse

Some users of mental health services have suffered physical and/or sexual abuse. The use of touch with such individuals is generally proscribed on the grounds that it will be associated with negative experiences. However, a number of practitioners and other workers have recommended touch therapy for that very reason: individuals who have suffered abuse need to overcome any resistance to or fear of touch; massage is seen to provide an appropriate means of achieving this end.

It is important for a space to be made where touch is not connected with violence, or a demand being made.

In some instances, physical abuse can also lead to problems of lowered self-esteem. Massage generally leads to an improved self-perception (p. 180) and can therefore provide a useful form of treatment in such cases.

It is interesting to note that some massage practitioners have described similarities between survivors of abuse and people who have what are described as eating disorders. Such disorders are said to involve similar problems of body perception.

PROFESSIONAL ISSUES

There are a number of complex issues involved in mental health work. Some of the background to the debate about models of care has already been discussed. Practitioners considering work in mental health settings should also be aware of common prejudices about mental ill health. For example, people with mental health problems are often thought to be unable to make decisions for themselves. One important aim of the user's movement has been to ensure that individuals are allowed to participate in the decisions that affect their lives. Practitioners may argue that they do always let clients make their own choices about treatment. However, choice and participation are complex issues and prejudices about an individual's ability to take decisions can be expressed in subtle ways. Another misconception, common in films and plays, is that the cause of mental illness is often simple, as long as it can be found buried somewhere deep in the patient's past.

Complementary practitioners working in mental health settings are likely to meet a very different client population from that found in private practice. Poverty and homelessness, which are both causes and consequences of mental ill health, are particularly prevalent. The range of ethnic origin and social background is also likely to be far greater.

A number of different professionals may liaise on the care of a person with a mental health problem. These may include a social worker, a community mental health nurse, an occupational therapist, a psychiatrist, a GP, 'key workers' and workers at day centres and other units. Though often logistically difficult, it is important for complementary practitioners to maintain effective relations with these individuals. An issue which is particularly pertinent to interdisciplinary working is that of emotional disclosure during massage. Complementary practitioners are not necessarily trained in counselling skills and it may not be appropriate for them to engage in counselling therapy. This is particularly true in mental health work, where the psychological issues are complex and may involve discussion of sensitive and difficult subjects such as sexual abuse. Workers at some units have expressed particular concern about disclosure of sensitive material during massage. In certain cases, practitioners are briefed about this possibility and are given guidance as to appropriate responses. Often, practitioners are encouraged to suggest to users that they might usefully discuss personal issues raised during a massage with another, specialist member of staff.

SUMMARY

The role of massage and aromatherapy in mental health appears to be:

- alleviation of stress, particularly at times of crisis;
- providing a concrete experience of relaxation;
- aiding the counselling process and psychosocial development;
- providing an alternative source of pleasure or relaxation to people with substance dependence;
- helping survivors of physical abuse to become comfortable with touch.

HOSPICE CARE

INTRODUCTION AND OVERVIEW OF PRACTICE

This section will discuss the use of massage and aromatherapy in hospice care. Patients are generally referred to hospices once the aim of their treatment becomes palliative rather than curative. Most are seen for the first time about a year before their death, though time between referral and death can, in practice, be as short as a few days or as long as several years. That said, there are no widely recognized criteria for deciding which patients are candidates for hospice care services.

Many individuals with cancer and AIDS are treated in hospices. For more specific information on the use of massage and aromatherapy with these two client groups, see pages 193–197 and 197–202.

Hospices provide both in- and out-patient services and may also engage in out-reach programmes. The modern hospice movement was established in the UK in the late 1960s by Dame Cicely Saunders and is based on the idea that medicine could be usefully extended to the care of the dying. Recently, hospices have evolved to provide a variety of non-medical services. These include arts and crafts, hair and beauty treatments and social events.

The use of massage and aromatherapy in hospices developed as much from the widespread use of volunteers to provide non-medical services as from any perceived health need. Many hospices first provided massage and aromatherapy services as a result of offers of free treatment from complementary practitioners. However, it is indicative of the growing recognition of the value of these therapies that some hospices are now employing complementary practitioners or nurses to practise massage. Wilkes (1992) reports that about 70% of UK hospices offer massage and aromatherapy services. In approximately two-thirds of these cases, treatment was primarily undertaken by nurses.

HEALTH ISSUES

Emotional and spiritual support in hospice care

Hospices have traditionally offered emotional and spiritual support to complement provision for patients' medical requirements. The use of massage and aromatherapy in hospice care is a natural extension of this attempt to meet a wide range of needs.

Massage is often seen primarily as a means to deal with the emotional stress associated with dying. As one hospice nurse put it: 'Dying is the most stressful event any of us are likely to go through.' Fear, despair, family dynamics and 'unfinished business', among other issues, can cause anxiety, tension and emotional upset in the dying patient. Gentle massage has been reported to aid relaxation and ease distress.

> The patients find the massage very calming and relaxing. This is sometimes of value even in clinically recognized conditions such as end-stage restlessness.

Though massage often takes the role of a general comfort measure, it has been claimed that it can play a deeper, more psychotherapeutic role. Many practitioners have made the link between physical and emotional release. Patients who are said to be 'rigid with emotion' are said to relax and 'let go' on the massage table. Privacy, time and individualized attention are said to be important in this respect. However, relaxation and feelings of warmth, safety and trust built up during massage are also important factors that aid the expression of feelings. It is reportedly common for patients to start talking, or even crying, during or shortly after massage. Such emotional release has been said to lead to enduring changes in some patients.

Some workers have also commented that massage can enable them to provide emotional support to a patient merely by their presence. One massage practitioner described her role as 'just being with a patient'. Most professional contact with a patient involves some kind of activity, administering a drug, rearranging the bedclothes or feeding. A nurse or complementary practitioner of massage need not have a particular role or reason for attending the patient. It is widely acknowledged that there is comfort for a dying person in just being with another individual: the most reassuring act can often be just a gentle, still touch held in silence.

In this respect, it is interesting that one nurse has commented: 'the practitioner's sense of peace, calmness and self-worth can be communicated to the patient via touch'. It is perhaps for this reason that massage is said to enhance relationships between patients and health professionals in hospices.

The feelings of pleasure and well-being which are said to result from a massage can also bring about important psychological benefits. Many hospice-care patients have problems of self-esteem and self-image. In some, this may even extend to a disgust of the body, particularly if they have undergone mutilating surgery. Patients who experience massage frequently make reference to physical pleasure: 'I feel as though I'm floating away'; 'I feel lighter' and 'I haven't been touched like that in years' are fairly typical comments. One medical director of a hospice claims that it was patient responses such as these which convinced him of the benefits of massage:

> It is clear that patients like massage and that it helps them to feel better. Massage is one of our most popular services.

It is of note that hairdressing is also a particularly popular service. The importance of pleasure and pampering in massage and aromatherapy should not be ignored.

Practitioners of massage and aromatherapy working in hospices are almost unanimous in their opinion that essential oils play only a minor role in treatment. The use of gentle touch is widely regarded to be of much greater importance. Many hospice patients are highly medicated and so, where essential oils are used at all, a relatively small number is chosen on the grounds of safety and suitability. Typically, oils with mild sedative effects are used in low dilution. Patients are generally asked to choose an oil or a ready-made mixture. One nurse has said that this can act as an 'ice breaker', a means of allowing a patient to accommodate to the idea of massage before hands-on work starts. In long-term patients who are massaged regularly, the smell of an essential oil can become associated with relaxation and thus act as a Pavlovian stimulus reinforcing the effects of the massage (see p. 165 for more on classical conditioning and smell).

Support for carers and staff

Dying can be a stressful and emotionally distressing time for family and friends. Moreover, the death of a patient can also be difficult for staff: the combination of long-term care and high staffing ratios often results in staff becoming attached to individuals in their care. The importance of adequate support for carers and staff has long been recognized and many hospices have developed a network of support services including respite care, support groups and counselling.

Massage and aromatherapy have also been reported to play a useful role: in some hospices, as many as 35–50% of treatments are given for carers and staff. Typically, staff and carers present to the massage service with an exacerbation of physical symptoms such as headache, arthritis or fatigue. However, talking and discussion often take up much of a session. Massage has been said to lead to the release of sometimes unacknowledged feelings, as has already been discussed. As one practitioner has remarked:

> Staff and carers 'unload' during massage. They'll generally express their worries, both professional and personal, without prompting.

This practitioner has also reported that staff usually come for massage 'when things get too much'. Staff in hospices are particularly keen to maintain a high quality of care and some have commented that massage has helped them to do so.

> Massage allows me to 'take in' so I can 'give out' when I need to.

Such comments suggest that massage is an appropriate form of support for carers and staff and indicate that this can have indirect benefits for patients.

Physical symptoms

There appears to be some disagreement about the extent to which massage and aromatherapy can be of benefit for physical symptoms common in dying patients. Some practitioners have been wary of claiming that they are able to treat, for example, insomnia or pain, particularly given the powerful medications available in hospices. That said, pain and sleep are both mediated by anxiety and practitioners of massage and aromatherapy may provide a useful service in aiding relaxation. Some workers have also commented that massage can distract a patient's attention away from pain. However, at least some of those working in hospices do believe that massage can have a direct impact on pain, particularly in the treatment of stiff or aching muscles. One hospice physician reported that: 'My patients tell me how surprised they are at the duration of the pain relief resulting from massage.' It also appears that massage can also provide a useful treatment for oedema in certain cases and this can be of benefit both for pain and mobility.

PROFESSIONAL ISSUES

Working with people who are dying raises a number of complex psychological issues. It has been said that practitioners who are frightened of death or dying will subconsciously transmit this fear to their patients. Certainly there is the rather tautological point that professionals who are uncomfortable about death or dying will be uncomfortable working in environments where death and dying is an everyday fact.

More generally, complementary practitioners who are unused to hospice settings have sometimes suffered feelings of inadequacy, particularly when patients or carers have talked about issues concerning death. This can be a particular problem because, as already discussed, massage seems to lead to the expression of emotions: patients, carers and staff may start talking about their fears, anxieties and worries during a massage. On occasion, revelations during massage have included particularly sensitive issues, such as sexual abuse. Complementary practitioners have reported that they often 'don't know what to say' to clients and that this has been a source of anxiety. Some have found other hospice professionals to be a useful resource. One commented that: 'I learnt just to listen and not to try and answer in order to make things better'. Conventional staff have often developed coping strategies, or established support structures, to deal with the profound professional difficulties associated with hospice care. These can usefully be extended to complementary practitioners.

Particular care needs to be taken in the physical procedures used in massage. Patients in hospices may be physically fragile and some are extremely sensitive to touch. It is important that only the most gentle massage techniques are used. As one nurse put it: 'All of my work consists of gentle stroking, holding and caressing; in fact, you might not want to describe what I do as massage at all.' In one hospice, problems were caused when a nurse who had undertaken a short course in massage worked too deeply in an attempt to loosen up stiff muscles and promote blood circulation. Great care must also be taken in moving or lifting patients. Most units have sought to discourage any changes of a patient's position for the purposes of massage and practitioners have generally worked on easily accessible areas such as the hands, feet and face.

Finally, given the high levels of medication used in hospices, and the relative lack of knowledge about interactions of essential oils, practitioners tend to limit the number of oils they use. Generally, four or five oils will be chosen and made up into premixed blends.

SUMMARY

The role of massage and aromatherapy in hospices appears to be:

- providing emotional support to the dying patient;
- general relaxation;
- relief from aches and pains and aiding sleep in some cases;
- support for carers and staff.

INTENSIVE CARE

Caroline Stevensen, MacMillan Clinical Nurse Specialist in Complementary Therapies, Royal London Homoeopathic NHS Trust, London, and Andrew Vickers

INTRODUCTION AND OVERVIEW OF PRACTICE

This section will focus on the use of massage and aromatherapy in the intensive care unit (ICU). Patients are admitted to the ICU if they require continuous monitoring and attention. Intensive therapy is also characteristic of the ICU: vital functions may be supported by machinery (as in artificial ventilation) and patients are often heavily medicated.

It is widely accepted that the environment of the ICU causes stress. ICUs are often noisy and harshly lit. The mere presence of machines, and the sometimes constant state of emergency among staff and patients, can also be significant stressors. Though the critical condition of ICU patients entails that stable physiological functioning takes priority over what might be seen as more subtle, psychological issues, there is growing awareness of the need to provide reassurance and emotional support. This has been at least partly responsible for the growth in the use of massage and aromatherapy in ICU.

Also important is what has been called 'technological distancing'. Nurses working in ICU may feel that their traditional caring role has been replaced by the technical task of ministering to machines. Massage and aromatherapy can be a means of rediscovering a more person-centred role by providing hands-on care.

HEALTH ISSUES

Isolation and communication

It is often difficult for carers, professional or otherwise, to see ICU patients as human beings. Patients tend to be sedated, and may have a limited ability to respond to social contact. The physical appearance of the patient – connected to machinery, often naked but for a sheet – may exacerbate this problem. In short, ICUs can lead to significant depersonalization of people and activities.

The use of touch and massage has been said to provide a means of overcoming depersonalization. For example, one woman described seeing her husband attached to a ventilator after heart surgery:

> It was as though a mechanical barrier was placed between us, making me afraid to touch him in case he would become disconnected from the oxygen and die. Only after encouragement was I able to hold his hand and stroke it soothingly. Then I knew I could help him get better.

Massage has been said to provide a suitable means of communication for carers. Verbal communication is often difficult, especially when patients are unresponsive, and carers have found that touch is the most satisfying and meaningful method of contact. Massage is also said to meet the need of carers to contribute to the care of the patient in some way, thereby reducing their own feelings of helplessness. This has been found to be particularly important in paediatric ICU, where parents have been helped to realize that they can still care for their children (p. 214).

Feelings of isolation are a common consequence of admission to an ICU. The lack of human contact may be exacerbated by anxiety and fear and by sterile procedures such as the wearing of masks, gowns and gloves by staff. Massage, particularly when given by carers, has been claimed to be an appropriate way of helping patients to overcome their sense of isolation. One nurse recalls that:

> One patient was in the ICU for 2 months. She was clearly frightened and this was exacerbated by the lack of any normal social

contact. Foot massage with tea-tree oil was incorporated into her daily care. She certainly looked less frightened after a treatment and often fell asleep. Later, she said that the massages had helped her greatly.

A number of nurses have encouraged carers to give appropriate touch and massage. By offering suitable advice and supervision, many carers have felt confident enough to touch and massage their loved ones and this has generally been of benefit to all concerned.

Noise and sleep

High levels of noise and sensory overload are suffered by patients in ICU. No doubt partly as a result, they often do not get adequate sleep. Frequent disturbances, as often occur in ICU, disrupt the quality of sleep, even though total sleep time is not always reduced.

The use of massage and aromatherapy is claimed to provide a means of distraction from the noise of ICU and can help some patients relax enough to fall asleep. Patients have reported their 'best ever night's sleep in hospital' following massage, despite the numerous disturbances that occur in ICU. A number of oils said to be sedative have been used by ICU staff to aid sleep.

One non-ventilated lady in her 70s found that a drop of rose oil on a tissue not only helped her to sleep, but 'took her to her own garden', which was full of roses.

In some cases, massage and aromatherapy can break the anxiety–insomnia–anxiety cycle. Some nurses have noticed that patients who would usually be upset by slight noises become noticeably calmer after treatment. This is turn aids sleep, leading to lower levels of anxiety the following day.

Emotional and psychological reactions

Patients in ICU are generally in a critical condition and may be anxious about a number of specific issues. These include death, disability, changes in family and social role, financial hardship, and loss of dignity, privacy and respect. It has been claimed that massage and aromatherapy are effective in lowering anxiety scores in ICU patients. This is supported by evidence from a clinical trial (p. 76).

Though the effects of massage and aromatherapy on anxiety seem to stem largely from general relaxation, the use of essential oils has been said to bring back feelings of comfort and security. It is said that the scent of lavender, for example, is often found to remind patients of their own homes or 'granny's garden'. The physical pleasure of aromatherapy massage can also provide a useful distraction from fear and worries about the future.

Physical effects of essential oils in ICU

A large number of claims have been made about the pharmacological properties of essential oils (p. 52). At least some of these properties are of potential value in ICU. For example, aromatherapists claim that lavender is of dramatic benefit in the treatment of burns. Other oils are said to be effective for constipation, or to have antibiotic, hypotensive or antiarrhythmic properties. However, the high levels of medication, the critical state of patients and the unproven nature of aromatherapy claims entail that such medically-oriented use of essential oils has been limited at the current time of writing.

PROFESSIONAL ISSUES

It is generally accepted that only conventional health professionals should offer aromatherapy and massage to patients in ICU. This is because the ICU environment presents a number of complex medical issues and it is unlikely that many non-medically-qualified therapists adequately understand the physiology and pharmacology of ICU patients.

One special problem of massage in ICU can be finding accessible body parts, free from tubes, lines or wires. Commonly, it is only the feet which are treated. This may, in any case, be the most appropriate form of treatment on the grounds that a full body massage may be too physiologically stimulating for an ICU patient. Extensive treatments may also be too time consuming to be feasible for ICU staff.

Given the intensive use of medication and the critical state of patients, the possibility of interactions or adverse effects from essential oils is a particular worry in ICU. As is the case for hospice care, one approach has been to use of a limited range of the safer oils. The issue of adverse effects is discussed at length in Chapter 11.

Consent for massage and aromatherapy can be a problem on the ICU when the patient is unconscious or under heavy sedation. In these situations, the issue of consent should be referred to the closest relative and documented as such in the medical notes. Practitioners claim that massage and aromatherapy may be of benefit even when a patient is not fully conscious.

SUMMARY

The role of massage and aromatherapy in intensive care appears to
be:

- reducing anxiety;
- alleviating feelings of isolation;
- helping relatives to feel involved in the care of a patient;
- aiding relaxation and sleep.

MASSAGE AND AROMATHERAPY: THE AUTONOMOUS PRACTITIONER

The previous sections of this book have discussed the use of massage and aromatherapy in a variety of conventional health settings.
There are notable differences between the practices described here
and those described in the standard massage and aromatherapy
textbooks. In the section on cardiovascular rehabilitation, for
example, aromatherapy is only mentioned in terms of stress reduction, a typical application being the use of essential oils for a
relaxing bath. This is in considerable contrast to the aromatherapy
textbooks, which claim that essential oils can be used to treat hypertension, poor circulation and even 'cardiac spasm'. The model of
practice for massage and aromatherapy found in the textbooks is
that of an autonomous practitioner working with sole responsibility
to treat a full range of symptoms. The model of practice described
in this book is generally of simple palliative care, often no more than
the relief of stress and anxiety. Though this is undoubtedly a fair
picture of what does typically take place in conventional health
settings in the UK, it is probable that many practitioners will balk at
what they may see as a 'relegation' of their profession to a marginal
therapeutic role.

There are various reasons for the differences between practitioners'
own model of care, that of the autonomous masseur or aromatherapist, and that described in this book. Firstly, working in
conventional health contexts means working in teams and sharing
both responsibility and decision-making. Practitioners have specific
roles in a team and this puts constraints on their ability to treat exactly
as they so choose. In oncology departments, for example, massage and
aromatherapy have been used in programmes of care primarily for the
purpose of alleviating anxiety and depression. It would be inappropriate for a practitioner independently to decide to use, say, orally
administered essential oils for an anti-tumour action, simply because
this would compromise a planned, integrated package of care for the

patient. One only has to imagine all members of a health care team – GP, oncologist, surgeon, radiologist, nurse, occupational therapist, social worker – simultaneously acting independently, beyond their agreed role, to see why constraints are necessary on individual members of a health team.

Conventional health-care settings also pose different medical problems from those normally encountered in a complementary practitioner's private clinic. An aromatherapist might feel relatively confident at treating, say, pain and poor circulation in a middle-aged man with mild arthritis. A highly medicated, unstable patient in an intensive care unit represents an entirely different set of problems. In this case, the scope of massage and aromatherapy practice is limited by uncertainty, particularly the possibility of adverse effects or drug interactions. In general, the patients typically described in textbooks are not similar to those found in the settings mentioned in this book. Tisserand (1988) for example, gives case histories including skin conditions, menstrual problems, vaginal infections, sprains and arthritis. This is in marked contrast to most of the patients described in this book, a significant proportion of whom (e.g. those in intensive care or those with profound disabilities) are highly unlikely to present at a massage or aromatherapy practitioner's surgery.

In addition, many of the practices previously described are unlike those found in traditional textbooks because they involve the use of simple techniques by conventional health professionals who do not have a full training. Some specialist practitioners of massage and aromatherapy are critical of this practice, just as homoeopaths and acupuncturists have criticized doctors for prescribing standard remedies or using 'formula' acupuncture in simple cases. Typically, practitioners contrast their extensive training, and the subtlety of their therapy, with the crude approach of the conventional professional 'on a weekend course'. Though one might be sympathetic to practitioners' claims that patients are getting a raw deal from 'ersatz' therapy, it surely does not seem necessary that all applications of a therapy require a maximally trained practitioner. For example, few would argue that one needs a surgeon to remove a small foreign body from a minor wound, even though this constitutes a form of surgery, or that one has to be a neurologist to prescribe aspirin for a mild headache. Similarly, one may not need to be a fully trained practitioner to use some simple, defined applications of massage and aromatherapy.

The following sections will describe the practices of masseurs and aromatherapists working autonomously in the community for two reasons. Firstly, it will provide an insight into the clinical background of practitioners working in the health service. Secondly, at least some independent practitioners are taking secondary and tertiary referrals from doctors and they generally work with relative clinical freedom.

MASSAGE

The clinical role and scope of massage as used by practitioners working autonomously in the community overlaps to a great extent with that described in this book. Much of a practitioner's time will be spent on general massage to alleviate stress and anxiety and to improve a patient's self-esteem and self-awareness. That said, certain practitioners may also attempt to bring about more specific changes in health. Some may learn special techniques of soft-tissue manipulation (p. 25) for the treatment of musculoskeletal disorders such as back pain, fibrositis or minor injuries. Others incorporate a passing knowledge of functional therapies such as Alexander technique or Feldenkrais (p. 9). Such practitioners see their role and scope as similar to that of osteopaths and chiropractors.

Practitioners who focus on the treatment of musculoskeletal disorders by using such techniques often try to distinguish themselves from other massage practitioners. They tend to do so by using titles such as 'remedial physical therapist' or 'sports massage therapist' and/or by describing their practice as a 'musculoskeletal injuries clinic' or the like. Few practitioners describing themselves as practising, for example, 'holistic massage' concentrate on using the techniques described above for the treatment of musculoskeletal disorders. See page 18 for a discussion of specific and non-specific massage.

Some practitioners of massage may learn techniques such as shiatsu or reflexology (p. 20), which, it is claimed, can bring about specific changes in health. It is possible that massage practitioners working autonomously in the community may decide to use such techniques to treat conditions such as asthma, or premenstrual syndrome. As pointed out at the start of Chapter 3, it is difficult to know the extent of such practice simply because there is a dearth of reliable information as to the patients seen and the techniques used by practitioners of massage.

AROMATHERAPY

Many aromatherapists restrict their practice to the sort of simple palliative techniques described in the middle sections of this book. That said, a significant number – estimates range between 30% and

60% – do use essential oils to treat the full range of symptoms in a variety of diseases, some of them relatively severe. Such practitioners see their role as similar to that of homoeopaths or herbalists – the use of individually tailored prescriptions to treat disease – and consider few medical problems to be truly outside the scope of aromatherapy. It can be difficult to identify just which practitioners commonly treat the full range of disease and which restrict their practice to palliative care. Some practitioners describe themselves as 'aromatologists' or even 'clinical aromatologists' to distinguish themselves from general aromatherapists. Though one is tempted to speculate that the use of the suffix '-ology' is no more than a crude attempt to sound scientific, and somehow more medical, the need felt to make distinctions between forms of aromatherapy is understandable.

A typical health problem treated by such aromatherapists might be acne or premenstrual syndrome. Given that aromatherapy involves rubbing antibacterial substances on the skin, something which undoubtedly promotes relaxation, such conditions are relatively obvious candidates for aromatherapy. Perhaps more surprising is that practitioners also say that they are able to treat conditions such as endometriosis, asthma or female infertility. They claim results such as a patient with endometriosis being pain-free within 2 months of treatment, or a woman becoming pregnant after 10 years of infertility. Practitioners explain these successes by claiming, for example, that treatment 'balances the hormone system', perhaps pointing to the oestrogenic properties of particular oils. Aromatherapists also often utilize naturopathic concepts of internal toxins and poor nutrition. For example, in the case of arthritis 'the toxic build up must be eliminated ... circulation to the affected joints must be improved, both to drain off the wastes and to improve nutrition to the affected tissues' (Davis, 1988: 36). Some also give a psychoneuroimmunological perspective, pointing out that if patients feel better mentally, they are likely to do better physically.

The techniques used by aromatherapists to treat such diseases are generally standard: application of essential oils by massage, baths and inhalation. Some practitioners also use deeper massages for specific parts of the body to ensure optimal delivery of essential oils. For example, they may give deep massage with diluted essential oils to the pelvic area in order to treat menstrual problems. They may also recommend that patients give themselves this type of massage using a premixed blend on a daily basis. Oral administration of essential oils is contentious and relatively rare in the UK and US. Certain practitioners who are particularly confident of their skills, such as those who describe themselves as clinical aromatologists, do prescribe oils by mouth and this is probably where aromatherapy most closely approaches the practices, role and scope of traditional medical herbalism.

Part Three
Management

Organizing massage and aromatherapy in conventional health settings

10

The use of massage and aromatherapy in conventional health settings is an innovation which, in some respects at least, involves a radical departure from conventional practices. For example, a nurse giving an aromatherapy treatment is administering, under his or her own direction, pharmacologically active substances not found in standard pharmacopoeias. Provision of the therapies may also involve specialist practitioners who do not have health-service experience.

Massage and aromatherapy have hitherto been introduced into the health service in a somewhat haphazard fashion. This is primarily because the use of these therapies has been provider-led. Typically, an individual nurse has become interested in using massage or aromatherapy, perhaps after going on a short course, and has started using the therapies on the ward, sometimes without sufficient consultation with other staff. Though this has not generally resulted in harm, it is clearly better to implement therapies in a planned and regulated manner. It has happened that senior clinicians discover, accidentally, that essential oils are being used on a ward without their knowledge. This has lead to outright bans, even when the very clinicians behind a ban may well have supported the practice had they been kept informed and consulted about its use.

There are three broad questions concerning the use of massage and aromatherapy in conventional health settings.

1) How can massage and aromatherapy be used safely and competently?
2) How can massage and aromatherapy be used appropriately and effectively?
3) How should massage and aromatherapy be introduced into new settings?

This chapter will discuss each of these three questions in turn. The aim is to raise and discuss general issues rather than to set out specific guidelines. Detailed protocols and procedures should be decided locally, by those individuals whose professional practice will be affected by the use of massage and aromatherapy. It is recommended that such policies should be written up formally and distributed to all interested parties. An example of a set of guidelines on the use of massage and aromatherapy is given by Wafer (1994). The discussion below is intended to be as comprehensive as possible. It is likely that some workers will be put off by the sheer volume and complexity of the management issues raised. It should be stated that not all management procedures need to be considered in all settings: see 'Limitations and Exceptions', below.

ENSURING SAFE AND COMPETENT USE OF MASSAGE AND AROMATHERAPY

Practitioners of complementary medicine are generally at pains to emphasize the safety of their therapy, especially when compared to conventional care. Though it is tempting to be sympathetic to such claims, it is important to avoid any false sense of security. It is probably true that, used properly, aromatherapy and, in particular, massage are highly unlikely to cause serious adverse effects. However, unless there are mechanisms to ensure that 'use' is 'proper' it is possible that harm may be caused. As it happens, there is evidence that this has already occurred. Price (1993: 137–139) reports three cases of adverse effects arising from the use of aromatherapy by improperly trained nurses. In two of these cases, undiluted essential oils were used (in one instance, drops of neat camomile oil were administered directly on to a patient's eye); in the third case, an extremely high dose of essential oil was added to a bath. Other cases have involved more subtle considerations. For example, in one instance, a young female nurse offered an elderly male patient a full body massage, an approach which was inappropriate in the circumstances and which embarrassed and upset the patient.

A number of issues pertinent to the safe use of massage and aromatherapy will be discussed in turn.

Competence of practitioners

Any individual wishing to practise massage or aromatherapy, be they a conventional health professional or a complementary therapist, should have appropriate training, experience and qualifications. At the current time of writing, there are few widely accepted qualifications for either massage or aromatherapy. This complicates the task of ensuring that practitioners are indeed competent. Advice from leading bodies within the conventional health professions (such as the Royal College of Nursing) is of only limited value: typically, codes of conduct state merely that a health professional 'should only undertake work for which he or she is trained and competent to practise' (United Kingdom Central Council for Nursing, Midwifery and Health Visiting, 1992). Advice for doctors or managers is generally that they should 'satisfy themselves' that any practitioner in their charge is competent. However, guidelines as to how anyone should check their own or another's competence are few and far between.

There are no easy answers to the problem of ensuring competence. That said, the following general questions may be useful.

- When and where was the practitioner trained?
- How long (in terms of classroom hours) was the course?
- What exactly is the practitioner intending to do?
- What does the practitioner see as outside his or her competence?
- Does the practitioner have professional indemnity insurance?

It can also be useful to get advice from an independent source conversant with the various schools and qualifications in massage and aromatherapy. As pointed out in Chapter 3, some institutions have rather grandiose names and issue impressive sounding diplomas for what may be insufficient courses. In the case of a complementary practitioner coming into a unit from outside the health service, it may be more appropriate for the appropriate manager or doctor to assess competence on the basis of an interview than to depend exclusively on qualifications. An initial probationary period can be a useful additional safeguard.

A further issue is the distinction between 'absolute' and 'appropriate' qualifications. In one view, any individual practising anything which could be described as massage or aromatherapy must have a particular therapy qualification (absolute qualification). Other workers, however, try to link qualifications with particular therapeutic activities (appropriate qualification). For example, whereas a nurse wishing to practise simple foot massage need not have an extensive training in massage, a practitioner wanting to prescribe essential oils therapeutically in, say, cancer care, would need to provide evidence that he or she was a fully qualified aromatherapist.

Quality of materials

Essential oils provided by some suppliers may be substandard. Many aromatherapists worry in particular about the adulteration of essential oils with synthetic substances. The quality of oils can also be compromised by lengthy or improper storage. Furthermore, the proportion of constituent compounds in an essential oil may change drastically depending on the particular variety of plant and stage of harvesting. It is therefore important that oils are precisely labelled. Though it is unknown whether substandard, mislabelled or adulterated oils have caused harm, it would be wise to ensure that supplies of essential oils are of high quality and again, advice from an independent source can be of particular value.

The treatment couches used for massage are a further safety consideration. A couch has collapsed during a treatment in at least one case. This may have resulted from the use of a doctor's examination table, which is not built to withstand the forces involved in massage. If patients are to receive massage on a treatment couch, this should be of sufficiently sturdy build.

Consultation and authorization

A general principle is that a practitioner should consult with the relevant doctor and obtain authorization from an appropriate manager before practice. Unfortunately, applying this principle is less simple than might at first appear. For example, does a practitioner have to consult with a doctor every time he or she wishes to give a patient a massage? Or just once for each patient? Or just once? Moreover, what form should consultation take? Similarly, does authorization have to be given by a manager for each and every massage? There are times when medical consultation and managerial authorization would seem overly cumbersome and bureaucratic. For example, a nurse places a hand on the shoulder of a patient who has become upset. This gradually evolves into a brief neck and shoulder rub. Should such behaviour be forbidden on the grounds that it does not involve consultation and authorization?

Consent

As for any therapy, informed consent from the patient, relative or carer should be obtained before massage or aromatherapy treatment. Though this is a relatively straightforward consideration, there needs to be agreement as to the form in which consent needs to be obtained and the degree to which there are exemptions or special circumstances, such as in the example of the shoulder rub given above.

An interesting issue associated with consent concerns respect for a patient's religious, cultural and spiritual beliefs. It is quite possible that a patient's beliefs about say, nudity, conflict with a practitioner's standard form of treatment and it can therefore be important for practitioners to state explicitly what they intend to do.

Documentation

The use of complementary therapy should be recorded in a patient's care plan and/or medical records. A proportion of complementary practitioners are not trained to keep notes and the need for careful documentation needs to be carefully explained and emphasized in such cases. The importance of confidentiality may also need to be stressed.

Limitations on practice

There need to be at least some formal constraints on what practitioners can do with patients. Advice from the professional organizations is that practitioners should not work outside the normal boundaries of their profession. This means that, for example, a nurse may use massage to help make a patient feel more comfortable before bedtime (a standard nursing duty) but should not use aromatherapy to treat, say, diabetes, as this falls outside the bounds of normal nursing practice.

It can be particularly important for practice guidelines to be established for complementary practitioners. In one somewhat extreme case, an aromatherapist working in a hospice took it upon herself to set up coloured lights and play music to patients to help them pass peacefully into the next world. The establishment of reasonable boundaries can help curb inappropriate practices and ensure fruitful co-working between all practitioners.

Some workers have recommended the establishment of peer-review groups of professionals which review one another's care. This gives practitioners 'ownership' over standards of practice and can prevent them feeling that such guidelines are handed down from a higher authority and are merely unwanted restrictions.

The issue of limitations on practice needs to be sensitively meshed with that of competence and training. Few would argue that a nurse who had completed one of the much maligned 'weekend courses' was not competent to give a simple, gentle foot massage in at least some cases. On the other hand, such an individual should clearly not be prescribing individualized essential oils for insomnia or depression. Matching specific health practices with particular levels of training and competence may be a rather detailed (and possibly intractable) task, but would appear to be a necessary element in any set of guidelines.

Clinical responsibility

It is important to determine lines of clinical responsibility, especially where complementary practitioners are involved.

Treatment protocols

Formal treatment protocols (see below) can be an important means of ensuring safety. Particular attention needs to be paid to the use of essential oils. Some units have specified a particular list of oils which can be used and have sometimes encouraged practitioners to make these up into premixed blends to guarantee appropriate dosing.

MANAGEMENT OF MASSAGE AND AROMATHERAPY IN DAY-TO-DAY PRACTICE

Massage and aromatherapy not only have to be practised at certain minimum standards of competence and safety, they also have to be used appropriately and effectively. This requires a degree of hands-on, day-to-day management. Though management can often seem rather ponderous and bureaucratic (especially to a complementary practitioner) simple mechanisms can often provide a powerful tool for ensuring optimal use of massage and aromatherapy. Because conventional health professionals are generally already subject to a degree of management, the needs of complementary practitioners will form the main focus of this section.

Supervision

Complementary practitioners are used to working autonomously in private practices in the community. They may therefore be unused to many features of health-service work. Issues which have presented problems to at least some complementary practitioners include the following:

- *Teamwork*. Many complementary practitioners are not used to sharing clinical responsibility for a patient, changing their practice to fit in with a team's overall activities or consulting with others before they decide on a course of action.
- *Documentation*. Practitioners of massage and aromatherapy often do not keep comprehensive notes. Even if they are used to note-taking, these may not be intelligible to other health professionals. Carefully written, legible records of treatment episodes and patient responses are required in health-service settings.

- *Therapeutic procedures.* There are few formal procedures in private complementary practice: practitioners do whatever they think is appropriate. This may involve, for example, using any oil they think suitable, or giving a particularly long massage if they feel that it would benefit the patient. There may be a need to specify particular therapeutic procedures in some conventional settings.
- *Accountability.* It is not clear in what ways and to whom complementary practitioners are accountable. If a practitioner in private practice harms or upsets a patient, for example, it is possible that the patient would not take matters further.

Careful and sympathetic supervision is needed to ensure that complementary practitioners understand the need for, and properly attend to, all standard procedures and practices of health-service work. In this respect, some workers have pointed to the value of early contact between a practitioner and a supportive, senior clinician. One medical director of a hospice insists on an preliminary interview with any member of staff – be they conventional health professional or complementary practitioner – who wishes to use massage or aromatherapy. The overall aim of the interview is to confirm the hospice's interest in and support of complementary therapies but to emphasize that there are certain ground rules: 'I stress that I think massage is great, but that this doesn't mean that anything goes.'

Supervision may also be required to help practitioners deal with the difficult professional issues sometimes posed by working in health-service settings. Practitioners may be unused to dealing with the range of ethnic origin and social class typical of conventional settings or the range and severity of health problems presented. Working with the dying, or chronically disabled, or those with mental health problems, may also be outside a practitioner's experience and can cause considerable professional and emotional difficulties. Moreover, private complementary therapists will, by definition, only have seen patients who have decided that they want and need therapy. In conventional health settings, patients may be referred or may enrol on a programme of which massage and aromatherapy is a part. Working with unwilling patients can cause difficulties. Supervision by an individual used to such problems can be of particular benefit.

However, it is important that supervision not is a means of preventing problems but is also seen as a positive aspect of a practitioner's professional development. Complementing expert supervision with peer supervision, in which practitioners of similar grade and expertise work together, can be a valuable means of ensuring this end.

It is important that clinical supervision is formalized in some way. Units at which supervision has been successfully introduced often have written procedures as to the precise nature of supervision procedures, appropriate topics to be discussed in supervision, how often supervision takes place and the times at which supervision procedures are to be reviewed.

Interdisciplinary meetings

The importance of inviting practitioners to attend interdisciplinary meetings cannot be overstated. If nothing else, meetings ensure that all practitioners feel involved in the common task of ensuring high-quality, integrated health care. In some units, practitioners have kept themselves to themselves, working quietly in a closed-off room and returning home at the end of the day without significant contact with other staff. Interdisciplinary meetings ensure that all clinicians can share observations about patients and can liaise appropriately so that the skills and strengths of the team are maximized.

A few representative examples will suffice to demonstrate the value of interdisciplinary collaboration.

- Regular team meetings at a primary-care centre have provided a forum for feedback on the appropriateness of referrals to and from complementary practitioners.
- Interdisciplinary meetings at an AIDS unit have enabled the dissemination of pertinent information, such as the death of a patient's partner, or a patient's history of mental health problems.
- Complementary practitioners working as volunteers in a hospice have discussed the appropriateness of different massage interventions with physiotherapists experienced in work with dying patients.
- Interdisciplinary meetings at a hospice have allowed discussion of problems common to all staff. These include emotional attachments to patients and revelation, by patients, of distressing personal experiences such as sexual abuse.
- Many practitioners who have worked without interdisciplinary collaboration and support have reported that this has resulted in professional stress.

Treatment protocols

The use of standard, formalized treatment protocols can often seem an unnecessary burden on practitioners, especially those without health-service experience. Protocols should address questions such as: which patients should receive treatment; contraindications; the approximate length of treatment; essential oils and dosages; the type of massage to be used. In some cases, protocols also may also need to make reference to patient choice and to the teaching of simple, self-help techniques to carers. Treatment protocols need not be overly prescriptive: for example, on the issue of which types of massage to use, a protocol might only state that this should be at the practitioner's discretion but that forceful manipulations should be avoided; similarly, protocols need not specify particular oils and dosages but might give a list of different oils and a suggested range of dilutions. Protocols also need to be flexible enough to allow for individual variation.

Review procedures

The use of massage and aromatherapy at a unit should be subject to regular review. Such a review should look at both the effectiveness of management procedures (e.g. treatment protocols) and at the outcomes of treatment (see 'Audit and Evaluation', below). Regular reviews can also play a positive role in re-emphasizing to all practitioners that management procedures are flexible and open to change. Presenting reviews as a two-way exchange of ideas, rather than as a panel sitting in judgement, can be useful in this respect. It can also be important for practitioners to be reviewed by professional peers and not just by senior clinicians or management.

Audit and evaluation

Complementary practitioners may be wary of audit and evaluation, not so much because they fear being 'shown up' but because they feel that standard assessment procedures may not detect what they see as subtle and sometimes unexpected types of change in a patient. There may also be an element of the fear of the unknown: most complementary practitioners are unfamiliar with audit and evaluation procedures. Audit needs to be sensitively presented to practitioners as a positive, rather than a threatening, aspect of health-service work. Appropriate advice and support can often be obtained from specially designated staff, such as a hospital quality assurance team.

Basic audit data can include: information on the number of patients seen; their presenting complaints; the source of referral (if applicable); the number of treatment sessions given; the therapies used (including any advice on self-help); and the reason for concluding treatment (if applicable). Evaluation of the outcome of treatment should be made using whatever means is standard in the unit concerned. Though this often involves simple questioning of the patient ('Do you feel better?') some units use more formal measures, such as health status question-naires.

Meeting practitioners' needs

Practitioners working in health-service settings have frequently complained about the inadequacy of their working environment. Massage and aromatherapy should ideally take place in a warm, quiet and private room, but often no special facilities are provided. One practitioner, for example, reported having to work in a corridor. Such problems may be considered to be part of a more general issue of job satisfaction: health-service work can often appear to bring more burdens (meetings, bureaucracy, restrictions on practice, etc.) than rewards. Effective management of massage and aromatherapy means meeting the needs of complementary practitioners. In other words, management should be a two-way process: not only the laying down of rules and guidelines, but the provision of an environment in which all practitioners feel they can work effectively.

INTRODUCING MASSAGE AND AROMATHERAPY INTO NEW SETTINGS

There are no hard and fast rules as to how complementary therapies should be introduced into conventional health-care settings. The fol-lowing sections will look at some general lessons suggested by those with suitable experience. Perhaps the key, overarching issue is that of openness: the introduction of new therapies should be done openly, with the consent and participation of all parties, rather than in an clan-destine manner.

Information

Information about proposed new services needs to be distributed as widely as possible. Interested parties include doctors, nurses, man-agers, pharmacy staff and physiotherapists. Means of information dis-tribution include introductory talks and demonstrations, staff meet-ings, bulletin boards, hospital magazines and flyers. Personalized let-ters, presentations and face-to-face interviews may be necessary with selected staff or staff groups. An information file, containing book ref-erences, research papers and the like, can be a useful back-up resource for those interested in learning more.

Consent

Appropriate consent for the introduction of massage and aromatherapy sometimes needs to be sought from higher authorities. For example, in a hospital setting, a drugs and therapeutics committee may need to sanction the use of essential oils on the grounds that they contain pharmacologically active substances. Practitioners should be aware that such committees are not always free from prejudice. One nurse commented that her proposal to use aromatherapy on a palliative care ward was seen 'as the thin end of the wedge, the start of a process which would end up with witchcraft'. That said, there is no need to be unduly suspicious: a defensive attitude may in itself hinder a successful implementation.

Practitioners

Massage and aromatherapy can be practised either by in-house health professionals or by complementary therapists. A decision needs to be taken at an early stage as to who should practise the therapies. Such a decision involves consideration of a number of issues, including current duties of staff, training, finances and the attitudes of other staff within a unit.

Time management

Time spent on massage and aromatherapy is time not spent on other duties. Health professionals wishing to change their practices to include complementary therapies may first need to discuss their time and responsibilities with an appropriate manager. It is worth remembering that massage and aromatherapy can often be given during quieter periods of the day or be integrated with existing care practices, for example, bathing.

Training

Who should bear the costs of training in complementary therapies? Massage and aromatherapy may not fall within a standard training budget, but one might be sympathetic to a nurse who felt unhappy about squeezing course fees from a restricted salary. Choosing a suitable course or training institution can also present significant problems. It is widely recognized that standards of training in massage and aromatherapy vary and that at least some courses are substandard. See the remarks about competence on page 240 and the comments about training institutions in Appendix A.

Establishing procedures

The procedures discussed above, for example, treatment protocols or supervision, need to be formally agreed and written up. This can often be one of the slowest and most difficult stages in any implementation. One means of speeding up this process is the drafting of broad, provisional proposals to be reviewed within a fixed period. It can often be difficult to make decisions about a therapy before it has actually been used in practice. A number of workers have advised that practice should be relatively limited at first and that it should build progressively. See McVey (1995) for more on developing policies on complementary therapies.

Costs

Essential oils, massage oils, towels and other materials incur costs. There needs to be a decision as to the budget from which these costs will be met. In some cases, complementary practitioners or nurses have bought their own materials. There are various reasons, quality control, for example, why this might be considered bad practice. Complementary practitioners may also need to be paid for their time. Practitioners have often worked for free, or for extremely low wages, and though this may be a necessary expedient in the initial stages of establishing a service, long-term low pay is not a good basis for ensuring mutual respect and equal power relations.

Inappropriate reactions

Implementation of massage and aromatherapy in conventional settings can provoke a variety of unhelpful reactions, ranging from the unnecessarily obstructive to the inappropriately enthusiastic. In some cases, complementary therapies have been seen as a form of panacea. This has led to the drawing up of plans for sweeping changes before any small-scale pilot schemes have been established and assessed. A simple rule-of-thumb, promoted by many, is: 'Start small, build carefully.' Another common mistake has been a desire to rush into the provision of massage and aromatherapy, on the grounds that any delay would be to deny patients a useful service. One nurse has described such an attitude as: 'Feet first, eyes shut.'

On the other hand, resistance to the introduction of massage and aromatherapy is also common. Detractors often do give reasonable arguments as to why the therapies should not be introduced or given official sanction. However, it should be recognized that opposition to the use of complementary therapies is often simply a gut reaction:

massage and aromatherapy represent practices, and possibly philosophies, that do not sit easily within some conventional practitioners'
personal understandings of health care. It is quite natural and understandable that those practitioners should feel uncomfortable with the
use of massage and aromatherapy within their professional environment. As such, it is incumbent upon advocates of these therapies to
avoid a moralistic and adversarial stance and to promote their beliefs
in a cautious and sensitive manner. Trying to defeat a detractor's
argument, and vigorously defend one's own position, may not always
be the most fruitful means of progress.

In practice, the problem is not so much direct opposition to massage
and aromatherapy – in the sense of trying to prevent their use – but a
general lack of cooperation and what one practitioner has described as
a 'non-verbal atmosphere' of hostility. Some complementary therapists have reported that they have been ignored and feel that this is an
attempt to let them 'wither on the vine'. Prolonged and consistent lack
of support and integration can make a practitioner's professional life
difficult, and sometimes unpleasant, and this may eventually lead to a
cessation of the activities causing the professional rejection.

As suggested above, the most effective means of overcoming
resistance to the use of massage and aromatherapy is generally not
adversarial argument. Most practitioners have found that attitudes
have changed slowly over time, primarily as a result of seeing patients
benefit, but also, in some cases, by personal experience of treatment.
Some practitioners have reported relatively dramatic changes in the
attitude of hitherto sceptical colleagues after an offer of a massage.
However, in most cases, change has been more gradual, a drip-feed
process fed by seeing the value to patients on a day-to-day basis.

Rankin-Box (1995b) suggests that successful introduction of complementary therapies to the workplace can be aided by highlighting
the familiar aspects of innovative techniques. For example, a gentle
hand massage at bedtime is analogous to nursing practices aiming to
make patients comfortable before sleep. A further issue is that of
'losing face'. Suggesting that, say, aromatherapy should be introduced
as a form of emotional support at a cancer unit can be taken to imply
that care has previously been inadequate. Practitioners need to be
sensitive to the criticism of current practice implicit in developing a
new service.

Drawing on experience

'Reinventing the wheel' seems to have become a particular problem in
the introduction of massage and aromatherapy to conventional settings. Many units have tried to solve all the problems associated with

an implementation from scratch. For example, some hospitals have discussed issues of training and competence at extraordinary lengths without drawing appropriately on the experience of others. An ideal situation is for a unit to find another which has already implemented massage and aromatherapy and use the procedures developed by that unit as an appropriate starting point. Organizations such as the Complementary Therapies Forum of the Royal College of Nursing, the British Holistic Medical Association, the National Association of Health Authorities and Trusts and the lead bodies of massage and aromatherapy, can sometimes be a useful source of suitable contact names and addresses (see the list of organizations in Appendix C). It is also worth remembering that massage and aromatherapy do not always constitute a 'special case' and general procedures can often be adapted. For example, many units have guidelines for the clinical supervision of nurses and it is likely that these can also be used for complementary practitioners.

LIMITATIONS AND EXCEPTIONS TO MANAGEMENT

The discussion of management procedures given above is intended to be as exhaustive as possible. Not every procedure mentioned need be implemented in every case. Aromatherapy massage of intensive care patients, for example, may very well require the adoption of most of the management procedures discussed above. The use of massage at a community mental health 'drop-in', on the other hand, might not require such a comprehensive management structure. There needs to be a reasonable evaluation of which procedures need to be considered by a unit.

In practice, it is rare for a complete set of management procedures to be in place before massage and aromatherapy are introduced to a unit. Generally, the adoption of a formal policy occurs after the therapies have been practised for a short while. This is not always to be dissuaded: it can be difficult to develop guidelines in the absence of practical experience simply because it is practical experience that provides the basis for effective policy. In most units, a fruitful interaction between management and practice has, over time, led to the development of an appropriate set of guidelines and procedures.

Another difficult issue results from the rather fuzzy boundaries of massage and aromatherapy. At what point does the use of comforting touch become massage? Does the vaporization of essential oils to provide a pleasant atmosphere constitute aromatherapy? There need to be at least some limits on the interference of management with everyday caring practices. To paraphrase a sentiment popular at the time of writing: government can get too big.

CONCLUSION

Massage and aromatherapy can only be successfully introduced into conventional settings if they are properly managed and organized. Though many, especially complementary practitioners, may balk at the sometimes tedious and constraining language of management, especially when contrasted to the intuitive and creative nature of massage and aromatherapy, some simple mechanisms can serve to ensure that patients receive safe and effective treatment:

Ensuring safe and competent use of massage and aromatherapy

Attention needs to be paid to:

- competence of practitioners;
- quality of materials;
- consultation and authorization;
- consent;
- documentation;
- limitations on practice;
- clinical responsibility.

Management of massage and aromatherapy in day-to-day practice

Attention needs to be paid to:

- supervision;
- interdisciplinary meetings;
- treatment protocols.
- review procedures;
- audit and evaluation;
- meeting practitioners' needs;

Introducing massage and aromatherapy into new settings

Attention needs to be paid to:

- information;
- consent;
- practitioners;
- time management issues;
- training;
- establishing procedures;
- costs;

- inappropriate reactions;
- drawing on experience.

Limitations and exceptions to management

Not all management procedures need to be implemented in all cases all of the time.

Safety of massage and aromatherapy

11

ADVERSE EFFECTS AND DRUG INTERACTIONS OF ESSENTIAL OILS

Essential oils contain pharmacologically active substances. The possibility that they might cause adverse effects or interact with prescribed medications is therefore a serious concern. It is not uncommon for aromatherapists or other clinicians to ask where they can obtain a 'list' of adverse effects and contraindications. This presupposes that some consensus has been reached as to the potentially harmful consequences of aromatherapy. Unfortunately, this has not occurred and, given the current lack of data, it appears unlikely that the situation will change in the foreseeable future.

This section will attempt to draw some tentative conclusions based on existing knowledge. The argument will consist of four main points.

- The likelihood and severity of adverse effects resulting from the use of essential oils is probably low.
- Adverse effects of essential oils have been reported.
- Aromatherapists have developed guidelines for the safe use of essential oils.
- The problem of adverse effects in aromatherapy is reducible to the question of professionalization.

THE LIKELIHOOD AND SEVERITY OF ADVERSE EFFECTS RESULTING FROM THE USE OF ESSENTIAL OILS IS PROBABLY LOW

There are a number of reasons to suppose that aromatherapy is probably a relatively safe treatment modality.

Chemical analysis of essential oils does not suggest high toxicity

The essential oils used by aromatherapists have been chemically analysed, primarily by gas chromatography (p. 29). The constituent compounds of essential oils are not thought to have particularly high toxicities.

Toxicity studies on rats give low toxicity values

Essential oils are widely used in the food and fragrance industries. It has been necessary for those industries to ensure the safety of their products by conducting toxicity studies on rats. In a typical study, rats are administered increasing doses of an essential oil until 50% are killed. This dose, known as an LD_{50}, can be used to estimate toxicity in humans. The LD_{50} values for the essential oils commonly used by aromatherapists suggest that they are unlikely to cause adverse reactions in humans (see, for example, International School of Aromatherapy, 1993).

Patch tests suggest that essential oils do not readily cause skin sensitivity or irritation

The fragrance industry has carried out research to test the allergic and irritation reactions from essential oils. In a typical study, an essential oil is diluted, applied to a patch of skin, covered by a gauze and left for a day or so. The area of skin is then examined for any signs of a reaction. These 'patch tests' generally involve about 25 volunteers. Patch tests of essential oils commonly used by aromatherapists suggest that they are unlikely to cause skin sensitivity or irritation (International School of Aromatherapy, 1993). Of note, however, is Bouhlal *et al.*'s (1989) demonstration that sensitivity to concretes and absolutes (p. 27) is higher than that to essential oils.

The doses used in aromatherapy are low

Only a few drops of essential oils are used in an aromatherapy massage of which only a small proportion actually enter the bloodstream through the skin. A typical aromatherapy treatment is likely to involve the absorption of no more than between 0.025 and 0.1 ml of essential oils (Tisserand and Balacs, 1995:25), a quantity unlikely to lead to adverse reactions, particularly given the apparently benign nature of essential oil constituents.

Aromatherapists do not appear to be harmed by essential oils

Practitioners of aromatherapy may be unique in that they take their own medicine as part of the actual treatment process: a practitioner will absorb oils through the skin of the hands and by inhalation of vapour while giving an aromatherapy massage. The quantity of essential oils absorbed by an aromatherapist over the course of a working week is likely to be much greater than that absorbed by a patient during a single treatment. However, aromatherapists do not appear (yet) to have been harmed by their profession.

Serious adverse effects arising from aromatherapy treatment have not been documented

The practice of aromatherapy is relatively widespread. If serious adverse effects of aromatherapy are anything other than extremely rare, one might expect them to have been documented more commonly in the medical literature (though see p. 262).

CERTAIN ADVERSE EFFECTS OF ESSENTIAL OILS HAVE BEEN REPORTED

There are a number of documented cases where essential oils have led to adverse effects. These have generally involved oral ingestion of relatively large quantities of oil. For example, in a case reported by Jacobs and Hornfeldt (1994), a 23-month-old boy became confused and was unable to walk after drinking less than 10 ml of tea tree oil. Though admitted to hospital, the child recovered within a few hours and was discharged after an overnight stay. A number of similar reports are given by Millet *et al.* (1981) and Tisserand and Balacs (1995). Reports of adverse effects arising from topical application or inhalation are not unknown, but these generally involve large quantities of oil, often in industrial settings. Parys (1983), for example, reports on a chemical burn experienced by a pharmaceutical worker who spilt peppermint oil on a hand that had previously undergone skin grafting due to injury. A particularly interesting paper is that of Villar *et al.* (1994) who report that animals treated topically for dermatological conditions with inappropriately high doses of tea tree oil showed signs of poisoning, such as weakness, uncoordination and muscle tremors. This is possibly the only report of a systemic adverse effect arising from dermal application of an essential oil.

In none of these cases did adverse effects result from an aromatherapy treatment. The implications for aromatherapy practice are therefore probably minor. Perhaps the only conclusion worth drawing is that essential oils can eventually be toxic, if given in high enough doses.

Documented adverse effects arising from aromatherapy treatment in humans are restricted, with one exception, to cases of contact dermatitis. Typical reports include a case of eczema due to Kamilosan, an ointment containing 10% oil of camomile (McGeorge and Steele, 1991); acute eczema to marigold oil in an aromatherapist (Bilsland and Strong, 1990) and a reaction to tea tree oil prescribed by an alternative clinic (de Groot and Weyland, 1992). Knight and Hausen (1994) investigated seven cases of contact dermatitis resulting from topical treatment with tea tree oil. Patients were patch tested with 1% tea tree oil and 15 solutions of 11 constituent compounds. The fraction most commonly causing an eczematous reaction was limonene. Interestingly, most patients reacted to more than one constituent compound. Given that certain individuals are sensitive to any number of natural and synthetic substances, reports such as these should not, perhaps, surprise us.

One of the few examples of an adverse effect resulting from an aromatherapy-type treatment involved a patient on warfarin anticoagulant therapy who suffered haematoma (accumulation of blood in the tissues) after receiving massage with wintergreen oil from his wife (Yeo, Choo and Tey, 1994). Wintergreen oil is 98% methyl salicylate and topical salicylates are known to increase the risk of bleeding in patients on warfarin. It may also be that trauma induced by massage was at least partly to blame. Aromatherapists will probably be quick to point out that this adverse effect did not result from a consultation with a registered practitioner. Nonetheless, the report does show that essential oils applied by massage can produce undesirable complications.

Other than this one case of haematoma, and the aforementioned cases of contact dermatitis, adverse effects of aromatherapy treatment in humans have apparently not been documented in the medical literature. This does not mean, however, that they have not occurred. There are anecdotal reports circulating of asthma attacks being provoked by essential oils and even one unconfirmed report of fatal anaphylactic shock. However, in no report is there an unambiguous link between the adverse event and a standard aromatherapy treatment. For example, in one story, an asthmatic episode followed an aromatherapy demonstration in which it appears that the vapours of a number of different oils were present in high concentration.

An area of particular interest is the possibility of minor, transient adverse effects following an aromatherapy treatment. Various individuals have reported feeling drowsy, lethargic, 'headachy', nauseous or even intoxicated after giving, receiving or observing an aromatherapy treatment. Such effects would be predicted from the purported psychological action of essential oils. If an oil has a sedative or stimulating action, and if the oil is used inappropriately, some form of minor psychological side-effect might be expected. This possibility is probably increased by the lack of reliable data as to the psychological actions of the oils (p. 58).

AROMATHERAPISTS HAVE DEVELOPED GUIDELINES FOR THE SAFE USE OF ESSENTIAL OILS

Aromatherapists are not unaware of the possibility of adverse effects arising from the use of essential oils. Training in the safe use of essential oils is a part of all reputable aromatherapy courses and most aromatherapy books do make mention of possible hazards. The safety issues that form a common part of aromatherapy discourse are as follows.

- *Administration of essential oils.* Oils should not be taken by mouth. They should not be applied to the skin without first diluting them in oil or water.
- *Avoidance of hazardous oils.* Certain essential oils (e.g. wormwood, pennyroyal) are known to have high toxicities and their use should be avoided.
- *Specific contraindications.* A number of oils are said to have properties which suggest that they should not be used in particular conditions. For example, certain oils are said to induce menstruation and hence are contraindicated in pregnancy; other oils are thought to trigger epilepsy in susceptible individuals; oils thought to have oestrogenic properties are contraindicated in oestrogen-dependent cancers.
- *General cautions.* Some oils are said to be phototoxic (they sensitize the skin to light) or photocarcinogenic (they promote the formation of tumours in the presence of light). Patients are advised not to expose themselves to sunlight after a treatment in which one of these oils was applied to the skin. Oils considered to be generally more toxic are contraindicated for young children, pregnant women, individuals with liver disease and others, such as the severely ill, likely to be especially sensitive.

There are two points worth making about this advice. Firstly, much of it is based on educated guesswork. For example, it is not clear whether any of the oils contraindicated in pregnancy have actually ever induced a miscarriage. And though some warnings, such as the avoidance of certain oils, are based on information such as LD_{50} tests, most are not.

Secondly, the contraindications given by different authors vary considerably. For example, Davis (1988: 118) suggests that fennel, hyssop, sage and rosemary may trigger epilepsy in susceptible individuals. Though Lawless (1994b) agrees, Tisserand says that rosemary is a treatment for epilepsy (1977: 283) and that fennel oil is of no danger (1977: 224). Neither Price (1993) nor the International School of Aromatherapy (1993) give any of these contraindications; Valnet (1980) agrees only with fennel and rosemary. Similarly, though Wildwood (1992: 30), Sadler (1991: 119) and Lawless (1994b: 166) state that marjoram should not be used in pregnancy, Price (1993) claims that adverse effects are 'unlikely'. Neither Tisserand (1977), Valnet (1980) nor Davis (1988) gives pregnancy as a contraindication for marjoram.

Possibly the most reliable source is Tisserand and Balacs (1995). This text is particularly good on the pharmacology of essential oils and gives a number of sensible general recommendations. Another worthwhile text, produced by the International School of Aromatherapy (1993), consists of a summary of a large amount of LD_{50} and sensitization data. There are, however, a number of errors. For example, the book states that 'the theoretical adult dose can be calculated by simply multiplying [a figure for rats] by 70'. It is untrue that a toxicity for a rat in terms of millilitres per kilogram will be the same as that for a human. This is because smaller animals have higher metabolic rates and thus break down and excrete toxic substances more rapidly than large animals. Conventionally, dosages are adjusted by a variable related to metabolic rate.

THE PROBLEM OF ADVERSE EFFECTS IN AROMATHERAPY IS REDUCIBLE TO THE QUESTION OF PROFESSIONALIZATION

Texts such as those by the International School of Aromatherapy (1993) and Tisserand and Balacs (1995) provide a useful insight into laboratory data on the toxicity of essential oils. That said, it is extremely difficult to draw conclusions about aromatherapy practice from either of these two books. This is because the possibility of interactions between essential oils and drugs is left completely unexplored by LD_{50} experiments and patch tests. Moreover, people who are ill often have lowered metabolism, poor nutritional status and compromised liver and kidney function. In addition, allergy is more common in those seeking medical help. Each of these factors is likely to increase any potential harmful effects of essential oils.

Aromatherapists and other health professionals need to know about the adverse effects of essential oils in practice: whether a particular oil is safe to use with a particular patient. Studies on rats and healthy volunteers can only provide a guidepost: reliable information on safety can only be developed from clinical data.

The fundamental problem for aromatherapy is the lack of a professional structure by which adverse effects of essential oils can be rigorously documented. There is no equivalent in aromatherapy of the 'yellow card system' by which British doctors record suspected adverse effects of conventional drugs. Moreover, there are a number of features of aromatherapy practice which suggest that adverse effects are unlikely to be reported.

In private practice, minor adverse effects, such as headache or lethargy, might be described as an 'exacerbation' or 'healing reaction'. This is said to be a feature of some complementary therapies and involves a worsening of symptoms (sometimes attributed to the mobilization and expulsion of toxins) as a prelude to a cure. Moreover, given that many individuals visit private aromatherapists for relaxation and general well-being, minor adverse effects may go unreported simply because a dissatisfied client will not return to the therapist. It is also possible that symptoms following an aromatherapy treatment are not attributed to the use of essential oils, especially as practitioners are often at pains to point out the safety of their 'natural' remedies compared to harmful drugs. Potentially more serious adverse effects, such as induction of an asthma attack, may go unreported in private practice for similar reasons.

In health care settings, minor adverse effects may be attributed to disease processes, drugs or the institutional environment. To give an example: a hospice patient receives an aromatherapy massage in the afternoon and develops a headache later that night. It is highly unlikely that nursing staff would attribute the headache to the use of essential oils. It is more probable that the headache would be seen as just a typical pain of a typical cancer patient.

A further complication concerns the long-term effects of aromatherapy. Though it appears that essential oils are eliminated relatively rapidly from the body (p. 144) it would be unwise to dismiss the possibility of long-term adverse effects from essential oils, particularly if oils are used consistently over significant periods of time. This problem might well invalidate the argument, given above, that essential oils are safe because aromatherapists do not appear to be affected by daily exposure.

However, perhaps the most crucial point is that even'if an unhappy patient did return to complain to a practitioner, or sought medical advice to deal with a symptom caused by treatment, or if a health professional in a conventional setting did correctly attribute a health problem to prior use of aromatherapy, it is not clear whether information about the possible adverse effects of the essential oils would be disseminated. As has been pointed out, no reliable mechanisms exist to ensure that this process takes place.

A hypothetical example should be sufficient to illustrate the difficulties involved in accurately assessing and disseminating information about the adverse effects of essential oils. Imagine that sandalwood oil interferes with certain prophylactic antiasthmatic agents. A London-based aromatherapist gives several treatments to an asthmatic patient. A number of oils are used, including sandalwood on certain occasions. The patient subsequently suffers an increase in asthma symptoms over the course of the following weeks. The patient may well fail to attribute this to the aromatherapy: it is perhaps more likely that stress, environmental factors and natural disease variations would be blamed. If the patient does, however, correctly link the aggravation with aromatherapy treatment, it is quite possible that he or she would fail to inform either the aromatherapist or a doctor. Furthermore, imagining that the aromatherapist and/or general practitioner were informed, it is not clear whether they would choose to share this information with others. In any event, how could they do so? How would an aromatherapist practising in, say, California come to learn about the possible dangers of sandalwood? The issue is further complicated by the fact that a number of cases would need to be collated to establish that it was sandalwood, out of a number of possible different oils, which was responsible for the exacerbation of asthma and that the mechanism for this effect was suppression of prophylaxis.

In summary, the reliability of safety data on essential oils is limited by the lack of established professional structures to collate and disseminate such data. If aromatherapy remains professionally immature, it is likely that the adverse effects, drug interactions and contraindications of essential oils will remain incompletely understood.

ADVERSE EFFECTS OF MASSAGE

Much of the previous discussion on essential oils is applicable to massage. Like essential oils, massage appears to be relatively safe. That said, adverse effects have been reported. And again, though practitioners have developed a number of sensible practice guidelines, these are not based upon carefully documented clinical evidence: the problem of adverse effects is, once more, essentially a question of professionalization.

It is worth briefly discussing cases of adverse effects arising from massage reported in the medical literature. Herskovitz, Strauch and Gordon (1992) report on a nerve injury following extremely vigorous shiatsu massage given by a traditional oriental practitioner in New York. The condition normalized after 8 weeks. Another case of problems arising from energetic shiatsu involved reappearance of herpes zoster (Mumm *et al.*, 1993). This was ascribed to the use of heavy pressure at the zoster site. Rahman, McAll and Chai (1987) and Becroft and Gunn (1989) also report on adverse effects resulting from traditional massage using deep pressure techniques.

These cases do not involve practices likely to be used in any of the settings described in this book. Their relevance for typical massage practice is therefore limited. Of possibly greater interest is that certain minor adverse effects have been anecdotally attributed to massage without this necessarily being documented. Headaches have been known to occur following treatment and this effect has yet to be adequately explained. Muscle soreness and even bruising can follow vigorous massage. Drowsiness and lethargy often result from massage, and though it is unclear whether this effect should really be considered 'adverse', it is worth bearing in mind if a patient intends to travel or return to work immediately following a treatment.

Contraindications to massage

Lists of contraindications to massage are in existence. Most of the contraindications are sufficiently obvious that one would expect a competent practitioner to recognize the inappropriateness of massage without having to remember and apply a clinical guideline. Such 'common sense' contraindications to massage include:

- acute infectious disease;
- unstable pregnancies;
- exacerbations of disorders affecting the musculoskeletal system, for example, rheumatoid arthritis;
- use of techniques likely to stimulate, such as vigorous strokes to increase blood circulation, in ill or weakened patients, for example, elderly people or those in hospice care;
- vigorous massage in conditions where skin or bones are weakened (e.g. cancer, fractures) or where bruising is likely (e.g. chemotherapy);
- massage to the feet or legs in deep vein thrombosis;
- phlebitis;
- undiagnosed signs or symptoms;
- massage strokes should avoid burns, broken skin and fungal infection.

It is also said that in the case of serious disease (e.g. hypertension, severe asthma, diabetes) massage should not be attempted without prior consultation with a doctor.

Two commonly given contraindications are worth discussing in more detail. Massage is said to be detrimental in patients with coronary disease, particularly in the immediate period following an MI. This is because changes in blood flow resulting from massage might be thought to put undue strain on a weak heart. Tyler *et al.* (1990) found that a 1-minute back rub slightly reduced venous oxygen saturation (from 67% to 63%) and increased heart rate (from 99 to 103 beats per minute) in post-cardiac-surgery patients in an intensive care unit. Measures returned to baseline within 4 minutes. The authors concluded that such minor changes do not support a blanket contraindication of massage in such patients. However, they do counsel that unduly vigorous and stimulating massage should be avoided and that patient responses should be monitored. Similarly, Bauer and Dracup (1987) found no significant physiological changes following a 6-minute back-rub in any of 25 patients with acute myocardial infarction.

Another widely discussed contraindication is cancer. It has long been thought that massage should be avoided in cancer on the grounds that it may cause metastasis, presumably by dislodging cells from established tumours. Clearly, it would be unwise for a practitioner to use very heavy pressure directly on the site of a tumour. That said, it seems extremely unlikely that the massage strokes generally used in the care of cancer patients would cause cells to break off from a primary tumour where this would not occur anyway as a result of everyday activity: it is hard to think of why gentle massage should be any more likely to spread cancer than say, walking or sitting.

SUMMARY: SAFETY OF MASSAGE AND AROMATHERAPY

- Adverse effects resulting from massage and aromatherapy appear to be neither common nor serious.
- Adverse effects of essential oils have occasionally been reported. These have not generally resulted from aromatherapy treatment.
- Some cases of contact dermatitis has been documented following aromatherapy.
- There are undocumented reports of allergic reactions to essential oils (e.g. asthma).
- There are a few cases of adverse effects resulting from massage, but these have involved techniques (e.g. extremely vigorous neck massage) unlikely to be used by practitioners working in conventional health settings.
- The use of massage and aromatherapy may lead to transient, minor symptoms such as headaches, lethargy, drowsiness or mild intoxication.

- Practitioners of massage and aromatherapists have developed guidelines for safe clinical practice, including both specific and general contraindications. These guidelines tend to be based on common sense and educated guesswork rather than on reliable clinical data.
- No professional mechanisms exist within aromatherapy and massage by which adverse effects can be documented, collated and disseminated to practitioners. This is a particular problem in aromatherapy, which involves the administration of pharmacologically active substances.

Epilogue

If you have never had a massage you perhaps have no business reading this book. Over the course of the last 250 pages or so, I have attempted to write an intellectually rigorous overview of massage and aromatherapy. I have made copious reference to the scientific literature and used standard techniques of analysis and argument to explore claims made by practitioners.

In the preface, I outlined my reasons for writing a book of this nature. What I would like to emphasize here is my belief in a plurality of discourses about massage and aromatherapy. Open a typical page of this text and you are likely to find, for example, a methodological critique of a study aiming to determine the psychophysiology of massage, or an analysis of the status of knowledge claims. Open a page of, say, George Downing's *The Massage Book*, and you are likely to find a description of massage given between friends, discussing, perhaps, the feelings of energy or 'aliveness' that result from massage. I did not use the former style of discourse because it is better than that used by Downing, I used it because it is different, important and currently underdeveloped.

I say that it is impossible to understand this book if you have never had a massage, because an academic discourse can only go some of the way towards describing something as basically human as touch or smell. I have written this book to expand the current discourse of massage and aromatherapy, not to replace it.

Finally, just so you know, I am a user of massage and aromatherapy. I regularly exchange massages with friends – often just a back rub through clothes – and I do sometimes use essential oils, mainly because I like their smell.

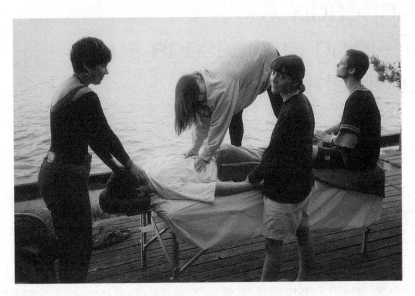

Figure E.1 The author (face down on table) undertaking research for this book.

Appendix A
Training in massage and aromatherapy

A large number of institutions claim to provide a training in massage and aromatherapy. A recent career guide (Maher, 1990) listed over 110 separate schools in the UK alone. This figure is likely to have grown over the course of the last few years.

Broadly speaking, training institutions are unregulated and there is often little similarity between either the courses taught or the mechanism by which a student is given a qualification. It is widely accepted that educational standards vary enormously. Though many practitioners are quick to malign the courses taught by just one or two individuals from their own homes, it is not entirely clear whether the training offered at some of the more established institutions necessarily results in more competent practitioners. This is because there is little agreement as to what determines competence in massage and aromatherapy. Simply put, if there is no generally accepted answer to the question 'What knowledge and skills does one need to be a competent practitioner?' there can be no standardization of training.

The situation does appear to be changing. There is a trend within complementary medicine for each therapy to establish a single national organization responsible for standards of training, qualification and registration. The recent establishment in the UK of the Aromatherapy Organisations Council, representing a number of the major aromatherapy bodies, is an example of this trend. A further encouraging development is the establishment of courses in massage and aromatherapy at university level. These are typically offered as optional modules on standard nursing courses, though there are some stand-alone degrees.

It is beyond the scope of this book to give a full list of training institutions in massage and aromatherapy. It is recommended that those interested in training contact a national organization (some important ones are listed below) and obtain details of individual institutions. These should be contacted for a prospectus.

A number of specialist courses have been established to cater for the needs of those already working as health professionals. These have been specially designed to be appropriate for both existing levels of knowledge and likely areas of practice. For example, aromatherapy courses for nurses concentrate on therapeutic techniques and do not include material, such as basic anatomy and physiology, with which nurses are already acquainted. Health professionals should contact their professional body for information and advice.

HOW TO CHOOSE A COURSE

In deciding between courses and training institutions, it may be useful to follow the guidelines set out below.

Objectives

Applicants need to ask themselves what they want out of training. They should consider how they intend to use their training and how they intend to practise. Particular attention should be paid to whether, and to what extent, training needs to be directed towards the treatment of specific disorders. Does the applicant wish to work autonomously, offering curative treatment for conditions such as back pain, acne or premenstrual syndrome? Or to provide non-specific palliative treatment?

Training needs

Applicants should identify their training needs by reflecting on their current level of skills and knowledge. They will also need to analyse what would be required to practise a therapy competently in the manner intended. Applicants should be aware that it is common to underestimate the skills and knowledge required to undertake a particular therapeutic activity.

Accreditation

Applicants need to be confident that the training offered by a particular institution is recognized and validated. They should be aware that training institutions almost always claim to be registered and recognized by impressive sounding national and international organizations and that very few will admit to being merely a prerogative of the teachers involved.

Qualifications

Applicants need to be confident that the qualifications offered by a training institution will be recognized outside that institution. Again they should be aware that many colleges attempt to obscure the value of the qualifications that they offer by giving them impressive sounding titles.

Practical issues

Applicants should consider the amount of time effort and money that they are prepared to invest in a course.

ADDRESSES

UNITED KINGDOM

Aromatherapy Organisations Council, 3 Latymer Close, Braybrooke, Market Harborough, Leicester LE16 8LN. Telephone: 01858 434242.

Massage Therapy Institute of Great Britain, PO Box 276, London NW2 4NR. Telephone: 0181 208 1607.

London and Counties Society of Physiologists, 330 Lytham Road, Blackpool FY4 1DW. Telephone: 01253 408443.

USA

Office of Alternative Medicine, National Institutes of Health, EPS-Suite 450, 6120 Executive Blvd, Rockville MD 20892. Telephone: 301 402 2466. A federally funded body. Can provide information on training courses.

American Massage Therapy Association, Suite 100, 820 Davis Street, Evanston, IL 60201-4444. Telephone: 708 864 0123.

National Association for Holistic Aromatherapy, 219 Carl Street, San Francisco, CA 94117. Telephone: 415 564 6785.

CANADA

Alberta Society of Professional Aromatherapists, 204 Queensland Place SE, Calgary, Alberta T2J 4E2. Telephone: 403 278 9788.

AUSTRALIA

International Federation of Aromatherapists, 83 Riverdale Road, Hawthorn, Victoria 3122.

Association of Massage Therapists, 3/33 Denham Street, Bondi NSW 2026.

NEW ZEALAND

New Zealand Register of Wholistic Aromatherapists, PO BOX 18399 Glen Innes, Auckland 6.

New Zealand Association of Therapeutic Massage Practitioners, PO Box 375, Hamilton.

SOUTH AFRICA

Lucile Bischoff, PO BOX 742, Galo Manor 2052.

Individuals residing in other countries should write to the Aromatherapy Organisations Council in the UK for details of a suitable contact.

Appendix B
Further reading

BOOKS ON MASSAGE AND TOUCH

There are many 'how-to' guides on massage. The majority are written for a non-professional audience and focus on massage given between friends. Downing (1974) remains my personal favourite. The book is particularly notable for its excellent illustrations and clear text. It also strikes an appropriate balance between precise descriptions of specific strokes and background discussion of the general principles of massage. Other well-known massage guides include Inkeles (1977, 1980) Lidell (1984) and Maxwell-Hudson (1988). Eyerman (1987) is of interest for its stunning photography and its emphasis on massage for dancers and athletes. Amongst a small number of books aimed at massage professionals are those of Juhan (1987) and Chaitow (1988). Juhan draws together a number of sources, including extensive reference to anatomy and physiology, to make general reflections on the role of massage and bodywork. Chaitow has a more practical aim and discusses the use of soft-tissue techniques in some detail.

For those interested in touch, there are three books of particular interest. Montagu's remarkable (1978) work *Touching: The Human Significance of the Skin* has no doubt been extremely influential in promoting the importance of the tactile sense. Montagu sometimes builds rather creatively from established data and his anthropology often veers towards the dangerously simplistic: traditional culture is seen as synonymous with simple truth, modern Western society is caricatured as monolithically scientistic and thereby isolated from wisdom. Montagu's cross-cultural comparisons also bear the stamp of a judgmental stance. That said, the book is a classic of its type and certainly worth a read. *Touch: An Exploration* (Autton, 1989) is also highly recommended. The work consists of wide-ranging reflections on the role and nature of touch and makes extensive reference to health issues. Autton draws heavily, if selectively, from the research literature with the result that the book is an excellent work of scholarship. Finally, Cardwell-Brown (1984) has edited an interesting and worthwhile collection of essays and research reports on touch entitled *The Many Facets Of Touch*.

BOOKS ON AROMATHERAPY AND THE SENSE OF SMELL

In Chapter 3, I offer a wide-ranging critique of the aromatherapy literature published to date. Few, if any, of these texts are worth recommending. However, at about the time that this book was going to press, two new works were published which represent a new departure for writing on aromatherapy. Price (1995) and Tisserand and Balacs (1995) are probably the first texts to be written especially for a professional audience. Both strive to be comprehensive, well-presented and well-argued. That said, the books are not without their flaws. Perhaps the main problem is that research (and science in general) is sometimes used to vindicate current practice, rather than critically to examine what that practice should be. Price, in particular, uses the scientific literature somewhat arbitrarily to support knowledge claims. For example, she reports on two uncontrolled trials of aromatherapy in labour which had positive results, but omits to mention Dale and Cornwell (1994), who conducted a methodologically rigorous study showing no difference between lavender oil and placebo treatment for perineal healing. In addition to Price, 1995 and Tisserand and Balacs (1995), *A Safety Guide on the Use of Essential Oils* (International School of Aromatherapy, 1993) is recommended for its comprehensive information on safety studies.

Those interested in the nature and role of the sense of smell are recommended to read two collections of research studies edited by Van Toller and Dodd (1991, 1992). Van Toller himself recommends Lake (1989) and Dorland (1993). Of general interest is Suskind's (1985) novel *Perfume: The Story of a Murderer*.

BOOKS FOR THE HEALTH PROFESSIONAL

Sanderson and Harrison (1991) is an excellent examination of massage and aromatherapy for people with learning difficulties. This is possibly the only text on these therapies aimed specifically at the health professional and might therefore be seen as a predecessor of this book.

Trevelyan and Booth (1994) and Rankin-Box (1995a) provide overviews of complementary medicine aimed specifically at nurses and midwives. The latter is written by nurses with experience of using complementary therapies in conventional health care settings and is particularly recommended.

GENERAL BOOKS ON COMPLEMENTARY MEDICINE

Two previous books by this author examine complementary therapies for people with disabilities. Both are written in a non-technical style and are appropriate for both the professional and general reader. Vickers (1993) is aimed primarily at disabled adults and includes discussion of conditions such as arthritis, multiple sclerosis, spinal injury and stroke. The second book, published in association with the Spastics Society (Vickers, 1994b) examines complementary therapies for cerebral palsy and related conditions. It concentrates primarily on children with disabilities.

The best introduction to the sociology of complementary medicine is Sharma (1991). The book is an open-minded exploration of the question: who uses or practises complementary medicine and why do they do so? Coward (1989) undertakes a brilliant analysis of the underlying ideology of complementary medicine. She looks at a number of the unexamined (and often unacknowledged) myths underpinning alternative health practices, for example, the concept of 'nature' and 'natural healing' and that of 'traditional' medicine. Pietroni (1990) presents a philosophical overview of general trends in medicine which attempts to explain and accommodate the rising interest in complementary therapies.

Appendix C
Other organizations

Research Council for Complementary Medicine, 60 Great Ormond Street, London WC1N 3JF. Telephone: 0171 833 8897; email: rccm@gn.apc.org. Provides information and advice for health professionals about research in complementary medicine. Can conduct literature searches of CISCOM, a specialist database of complementary medicine research.

British Holistic Medical Association, Trust House, Royal Shrewsbury Hospital South, Shrewsbury SY3 8XF. Organization for professionals interested in holistic medicine.

National Association of Health Authorities and Trusts, Birmingham Research Park, Vincent Drive, Birmingham B15 2SQ. Representative body for purchasers. May be able to offer advice on purchasing or providing complementary medicine.

Royal College of Nursing, Complementary Therapies Special Interest Group, 20 Cavendish Square, London W1M 0AB. Contact point for nurses interested in massage and aromatherapy.

References

Abraham, M., Sarada Devi, N., Sheela, R. (1979) Inhibiting effect of Jasmine flowers on lactation. *Indian J. Med. Res.*, **69**, 88–92.

Ackerman, D. (1990) *A Natural History of the Senses*, Chapmans, London.

Acolet, D., Modi, N., Giannakoulopoulos, X. *et al.* (1993) Changes in plasma cortisol and catecholamine concentrations in response to massage in preterm infants. *Arch. Dis. Child.*, **68**(1 Suppl), 29–31.

Aguilera, D. (1967) The relationship between physical contact and verbal interaction between nurses and patients. *J. Psychiat. Nurs.*, **5**, 5–21.

Albert-Puleo, M. (1980) Fennel and anise as estrogenic agents. *J. Ethnopharmacol.*, **2**(4), 337–344.

al-Hader, A. A., Hasan, Z. A. and Aqel, M. B. (1994) Hyperglycemic and insulin release inhibitory effects of Rosmarinus officinalis. *J. Ethnopharmacol.*, **43**(3), 217–221.

Altman, J., Das, G. D., Anderson, W. J. and Wallace, R. B. (1968) Behaviorally induced changes in the length of cerebrum in rats. *Devel. Psychobiol.*, **1**(2), 112–117.

Altman, J., Das, G. D. and Anderson, W. J. (1968) Effects of infantile handling on morphological development of the rat brain: an exploratory study. *Devel. Psychobiol.*, **1**(1), 10–20.

Aqel, M. B. (1991) Relaxant effect of the volatile oil of Rosmarinus officinalis on tracheal smooth muscle. *J. Ethnopharmacol.*, **33**(1–2), 57–62.

Aqel, M. B. (1992) A vascular smooth muscle relaxant effect of *Rosmarinus officinalis*. *Int. J. Pharmacol.*, **30**(4), 281–288.

Arkko, P. J., Pakarinen, A.J. and Kari-Koskinen, O. (1983) Effects of whole body massage on serum protein, electrolyte and hormone concentrations, enzyme activities and hematological parameters. *Int. J. Sports Med.*, **4**, 265–267.

Arnould-Taylor, W. E. (1981) *Aromatherapy for the Whole Person*, Stanley Thornes, Cheltenham.

Arnould-Taylor, W. E. (1992) *A Textbook of Holistic Aromatherapy*, Stanley Thornes, Cheltenham.

Autton, N. (1989) *Touch: An Exploration*, Darton, Longman & Todd, London.

Baker, R. T. and Smith, H. G. (1920) *A Research on the Eucalyptus*, Government of New South Wales, Sydney, Australia.

Balacs, T. (1991) Essential issues. *Int. J. Aromather.*, **3**(4), 23–25.

Balacs T. (1992) Peppermint pharmacology. *Int. J. Aromather.*, **4**(2), 22–5.

Baldry, P. E. (1993). *Acupuncture, Trigger Points and Musculoskeletal Pain,*

Churchill Livingstone, Edinburgh.

Balke, B., Anthony, J. and Wyatt, F. (1989) The effects of massage treatment on exercise fatigue. *Clin. Sports Med.*, **1**, 189–196.

Barnett, K. (1972) A survey of the current utilization of touch by health team personnel with hospitalized patients. *Int. J. Nurs. Studies*, **9**, 195–209.

Barr, J. S. and Taslitz, N. (1970) The influence of back massage on autonomic functions. *Physical Ther.*, **50**(12), 1679–1691.

Barsoum, G., Perry, E. P. and Fraser, I. A. (1990) Postoperative nausea is relieved by acupressure. *J. Roy. Soc. Med.*, **83**(2), 86–89.

Bassett, I. B, Pannowitz, D. L. and Barnetson, R. S. (1990) A comparative study of tea-tree oil versus benzoylperoxide in the treatment of acne. *Med. J. Aust.*, **153**(8), 455–458.

Bauer, W.C. and Dracup, K. A. (1987) Physiologic effects of back massage in patients with acute myocardial infarction. *Focus Crit. Care*, **14**(6), 42–46.

Beck, M. (1988). *The Theory and Practice of Therapeutic Massage*, Milady, New York.

Becroft, D. M. and Gunn, T. R. (1989) Prenatal cranial haemorrhages in 47 Pacific Islander infants: is traditional massage the cause? *N. Z. Med. J.*, **102**(867), 207–210.

Bell, A. J. (1964) Massage and the physiotherapist. *Physiotherapy*, **50**, 406–408.

Bell, G. D. and Doran, J. (1979) Gallstones dissolution in man using an essential oil preparation. *Br. Med. J.*, **i**, 24.

Bell, L. (1992) Looking at the effects of two different essential oils, lavender and geranium, compared to a carrier oil only. Unpublished MS, Louise Bell, Southend Hospital, Essex, UK.

Belluomini, J., Litt, R. C., Lee, K. A. and Katz, M. (1994) Acupressure for nausea and vomiting of pregnancy: a randomized, blinded study. *Obs. Gynecol.*, **84**(2), 245–248.

Benson, H. (1988) *The Relaxation Response*, Collins, London.

Berger, H., Jarosch, E. and Madreiter W. (1978a) Effect of VapoRub and petrolatum on frequency and amplitude of breathing in children with acute bronchitis. *J. Int. Med. Res.*, **6**, 483–486.

Berger, H., Jarosch, E. and Madreiter W. (1978b) Effects of VapoRub and petrolatum on restlessness in children with acute bronchitis. *J. Int. Med. Res.*, **6**, 491–493.

Berger, H., Orgler, W., Jarosch, E. and Madreiter W. (1978) Effect of VapoRub and petrolatum on skin and rectal temperature in children with acute bronchitis. *J. Int. Med. Res.*, **6**, 487–490.

Bernstein, L. (1957) The effects of variation in handling upon learning and retention. *J. Comp. Physiol. Psychol.*, **50**, 162–167.

Beylier, M. F. (1979) Bacteriostatic activity of some Australian essential oils. *Perfumer Flavorist*, **4**(2), 23–25.

Bierman, W. (1960) Influence of cycloid vibration massage on trunk flexion. *Am. J. Phys. Med.*, **39**, 219–224.

Bilsland, D. and Strong, A. (1990) Allergic contact dermatitis from the essential oil of French marigold (Tagetes patula) in an aromatherapist. *Contact Dermatitis*, **23**(1), 55–56.

Boone, T., Cooper, R. and Thompson, W. R. (1991) A physiological evaluation of the sports massage. *Athletic Training*, **26**, 51–54.

Bordia, P. *et al.* (1990) Responsiveness to olfactory stimuli presented in sleep.

Physiol. Behav., **48**, 87–90.

Bork, K., Korting, G. W. and Faust, G. (1972) Increase of certain serum enzyme levels (GOT, LDH, CPK, MK) after body massage and its significance in dermatomyositis. *Klin. Wochenschr.*, **50**(6), 332–333.

Bouhlal, K. *et al.* (1989) The cutaneous effects of the common concretes and absolutes used in the perfume industry. *J. Essential Oil Res.*, **1**, 169–195.

Boyd, E. M. and Hicks, R. N. (1955) Anethole and respiratory tract fluid. *Fed. Proc.*, **14**, 321.

Boyd, E. M. and Pearson, G. L. (1946) On the expectorant action of volatile oils. *Am. J. Med. Sci.*, **211**, 602–610.

Boyd, E. M. and Sheppard, E. P. (1966) Friar's Balsam and respiratory tract fluid. *Am. J. Dis. Child.*, **111**, 630–634.

Boyd, E. M. and Sheppard, E. P. (1968) The effect of steam inhalation of volatile oils on the output and composition of respiratory tract fluid. *J. Pharmacol. Exp. Therap.*, **163**(1), 250–256.

Boyd, E. M. and Sheppard, E. P. (1970) The effect of inhalation of citral and geraniol on the output and composition of respiratory tract fluid. *Arch. Int. Pharmacodyn. Ther.*, **188**, 5–13.

Bräunig, B., Dorn, M. and Knick, E. (1992) Echinaceae purpureae radix: zur Stärkung der körpereigenen Abwehr bei grippalen Infekten. *Z. Phytotherapie*, **13**(1), 7–13.

Bright, T., Bittick, K. and Fleeman, B. (1981) Reduction of self-injurious behavior using sensory-integrative techniques. *Am. J. Occup. Ther.*, **35**, 167–172.

Brocklehurst-Woods, J. (1990) The use of tactile and vestibular stimulation to reduce stereotypic behaviors in two adults with mental retardation. *Am. J. Occup. Ther.*, **44**(6), 536–541.

Bronough, R. L. (1990) In vivo percutaneous absorbtion of fragrance ingredients in rhesus monkeys and humans. *Food Chem. Toxicol.*, **28**(5), 369–374.

Buchbauer, G., Jirovetz, L., Jäger, W. *et al.* (1993) Fragrance compounds and essential oils with sedative effects upon inhalation. *J. Pharm. Sci.*, **82**(6), 660–664.

Buck, D. S., Nidorf, D. M. and Addino, J. G. (1994) Comparison of two topical preparations for the treatment of onychomycosis: *Melaleuca alternifolia* (tea tree) oil and clotrimazole. *J. Fam. Practice*, **38**(6), 601–605.

Buckle, J. (1993) Aromatherapy: Does it matter which lavender oil is used? *Nurs. Times*, **89**(20), 32–35.

Burnside, I. (1973) Touching is talking. *Am. J. Nurs.* 2060–2063.

Cafarelli, E., Sim, J., Carolan, B. and Liebesman, J. (1990) Vibratory massage and short-term recovery from muscular fatigue. *Int. J. Sports Med.*, **11**(6), 474–478.

Calabrese, J. *et al.* (1987) Alterations in immunocompetence during stress, bereavement, and depression: focus on neuroendocrine regulation. *Am. J. Psychiat.*, **144**, 1123–1134.

Cannard, G. (1993) A study on the effectiveness of aromatherapy for sleep disturbances in the elderly. Unpublished MS, available from the author.

Cardwell-Brown, C. (ed.) (1984) *The Many Facets of Touch*, Johnson & Johnson Baby Products Co., Pediatric Round Table Series.

Carson, C. F. and Riley, T. V. (1993) Antimicrobial activity of the essential oil of *Melaleuca alternifolia*. *Lett. Appl. Microbiol.*, **16**(2), 49–55.

Carson, C. F. and Riley, T. V. (1994) The antimicrobial activity of tea tree oil. *Med.*

J. Aust., **160**(4), 236.

Cassidy, J. D., Lopes, A. A. and Yong-Hing, K. (1992) The immediate effect of manipulation versus mobilization on pain and range of motion in the cervical spine: a randomized controlled trial. *J. Manipulative Physiol. Therapeut.*, **15**(9), 570–575.

Chadha, A. and Madyastha, K. M. (1984) Metabolism of geraniol and linalool in the rat and effects on liver and lung microsomal enzymes. *Xenobiotica*, **14**(5), 365–374.

Chaitow, L. (1988) *Soft Tissue Manipulation*, Thorsons, Wellingborough.

Chalchat, J. C. *et al.* (1993) Essential oils of rosemary (*Rosmarinus officinalis L.*). The chemical composition of oils of various origins (Morocco, Spain, France). *J. Essential Oil Res.*, **5**, 613–618.

Chalmers, I. and Altman, D. G. (eds). (1995) *Systematic reviews*, BMJ Publishing, London.

Chialva, F. *et al.* (1982) Qualitative evaluation of aromatic herbs by direct headspace GC analysis. *J. High Res. Chromat. Commun.*, **5**(4), 182–188.

Chien, Y. W. (ed.) (1985) *Transnasal Systemic Medications*, Elsevier, Oxford.

Clegg, R. J., Middleton, B., Bell, G. D. and White, D. A. (1980) Inhibition of hepatic cholesterol synthesis and S-3-hydroxy-3-methylglutaryl-CoA reductase by mono and bicyclic monoterpenes administered *in vivo*. *Biochem. Pharmacol.*, **29**(15), 2125–2127.

Coates, T. J., McKusic, L., Kuno, R. and Stites, D. P. (1989) Stress reduction training changed number of sexual partners but not immune function in men with HIV. *Am. J. Public Health*, **79**, 855–857.

Cohen, B. M. (1982) Acute aromatics inhalation modifies the airways effects of the common cold. *Respiration*, **43**, 285–293.

Collins, A. J., Notarianni, L. J., Ring, E. F. and Seed, M. P. (1984) Some observations on the pharmacology of 'Deep-Heat', a topical rubefacient. *Ann. Rheum. Dis.*, **43**(3), 411–415.

Cordland, D. K. and Mason, W. A. (1968) Infant monkey heart rate: habituation and effects of social substitutes. *Dev. Psychobiol.*, **1**(4), 254–256.

Corley, M. C., Ferriter, J., Zeh, J. and Gifford, C. (1995) Physiological and psychological effects of back rubs. *Appl. Nurs. Res.*, **8**(1), 39–42.

Cornelius, W. L., Ebrahim, K., Watson, J. and Hill, D. W. (1992)The effects of cold application and modified PNF stretching techniques on hip joint flexibility in college males. *Res. Q Exercise Sport*, **63**(3), 311–314.

Corner, J., Cawley, N. and Hildebrand S. (1995) An evaluation of the use of massage and essential oils on the wellbeing of cancer patients. *Int. J. Palliative Nurs.*, **1**(2), 67–73.

Cornwell, P. A. and Barry, B. W. (1994) Sesquiterpene components of volatile oils as skin penetration enhancers for the hydrophilic permeant 5-fluorouracil. *J. Pharm. Pharmacol.*, **46**(4), 261–269.

Cottingham, J. T., Porges, S. W. and Richmond, K. (1988) Shifts in pelvic inclination angle and parasympathetic tone produced by Rolfing soft tissue manipulation. *Physical Ther.*, **68**(9), 1364–1370.

Cottingham, J. T., Porges, S. W. and Lyon, T. (1988) Effects of soft tissue mobilization (Rolfing pelvic lift) on parasympathetic tone in two age groups. *Physical Ther.*, **68**(3), 352–356.

Coward, R. (1989). *The Whole Truth: The Myth of Alternative Medicine*, Faber & Faber, London.

Crosman, L. J., Chateauvert, S. R. and Weisberg, J. (1984) The effects of massage to the hamstring muscle group on range of motion. *J. Orthopaed Sports Physical Ther.*, **Nov/Dec**, 168–172.

Cullition, B. J. (1987) Take two pets and call me in the morning. *Science*, **237**(4822),1560–1561.

Cyriax, J. (1985) Clinical applications of massage, in *Manipulation, Traction and Massage*, (ed. J. V. Basmajian), Williams & Wilkins, Baltimore, MD.

Dale, A. and Cornwell S. (1994) The role of lavender oil in relieving perineal discomfort following childbirth: a blind, randomised clinical trial. *J. Adv. Nurs.*, **19**, 89–96.

Danneskiold-Samsoe, B., Christiansen, E., Lund, B. and Anderson, R. B. (1982) Regional muscle tension and pain ('fibrositis'). Effect of massage on myoglobin in plasma. *Scand. J. Rehab. Med.*, **15**, 17–20.

Danneskiold-Samsoe, B., Christiansen, E. and Bach Andersen, R. (1986) Myofascial pain and the role of myoglobin. *Scand. J. Rheumatol.*, **15**(2), 174–178.

Davis, P. (1988) *Aromatherapy: An A–Z*, C. W. Daniel, Saffron Walden.

Davis, P. (1991) *Subtle Aromatherapy*, C. W. Daniel, Saffron Walden.

Davis, P. (1994) A healing partnership. *Int. J. Alt. Comp. Med.*, **12**(4), 9–12 (reprinted from *Aromather. Q.*).

Day, J. A., Mason, R. R. and Chesrown, S. E. (1987) Effect of massage on serum level of beta-endorphin and beta-lipotropin in healthy adults. *Physical Ther.*, **67**(6), 926–930.

De Aloysio, D., Penacchioni P. (1992) Morning sickness control in early pregnancy by Neiguan point acupressure. *Obs. Gynecol.* **80**(5), 852–4.

Deans, S. G. and Svoboda, K. P. (1990) The antimicrobial properties of marjoram (*Origanum marjorana* L.) volatile oil. *Flavour Fragrance J.*, **5**(3), 187–190.

Debelmas, A. M. and Rochat, J. (1967) Etude pharmacologique des huiles essentielles. Activité antispasmodique étudiée sur une cinquantaine d'échantillons différents. *Plantes Médicinales Phytothér.*, **1**, 23–27.

De Blasi, V., Debrot, S., Menoud, P. A. *et al.* (1990) Amoebicidal effect of essential oils *in vitro*. *J. Toxicol. Clin. Exp.*, **10**(6), 361–373.

Deethardt, J. F. and Hines, D. G. (1983) Tactile communication and personality differences. *J. Nonverbal Behav.*, **8**, 143–156.

De Groot, A. C. and Weyland, J. W. (1992) Systemic Contact Dermatitis from tea tree oil. *Contact Dermatitis*, **27**(4), 279–280.

DeLuze, C., Bosia, L., Zirbs, A. *et al.* (1992) Electroacupuncture in fibromyalgia: results of a controlled trial. *Br. Med. J.*, **305**(6864), 1249–1252.

Dew, M., Evans, B. J. and Rhodes, J. (1984) Peppermint oil for the irritable bowel syndrome: a multicentre trial. *Br. J. Clin. Prac.*, **38**, 45–48.

DeWever, M. K. (1977) Nursing home patients' perception of nurses' affective touching. *J. Psychol.*, **96**, 163–171.

Dicke, E. *et al.* (eds) (1978) *A Manual of Reflexive Therapy of the Connective Tissues*, Sidney S. Simon, Sarsdale, NY.

Dickson, P. R. (1984) Effect of a fleecy woollen underlay on sleep. *Med. J. Aust.*, **140**, 87–89.

Dickstein, R., Hocherman, S., Pillar, T. and Shaham, R. (1986) Stroke rehabilitation. Three exercise therapy approaches. *Physical Ther.*, **66**(8), 1233–1238.

Diliberto, J. J., Srinivas, P., Overstreet, D. *et al.* (1990) Metabolism of citral, an alpha,beta-unsaturated aldehyde, in male F344 rats. *Drug Metab.*

Disposition, **18**(6), 866–875.

Diliberto, J. J., Usha, G. and Birnbaum, L. S. (1988) Disposition of citral in male Fischer rats. *Drug Metab. Disposition* **16**(5), 721–727.

Doran, J., Keighley, M. R. B. and Bell, G. D. (1979) Rowachol – a possible treatment for cholesterol gallstones. *Gut*, **20**, 312.

Dorland, G. J. (1993) *Scents Appeal: The Silent Persuasion of Aromatic Encounters*, Wayne Dorland Co, Mendham, NJ.

Dossetor, D. R., Couryer, S. and Nicol, A. R. (1991) Massage for very severe self-injurious behaviour in a girl with Cornelia de Lange syndrome. *Dev. Med. Child Neurol.*, **33**(7), 636–640.

Downing, G. (1974) *The Massage Book*, Penguin, Harmondsworth.

Drescher, V. M., Gantt, W. H. and Whitehead, W. E. (1980) Heart rate response to touch. *Psychosomatic Med.*, **42**(6), 559–565.

Drews, T., Kreider, R. B., Drinkard, B. *et al.* (1990) Effects of post event massage therapy on repeated endurance cycling. *Int. J. Sports Med.*, **11**, 407.

Dube, S., Upadhyay, P. D. and Tripath, S. C. (1989) Antifungal, physiochemical and insect-repelling activity of the essential oil of *Ocimum basilicum*. *Can. J. Botany*, **67**(7), 2085–2087.

Duncan, S. (1969) Nonverbal communication. *Psychol. Bull.*, **72**, 118–137.

Dundee, J. W., Sourial, F. B., Ghaly, R. G. and Bell, P. F. (1988) P6 acupressure reduces morning sickness. *J. Roy. Soc. Med.*, **81**(8), 456–457.

Dunn, C., Sleep, J. and Collett, D. (1995) Sensing an improvement: an experimental study to evaluate the use of aromatherapy, massage and periods of rest in an intensive care unit. *J. Adv. Nurs.*, **21**(1), 34–40.

Ebner, M. (1985). *Connective Tissue Manipulations*, Robert E. Kreiger, Florida.

Ehrlichman, H. and Halpern, J. N. (1988) Affect and memory: effects of pleasant and unpleasant odors on retrieval of happy and unhappy memories. *J. Personality Social Psychol.*, **55**, 769–779.

Eichelberger, G. (1993) Study on foot reflex zone massage. Alternative to tablets. *Krankenpflege – Soins Infirmiers*, **86**(5), 61–63.

Eisenberg, D. M., Kessler, R. C., Foster, C *et al.* (1993) Unconventional medicine in the United States: prevalence, costs, and patterns of use. *N. Engl. J. Med.*, **328**(4), 246–252.

Ek, A. C., Gustavsson, G. and Lewis, D. H. (1985) The local skin blood flow in areas at risk for pressure sores treated with massage. *Scand. J. Rehab. Med.*, **17**(2), 81–86.

Elkins, E. C., Herrick, J. F., Grindlay, J. H *et al.* (1963) Effect of various procedures on the flow of lymph. *Arch. Physical Med.*, **34**, 31–39.

Ellis, W. R. and Bell, G. D. (1981a) Treatment of biliary duct stones with a terpene preparation. *Br. Med. J.*, **282**, 611.

Ellis, W. R. *et al.* (1980) Radio-opaque gallstones – reduction in size and calcium content on treatment with Rowachol. *Gut*, **21**, 910.

Ellis, W. R. *et al.* (1981b) Mechanisms for adjuvant cholelitholytic properties of the monoterpene *Rowachol*. *Clin. Sci.*, **61**, 38.

Ellis, W. R. *et al.* (1984) Pilot study of combination treatment for gallstones with medium dose chenodeoxycholic acid and a terpene preparation. *Br. Med. J.*, **289**, 153–156.

Ellison, M., Goehrs, C., Hall, L. *et al.* (1992) Effect of retrograde massage on muscle soreness and performance. *Physical Ther.*, **72**, 100.

Elson, C. E., Underbakke, G. L., Hanson, P. *et al.* (1989) Impact of lemongrass oil, an essential oil, on serum cholesterol. *Lipids*, **24**(8), 677–679.

Eltze, C. H., Hildebrandt, G. and Johanson, M. (1982) Uber die Wirksamkeit der Vibrationsmassage beim Muskelkater. *Z. Phys. Med. Balm Med. Klimatol.*, **11**, 366–376.

Endresen, I. M. *et al.*(1987) Psychological stress factors and concentration of immunoglobulins and components in Norwegian nurses. *Work Stress*, **1**, 365–375.

Engelstein, D., Kahan, E. and Servadio, C. (1992) Rowatinex for the treatment of ureterolithiasis. *J. Urologie*, **98**(2), 98–100.

England, A. (1993) *Aromatherapy for Mother and Baby*, Vermilion, London.

Ernst, E., Matrai, A., Magyarosy, I. *et al.* (1987) Massages cause changes in blood fluidity. *Physiotherapy*, **73**(1), 43–47.

Estabrooks, C. A. (1989) Touch: a nursing strategy in the intensive care unit. *Heart Lung*, **18**(4), 392–401.

Etnyre, B. R. and Abraham, L. D. (1986a) Gains in range of ankle dorsiflexion using three popular stretching techniques. *Am. J. Physical Med.*, **65**(4), 189–196.

Etnyre, B. R. and Abraham, L. D. (1986b) H-reflex changes during static stretching and two variations of proprioceptive neuromuscular facilitation techniques. *Electroencephalog. Clin. Neurophysiol.*, **63**(2), 174–179.

Evonuk, G. E., Kuhn, C. M. and Schanberg, S. M. (1979) The effect of tactile stimulation on serum growth hormone and tissue ornithine decarboxylase activity during maternal deprivation in rat pups. *Comm. Psychopharmacol.*, 363–70.

Eyerman, K. (1987) *Massage*, Sidgwick & Jackson, London.

Eysenck, H. (1988) Personality, stress and cancer prediction and prophylaxis. *Br. J. Med. Psychol.*, **61**, 57–75.

Fakouri, C. and Jones P. (1987) Relaxation RX: slow stroke back rub. *J. Gerontol. Nurs.*, **13**(2), 32–35.

Falk, A. *et al.* (1990) Uptake, distribution and elimination of alphapinene in man after exposure by inhalation. *Scand. J. Work Environ. Health*, **16**, 372–378.

Falk-Filipsson, A. (1993) D-limonene exposure to humans by inhalation: uptake, distribution, elimination and effects on the pulmonary system. *J. Toxicol. Environ. Health*, **38**, 77–88.

Fang, H. J., Su, X. L., Liu, H. Y. *et al.* (1989) Studies on the chemical components and anti tumour action of the volatile oils from *Pelargonium graveolens*. *Yao Hsueh Hsueh Pao*, **24** (5), 366–371.

Ferguson, H. C. (1966) Effect of red cedar chip bedding on hexobarbital and pentobarbital sleep time. *J. Pharm. Sci.*, **55**, 1142.

Ferley, J. P., Poutignat, N., Zmirou, D. *et al.* (1989) Prophylactic aromatherapy for supervening infections in patients with chronic bronchitis. Statistical evaluation conducted in clinics against a placebo. *Phytother. Res.*, (3), 97–100.

Fernandez, D. (1988) Immunocompetence during stress. *Am. J. Psychiat.*, **145**, 536–537.

Ferrell-Torry, A. T. and Glick, O. J. (1993) The use of therapeutic massage as a nursing intervention to modify anxiety and the perception of cancer pain. *Cancer Nurs.*, **16**(2), 93–101.

Field, T. (1980) Supplemental stimulation of preterm neonates. *Early Hum. Dev.*, **4**, 301–314.

Field, T. (1990) Alleviating stress in newborn infants in the intensive care unit. *Clinics Perinatol.*, **17**(1), 1–9.

Field, T., Morrow, C., Valdeon, C. *et al.* (1992) Massage reduces anxiety in child and adolescent psychiatric patients. *J. Am. Acad. Child Adolesc. Psychol.*, **31**(1), 125–131.

Field, T., Scafidi, F. and Schanberg S. (1987) Massage of preterm newborns to improve growth and development. *Paediat. Nurs.*, **13**(6), 385–387.

Field, T. M., Schanberg, S. M., Scafidi, F. *et al.* (1986) Tactile/kinesthetic stimulation effects on preterm neonates. *Pediatrics*, **77**(5), 654–658.

Finkelstein, P., Yost, K. G. and Grossman, E. (1990) Mechanical devices versus antimicrobial rinses in plaque and gingivitis reduction. *Clin. Prevent. Dent.*, **12**(3), 8–11.

Fisher, J. D., Rything, M. and Heslin, P. (1976). Hands touching hands: affective and evaluative effects of an interpersonal touch. *Sociometry*, **31**, 416–421.

Fischer-Rizzi, S. (1990) *Complete Aromatherapy Handbook: Essential Oils for Radiant Health*, Sterling Publishing, New York.

Flowers, K. R. (1988) String wrapping versus massage for reducing digital volume. *Physical Ther.*, **68**(1), 57–59.

Formacek, V. and Kubeczka, K. H. (1982) *Essential Oils Analysis by Capillary Gas Chromatography and Carbon-13 NMR Spectroscopy*, John Wiley, Chichester.

Fornell, J., Sundin, Y. and Lindhe, J. (1975) Effect of Listerine on dental plaque and gingivitis. *Scand. J. Dent. Res.*, **83**, 18–23.

Forsythe. E. (1988). *Multiple Sclerosis: Exploring Sickness and Health*, Faber & Faber, London.

Fraser, J. and Kerr, J. R. (1993) Psychophysiological effects of back massage on elderly institutionalized patients. *J. Adv. Nurs.*, **18**(2), 238–245.

Freeman, E. (1969) The effects of interpesonal stimulation on growth and development of premature infants. Unpublished PhD thesis, University of Florida.

Freeman, L. (1987) Expanding the investigation and treatment modalities in a cardiology department. *Complementary Med. Res.*, **2**(2), 161–167.

Fuller, J. L. (1967) Experiential deprivation and later behaviour. *Science*, **158**, 1645–1652.

Gabbrielli, G., Loggini, F., Cioni, P. L. *et al.* (1988) Activity of lavandino essential oil against non-tubercular opportunistic rapidly grown Mycobacteria. *Pharmacol. Res. Commun.*, **20**(5), 37–40.

Gershbein, L. L. (1977) Regeneration of rat liver in the presence of essential oils and their components. *Food Cosmetics Toxicol.*, **15**, 173–181.

Getchell, T. V., Doty, R. L., Bartoshuk, L. M. and Snow, J. B. (1991) *Smell and Taste in Health and Disease*, Raven Press, New York.

Giachetti, D., Taddei, E. and Taddei, I. (1988) Pharmacological activity of essential oils on Oddi's sphincter. *Planta Med.*, **54**(5), 389–392.

Gieron, C., Wieland, B., von der Laage, D. and Tolksdorf, W. (1993) Acupressure in the prevention of postoperative nausea and vomiting. *Anaesthetist*, **42**(4), 221–226.

Ginsberg, F. and Famaey, J. P. (1987) A double blind study of topical massage with rado-salil ointment in mechanical low back pain. *J. Int. Med. Res.*, **15**, 148–153.

Glick, M. S. (1986) Caring touch and anxiety in myocardial infarction patients in the intermediate cardiac care unit. *Intensive Care Nurs.*, **2**, 61–66.

Göbel, H., Schmidt ,G. and Soyka, D. (1994) Effect of peppermint and eucalyptus oil preparations on neurophysiological and experimental algesimetric headache parameters. *Cephalalgia, 14*(3), 228–234.

Goldberg, J., Sullivan, S. J. and Seaborne, D. E. (1992) The effect of two intensities of massage on H-reflex amplitude. *Physical Ther., 72*(6), 449–457.

Goldberg, J., Seaborne, D. E., Sullivan, S. J. and Leduc, B. E. (1994) The effect of therapeutic massage on H-reflex amplitude in persons with a spinal cord injury. *Physical Ther., 74*(8), 728–737.

Gomez, E. T. and Turner, C. W. (1939) The effect of anol on the growth of the mammary gland. *Am. J. Cancer, 37*, 108–113.

Goodykoontz, L. (1979) Touch: attitudes and practice. *Nurs. Forum, 18*, 4–17.

Gordon, J. M., Lamster, I. B. and Seiger, M. C. (1985) Efficacy of Listerine antiseptic in inhibiting the development of plaque and gingivitis. *J. Clin. Periodontol., 12*, 697–704.

Gorski, P. A. *et al.* (1984) Caring for immature infants – a touchy subject, in *The Many Facets of Touch*, (ed. C. Cardwell-Brown), Johnson & Johnson Baby Products Company, Pediatric Round Table Series.

Gottfried, A. W. (1984) Touch as an organizer for learning and development, in *The Many Facets of Touch*, (ed. C. Cardwell-Brown), Johnson & Johnson Baby Products Company, Pediatric Round Table Series.

Grayson, J. (1993) *The Fragrant Year: Seasonal Meditations with Aromatherapy Oils*, Aquarian/Thorsons, London.

Green, R. G., Green, M. L. (1987) Relaxation increases salivary immunoglobulin A. *Psychol. Rep., 61*(2), 623–629.

Greenberg, B. M. (1972) Therapeutic effects of touch on alteration of psychotic behaviour in institutionalized elderly patients. Unpublished MSc Thesis, Duke University, North Carolina.

Groër, M., Mozingo, J., Droppleman, P. *et al.* (1994) Measures of salivary secretory immunoglobulin A and state anxiety after a nursing back rub. *Appl. Nurs. Res., 7*(1), 2–6.

Guillemain, J., Rousseau, A. and Delaveau, P. (1989) Neurodepressive effects of the essential oil of *Lavandula angustifolia* Mill. *Ann. Pharmaceut. Françaises, 47*(6), 337–343.

Hammerschmidt, F. J., Clark, A. M., Soliman, F. M. *et al.* (1993) Chemical composition and antimicrobial activity of essential oils of *Jasonia candicans* and *J. montana*. *Planta Med., 59*(1), 68–70.

Hanau, P. *et al.* (1983) The influence of limonene on induced delayed hypersensitivity to citral in guinea pigs. *Acta Dermato Venereol., 63*, 1–7.

Hansen, T. I. and Kristensen, J. H. (1973) Effect of massage, shortwave diathermy and ultrasound upon ^{133}Xe disappearance rate from muscle and subcutaneous tissue in the human calf. *Scand. J. Rehab. Med., 5*(4), 179–182.

Hanten, W. P. and Chandler, S. D. (1994) Effects of myofascial release leg pull and sagittal plane isometric contract–relax techniques on passive straight-leg raise angle. J. Orthopaed Sports *Physical Ther., 20*(3), 138–144.

Hardy, M. (1991) Sweet scented dreams. *Int. J. Aromather., 3*(1), 12–13.

Harlow, H. F. and Zimmermann, R. R. (1958) The development of affectional responses in infant monkeys. *Proc. Am. Philos. Soc., 102*, 501–509.

Harmer, P. A. (1991) The effects of pre-performance massage on stride frequency in sprinters. *Athletic Training, 26*, 55–59.

Harris, B. and Lewis, R. (1994) The use of massage and touch in stress management. *Int. J. Alt. Complement. Med.*, **4**, 12.

Hasselmeyer, E. G. (1964) The premature neonate's response to handling. *J. Am. Nurses Assoc.*, **2**, 14–15.

Hawthorn, M. *et al.* (1988) The actions of peppermint oil and menthol on calcium channel dependent processes in intestinal, neuronal and cardiac preparations. *Aliment. Pharmacol. Ther.*, **2**, 108–118.

Helders, P. J., Cats, B. P. and Debast, S. (1989) Effects of a tactile stimulation/range-finding programme on the development of VLBW-neonates during the first year of life. *Child: Care Health Devel.*, **15**(6), 369–380.

Henley, G. (1973) Status and sex. *Bull. Psychosom. Soc.*, **2**, 91–93.

Henneman, E. (1989) The effect of nursing contact on the stress response of patients being weaned from mechanical ventilation. *Heart Lung*, **18**(5), 483–489.

Herskovitz, S., Strauch, B. and Gordon, M. J. (1992) Shiatsu massage-induced injury of the median recurrent motor branch. *Muscle Nerve*, **15**(10), 1215.

Hills, J. M. and Aaronson, P. I. (1991) The mechanism of action of peppermint oil on gastrointestinal smooth muscle. An analysis using patch clamp electrophysiology and isolated tissue pharmacology in rabbit and guinea pig. *Gastroenterology*, **101**(1), 55–65.

Hirsjarvi, P. A., Junnila, M. A. and Valiaho, T. U. (1990) Gentled and non-handled rates in a stressful open-field situation; differences in performance. *Scand. J. Psychol.*, **31**(4), 259–265.

Hoefler, C., Fleurentin, J., Mortier, D. *et al.* (1987) Comparative choleretic and hepatoprotective properties of young sprouts and total plant extracts of *Rosmarinus officinalis* in rats. *J. Ethnopharmacol.*, **19**(2), 133–143.

Hollis, M. (1987) *Massage for Therapists*, Blackwell, Oxford.

Hopkins, C. (1991) *The Joy of Aromatherapy*, Harper-Collins, London.

Houghton, P. (1994) *Valerian. Pharm. J.*, **252**(6798), 95–96.

Hovind, H. and Nielsen, S. L. (1974) Effect of massage on blood flow in skeletal muscle. *Scand. J. Rehab. Med.*, **6**(2), 74–77.

Igima, H. *et al.* (1976) The use of D-limonene preparation as a dissolving agent of gallstones. *Dig. Dis.*, **21**, 926–939.

Igima, H. *et al.* (1991) Medical dissolution of gallstones. *Dig. Dis. Sci.*, **36**(2), 200–208.

Inkeles, G. (1977) *The Art of Sensual Massage*, Unwin, London.

Inkeles, G. (1980) *The New Massage*, Unwin, London.

International School of Aromatherapy (1993) *A Safety Guide on the Use of Essential Oils*, Natural by Nature, London.

Jacobs, M. R. and Hornfeldt, C. S. (1994) Melaleuca oil poisoning. *J. Toxicol. Clin. Toxicol.*, **32**(4), 461–464.

Jäger, W., Buchbauer, G., Jirovetz, L. and Fritzer, M. (1992a) Percutaneous absorption of lavender oil from a massage oil. *J. Soc. Cosmet. Chem.*, **43**, 49–54.

Jäger, W. *et al.* (1992b) Evidence of the sedative effect of neroli oil, citronellal and phenylethyl acetate on mice. *J. Essential Oil Res.*, **4**, 387–394.

Janssen, A. M., Scheffer, J. J. and Svendsen, A. B. (1987) Antimicrobial activity of essential oils: 1976–1986 literature review. Aspects of the test methods. *Planta Med.*, **53**(5), 395–398.

Janssens, J., Laekeman, G. M., Pieters, L. A. *et al.* (1990) Nutmeg oil: identification and quantitation of its most active constituents as inhibitors of platelet aggregation. *J. Ethnopharmacol.*, **29**(2), 179–188.

Jellinek, J. S. (1994) Aroma-chology: a status review. *Cosmet. Toiletries Mag.*, **109**, 83–101.

Jirovetz, L., Buchbauer, G. *et al.* (1992) Analysis of fragrance compounds in blood samples of mice by gas chromatography, mass spectrometry, GC/FTIR and GS/AES after inhalation of sandalwood oil. *Biomed. Chromatog.*, **6**(3), 133–134.

Joachim, G. (1983). Step by step massage techniques. *Can. Nurse*, **4 Dec**, 32–35.

Jori, A. *et al.* (1969) Effects of essential oils on drug metabolism. *Biochem. Pharmacol.*, **18**, 2081–2085.

Jori, A., Bianchetti, A., Prestini, P. E. and Gerattini, S. (1970) Effect of eucalyptol (1,8-cineole) on the metabolism of other drugs in rats and in man. *Eur. J. Pharmacol.*, **9**(3), 362–366.

Jourard, S. M. and Rubin, S. E. (1968) Self-disclosure and touching: a study of two modes of interpersonal encounter and their inter-relation. *J. Humanistic Psychol.*, **8**, 39–48.

Juhan, D. (1987) *Job's Body: A Handbook for Bodywork*, Station Hill Press, New York.

Juven, B. J., Kanner, J., Schved, F. and Weisslowicz, H. (1994) Factors that inter-act with the antibacterial action of thyme essential oil and its active con-stituents. *J. Appl. Bacteriol.*, **76**(6), 626–631.

Kaada, B. and Torsteinbo, O. (1987) Vasoactive intestinal polypeptides in con-nective tissue massage. *Gen. Pharmacol.*, **18**, 379–383.

Kaada, B. and Torsteinbo, O. (1989) Increase of plasma beta-endorphins in con-nective tissue. *Gen. Pharmacol.*, **20**(4), 487–489.

Kaba, H. and Keverne, E. B. (1988) The effects of microinfusions of drugs into the accessory olfactory-bulb on the olfactory block to pregnancy. *Neuro-science* **25**(3), 1007–1011.

Kanamura, A., Kawasaki, M., Indo, M. *et al.* (1988) Effects of odours on the con-tingent negative variation and the skin potential level. *Chem. Senses*, **13**, 326.

Karamat, E., Ilmberger, J., Buchbauer, G. *et al.* (1992) Excitatory and sedative effects of essential oils on human reaction time performance. *Chem. Senses*, **17**, 847.

Kattwinkel, J., Nearman, H. S., Fanaroff, A. A. *et al.* (1975). Apnea of pre-maturity: comparative therapeutic effects of cutaneous stimulation and nasal continuous positive airway pressure. *J. Pediat.*, **86**, 588–592.

Kaufman, M. A. (1964) Autonomic responses as related to nursing comfort measures. *Nurs. Res.*, **13**(1), 45–55.

Keeble, S. (1995a) *Experimental Research 1: An Introduction to Experimental Design*, Churchill Livingstone, Edinburgh.

Keeble, S. (1995b) *Experimental Research 2: Conducting and Reporting Experimental Research*, Churchill Livingstone, Edinburgh.

Kennel, J. H. *et al.* (1974) Maternal behavior one year after early and extended post-partum contact. *Dev. Med. Child Neurol.*, **16**, 172–179.

Kho, H. G., Kloppenborg, P. W. and van Egmond, J. (1993) Effects of acupunc-ture and transcutaneous stimulation analgesia on plasma hormone levels during and after major abdominal surgery. *Eur. J. Anaesthesiol.*, **10**(3), 197–208.

Kikuchi, A. *et al.* (1991) JASTS XXIV Abstract 7: Effect of odors on cardiac response patterns in a reaction time task. *Chem. Senses*, **16**(2), 183.

King, J. R. (1991) Anxiety reduction using fragrances, in *Perfumery: The Psychology and Biology of Fragrance*, (eds S. Van Toller and G. H. Dodd), Chapman & Hall, London.

Kirk-Smith, M. D. (1983) Unconscious odour conditioning in human subjects. *Biol. Psychol.*, **17**, 221–231.

Kisner, C. D. and Taslitz, N. (1968) Connective tissue massage: influence of the introductory treatment on autonomic functions. *Physical Ther.*, **48**(2), 107–119.

Klauser, A. G., Flaschentrager, J., Gehrke, A. and Muller-Lissner, S. A. (1992) Abdominal wall massage: effect on colonic function in healthy volunteers and in patients with chronic constipation. *Z. Gastroenterol.*, **30**(4), 247–251.

Knasko, S. C. (1992) Ambient odors effect on creativity, mood and perceived health. *Chem. Senses*, **17**(1), 27–35.

Knasko, S. C. (1993) Performance, mood and health during exposure to intermittent odors. *Arch. Environ. Health*, **48**(5), 3058.

Knasko, S. C., Gilbert, A. N. and Sabini, J. (1990) Emotional state, physical well-being and performance in the presence of feigned ambient odor. *J. Appl. Soc. Psychol.*, **20**, 1345–1347.

Knight, T. E. and Hausen, B. M. (1994) Melaleuca oil (tea tree oil) dermatitis. *J. Am. Acad. Dermatol.*, **30**(3), 423–427.

Knoblock, K. *et al.* (1989) Antibacterial and antifungal properties of essential oil components. *J. Essential Oil Res.*, **1**, 119–128.

Kodama, R., Inoue, H., Noda, K. *et al.* (1976) Effect of d-limonene and related compounds on bile flow and biliary lipid composition in rats and dogs. *Life Sci.*, **19**(10), 1559–1567.

Korting, H. C., Schafer-Korting, M., Hart, H. *et al.* (1993) Anti-inflammatory activity of hamamelis distillate applied topically to the skin. Influence of vehicle and dose. *Eur. J. Clin. Pharmacol.*, **44** (4), 315–318.

Kovar, K. A., Gropper, B., Friess, D. and Ammon, H. P. (1987) Blood levels of 1,8-cineole and locomotor activity of mice after inhalation and oral administration of rosemary oil. *Planta Med.*, **53**(4), 315–318.

Kraft, G. H., Fitts, S. S. and Hammond, M. C. (1992) Techniques to improve function of the arm and hand in chronic hemiplegia. *Arch. Physical Med. Rehab.*, **73**(3), 220–227.

Kuhn, C. M. *et al.* (1978) Selective depression of serum growth hormone during maternal deprivation in rat pups. *Science*, **201**, 1034–1036.

Kuhn, C. M., Schanberg, S. M., Field, T. *et al.* (1991) Tactile-kinesthetic stimulation effects on sympathetic and adrenocortical function in preterm infants. *J. Pediat.*, **119**(3), 434–440.

Lacroix, N. (1991) *Massage for Total Relaxation*, Dorling Kindersley, London.

Lafuente, A., Noguera, M., Puy, C. *et al.* (1990) Effekt der Reflexzonenbehandlung am Fuß bezuglich der prophylaktischen Behandlung mit Flunarizin bei an Cephalea-Kopfschmerzen leidenden Patienten. *Erfahrungsheilkunde*, **39**(11), 713–715.

Lake, M. (1989) *Scents and Sensuality: The Essence of Excitement*, John Murray, London.

Lallement-Guilbert, N. and Benzanger-Beauesne, L. (1970) Recherche sur les flavonoides de quelques labiées médicinales. *Plantes Médicinales Phytothér.*, **4**(2), 92–107.

Lamster, I. B., Alfano, M. C., Seiger, M. C. and Gordon, J. M. (1983) The effect of Listerine antiseptic on reduction of existing plaque and gingivitis. *Clin. Prevent. Dent.*, **5**, 12–16.

Langland, R. M. and Panicucci, E. (1982) Effects of touch on communication with elderly confused patients. *J. Gerontol. Nurs.*, **8**(3), 152–155.

Larsen, J. H. (1990) Infants' colic and belly massage. *Practitioner*, **234** (1487), 396–397.

Larsen, K. S. and Leroux, J. (1984) A study of same sex touching attitudes: scale development and personality predictors. *J. Sexual Res.*, **20**, 264–278.

Lautié, R. and Passebecq, A. (1979). *Aromatherapy: The Use of Plant Essences in Healing*, Thorsons, Wellingborough.

Lawless, J. (1994a) *Lavender Oil*, Thorsons, London.

Lawless, J. (1994b) *Aromatherapy and the Mind*, Thorsons, London.

Lech, Y., Olesen, K. M., Hey, H. *et al.* (1988) Treatment of irritable bowel syndrome with peppermint oil A double-blind study with a placebo. *Ugeskrift For Laeger.* **150**(40), 2388–9.

Leicester, R. J. and Hunt, R. H. (1982) Peppermint oil to reduce colonic spasm during endoscopy. *Lancet*, ii, 989.

Leuschner, M., Leuschner, U., Lazarovici, D. *et al.* (1988) Dissolution of gall stones with an ursodeoxyicholic acid menthol preparation: a controlled prospective double blind trial. *Gut*, **29**, 428–432.

Leuschner, U. *et al.* (1987) Methyl-tert-butyl-ether (MTBE) treatment of cholesterol stones: toxicity and dissolution of stone debris. *Gastroenterology*, **92**, 1750.

Levin, S. R. (1990). Acute effects of massage on the stress reponse. Unpublished MSc Thesis, University of North Carolina.

Levine, S. (1960) Stimulation in infancy. *Scientific Am.*, **202**, 81–86.

Licht, E. (1963) *Massage, Manipulation and Traction*, E. Licht, Connecticut.

Lidell, L. (1984) *The Book of Massage*, Ebury, London.

Lindahl, O. and Lindwall, L. (1989) Double blind study of a valerian preparation. *Pharmacol. Biochem. Behav.*, **32**(4), 1065–1066.

Linkous, L. W. and Stutts, R. M. (1990) Passive tactile stimulation effects on the muscle tone of hypotonic, developmentally delayed young children. *Perceptual Motor Skills*, **71**(3 Pt 1), 951–954.

Linsenmann, P. and Swoboda, M. (1986) Therapeutische Wirksamkeit ätherischer Öle bei chronisch-obstruktiver Bronchitis. *Therapiewoche*, **36**, 1162–1166.

Longworth, J. C. (1982) Psychophysiological effects of slow stroke back massage in normotensive females. *Adv. Nurs. Sci.*, **4**(4), 44–61.

Lorenzetti, B. B., Souza, G. E., Sarti, S. J. *et al.* (1991) Myrcene mimics the peripheral analgesic activity of lemongrass tea. *J. Ethnopharmacol.*, **34**(1), 43–48.

Lorig, T. S. (1992). Cognitive and non-cognitive effects of odour exposure, in *Fragrance: The Psychology and Biology of Perfume*, (eds S. Van Toller and G. H. Dodd), Elsevier, Barking.

Lorig, T. S. and Roberts, M. (1990) Odour and cognitive alteration of the contingent negative variation. *Chem. Senses*, **15**, 537–545.

Lorig, T. S. and Schwartz, G. E. (1989) EEG during relaxation and food imagery. *Imagination, Cognition Personality*, **8**, 201–208.

Lowen, A. (1971) *The Langugage of the Body*, Collier, New York.

Lowen, A. (1976). *Bioenergetics*, Penguin, Harmondsworth.

Lucas, R. C. and Koslow, R. (1984) Comparative study of static, dynamic, and proprioceptive neuromuscular facilitation stretching techniques on flexibility. *Perceptual Motor Skills*, **58**(2), 615–618.

Ludvigson, H. W. and Rottman, T. R. (1989) Effects of ambient odors of lavender and cloves on cognition, memory, affect and mood. *Chem. Senses*, **14**(4), 525–536.

Lundeberg, T., Nordemar, R. and Ottoson, D. (1984a) Pain alleviation by vibratory stimulation. *Pain*, **20**, 25–44.

Lundeberg, T. (1984b) Long-term results of vibratory stimulation as a pain-relieving measure for chronic pain. *Pain*, **20**, 13–23.

Lynch, J. J. and McCarthy, J. F. (1967) The effect of petting on a classically conditioned emotional response. *Behav. Res. Ther.*, **5**, 55–62.

Lynch, J. J. and McCarthy, J. F. (1969). Social responding in dogs: heart rate changes to a person. *Psychophysiology*, **5**, 389–393.

Lynch, J. J. *et al.* (1974a) Effects of human contact on the heart activity of curarized patients in a shock-trauma unit. *Am. Heart J.*, **88**(2), 160–168.

Lynch, J. J. *et al.* (1974b) The effects of human contact on cardiac arrythmia in coronary care patients. *J. Nerv. Ment. Dis.*, **158**(2), 88–99.

McConway, K. (ed.) (1994). *Studying Health and Disease*, Open University Press, Buckingham.

McCorkle, R. (1974) Effects of touch on seriously ill patients. *Nurs. Res.*, **23**, 125–132.

McGeorge, B. C. and Steele, M. C. (1991) Allergic Contact Dermatitis of the nipple from Roman chamomile ointment. *Contact Dermatitis*, **24** (2), 139–140.

McKechnie, A. A., Wilson, F., Watson, N. and Scott, D. (1983) Anxiety states: a preliminary report on the value of connective tissue massage. *J. Psychosom. Res.*, **27**(2), 125–129.

McKenzie, W. T., Forgas, L., Vernino, A. R. *et al.* (1992) Comparison of a 0.12% chlorhexidine mouthrinse and an essential oil mouthrinse on oral health in institutionalized, mentally handicapped adults: one-year results. *J. Periodontol.*, **63**(3), 187–193.

Mackereth, P. (1993). *Aromatherapy, Massage and Touch*, Grampian Health Board: Consensus Conference on Complementary Medicine, Aberdeen.

McNeely, D. A. (1987). *Touching: Body Therapy and Depth Psychology*, Inner City Books, Toronto.

McVey, M. (1995) Policy development, in *The Nurses' Handbook of Complementary Therapies*, (ed. D. Rankin-Box), Churchill Livingstone, Edinburgh.

Maher, G. (1990) *Start a Career in Alternative Medicine*, Tackmark, Middlesex.

Maiche, A. G., Grohn, P. and Maki Hokkonen, H. (1991) Effect of chamomile cream and almond ointment on acute radiation skin reaction. *Acta Oncol.*, **30**(3), 395–396.

Major, B. (1981) Gender patterns in touching behavior, *Gender and Nonverbal Behavior*, (eds C. Mayo and N. M. Henley), Springer-Verlag, New York, p. 15–37.

March, B. E. and Macmillan, C. (1987) Plasma corticostrone concentrations in growing chickens fed diets formulated to promote different rates of growth. *Poultry Sci.*, **66**(8), 1358–1366.

Markos, P. D. (1979) Ipsilateral and contralateral effects of proprioceptive neuromuscular facilitation techniques on hip motion and electromyographic activity. *Physical Ther.*, **59**(11), 1366–1373.

Marotti, M. *et al.* (1994) Effects of variety and ontogenic stage on the essential oil composition and biological activity of fennel (*Foeniculum vulgare* Mill). *J. Essential Oil Res.*, **6**(1), 57–62.

Marquardt, H. (1983) *Reflex Zone Therapy of the Feet*, Thorsons, Wellingborough.

Martin, G. (1989) *Aromatherapy*, Optima, London.

Maxwell-Hudson, C. (1988) *The Complete Book of Massage*, Dorling-Kindersley, London.

Meek, S. S. (1993) Effects of slow stroke back massage on relaxation in hospice clients. *Image*, **25**(1), 17–21.

Melzack, R. and Wall, D. (1965) Pain mechanism: a new theory. *Science*, **150**, 971.

Melzig, M. and Teuscher, E. (1991) Investigations of the influence of essential oils and their main components on the adenosine uptake by cultivated endothelial cells. *Planta Med.*, **57**(1), 41–42.

Millet, Y. *et al.* (1981) Toxicity of some essential plants oils. Clinical and experimental study. *Clin. Toxicol.*, **18**(12), 1485–1498.

Mills, M. E., Thomas, S. A. and Lynch, J. J. (1976) Effect of pulse palpation on cardiac arrhythmia in coronary care patients. *Nurs. Res.*, **25**, 378–382.

Mitchell, S. (1993) Dementia: aromatherapy's effectiveness in disorders associated with dementia. *Int. J. Aromather.*, **3**(2), 20–23.

Miyake, Y. *et al.* (1991) JASTS XXIV Abstract 6: Effect of odors on humans (I). Effects on sleep latency. *Chem. Senses*, **16**(2), 183.

Moleyar, V. and Narasimham, P. (1992) Antibacterial activity of essential oil components. *Int. J. Food Microbiol.*, **16**(4), 337–342.

Mongold, J. J., Camillieri, S., Susplugas, P. *et al.* (1991) Activité cholagogue-choleretique d'un extrait lyophilisé de *Rosmarinus officinalis* L. *Plantes Médicinales Phytothér.*, **25**(1), 6–11.

Montagu, A. (1978) *Touching: The Human Significance of the Skin*, Harper & Row, New York.

Moore, M. A. and Kukulka, C. G. (1991) Depression of Hoffmann reflexes following voluntary contraction and implications for proprioceptive neuromuscular facilitation therapy. *Physical Ther.*, **71**(4), 321–329.

Moran, A., Martin, M. L., Montero, M. J. *et al.* (1989) Analgesic, antipyretic and anti-inflammatory activity of the essential oil of Artemisia caerulescens subsp. gallica. *J. Ethnopharmacol.* **27**(3), 307–317.

Moran, J., Addy, M. and Roberts, S. (1992) A comparison of natural product, triclosan and chlorhexidine mouthrinses on 4 day plaque regrowth. *J. Clin. Periodontol.*, **19**(8), 578–582.

Morelli, M., Seaborne, D. E. and Sullivan, S. J. (1990) Changes in H-Reflex amplitude during massage of triceps surae in healthy subjects. *J. Orthopaed. Sports Physical Ther.*, **12**(2), 55–59.

Morelli, M., Seaborne, D. E. and Sullivan, S. J. (1991) H-reflex modulation during manual muscle massage of human triceps surae. *Arch. Physical Med. Rehab.*, **72**(11), 915–919.

Mörsdorf, K. (1966) Cyclische Terpene und ihre chloretische Wirkung. *Chim. Therapeut.*, **7**, 442–443.

Mortimer, P. S., Simmonds, R., Rezvani, M. *et al.* (1990) The measurement of skin lymph flow by isotope clearance–reliability, reproducibility, injection dynamics, and the effect of massage. *J. Invest. Dermatol.*, **95**(6), 677–682.

Mukamel, E., Engelstein, D., Simon, D. and Servadio, C. (1987) The value of Rowatinex in the treatment of ureterolithiasis. *J. Urol.* (Paris), **31**, 31.

Mumm, A. H., Morens, D. M., Elm, J. L. and Diwan, A. R. (1993) Zoster after shiatsu massage. *Lancet*, **341**(8842), 447.

Nagai, H. *et al.* (1991) JASTS XXIV Abstract 49: Effect of odors on humans (II). Reducing effects of mental stress and fatigue. *Chem. Senses*, **16**(2), 183.

Naliboff, B. D. and Tachiki, K. H. (1991) Autonomic and skeletal muscle responses to nonelectrical cutaneous stimulation. *Percept. Motor Skills*, **72**(2), 575–584.

Nash, P. *et al.* (1986) Peppermint oil does not relieve the pain of irritable bowel sydrome. *Br. J. Clin. Pract.*, **40**, 292–293.

Nelson, D., Heitman, R. and Jennings, C. (1986) Effects of tactile stimulation on premature infant weight gain. *J. Obs. Gynecol. Neonat. Nurs.*, **15**(3), 262–267.

Nichols, S. (ed.) (1992) *Aromatherapy*, Moscovitch & Co, London.

Nikolaevskii, V. V., Kononova, N. S., Pertsovskii, A. I. and Shinkarchuk, I. F. (1990) Effect of essential oils on the course of experimental atherosclerosis. *Patol. Fiziol. Eksp. Ter.*, **Sep–Oct**(5), 52–53.

Nordschow, M. and Bierman W. (1962) The influence of manual massage on muscle relaxation. *J. Am. Physical Ther. Assoc.*, **42**, 653–657.

Nwaiwu, J. I. and Akah, P. A. (1986) Anticonvulsant activity of the volatile oil from the fruit of Tetrapleura tetraptera. *J. Ethnopharmacol.*, **18**(2), 103–107.

O'Brien, J. (1986) In *An Alternative Curriculum for Youths and Adults with Severe Learning Difficulties*, (eds J. T. Bellamy and B. Wilcox), Paul Brooks, Baltimore, MD.

Ocete, M. A., Risco, S., Zarzuelo, A. and Jimenez, J. (1989) Pharmacological activity of the essential oil of Bupleurum gibraltaricum: anti-inflammatory activity and effects on isolated rat uteri. *J. Ethnopharmacol.*, **25**(3), 305–313.

Ogunlana, E. O., Hoglund, S., Onawunmi, G. and Skold, O. (1987) Effects of lemongrass oil on the morphological characteristics and peptidoglycan synthesis of Escherichia coli cells. *Microbios*, **50**(202), 43–59.

Oleson, T. and Flocco, W. (1993) Randomized controlled study of premenstrual symptoms treated with ear, hand, and foot reflexology. *Obs. Gynecol.*, **82**(6), 906–911.

Oliveri, D. J., Lynn, K. and Hong, C. Z. (1989) Increased skin temperature after vibratory stimulation. *Am. J. Physical Med. Rehab.*, **68**(2), 81–85.

Olson, B. (1989) Effects of massage for prevention of pressure ulcers. *Decubitus*, **2**(4), 32–37.

Onawunmi, G. O., Yisak, W. A. and Ogunlana, E. O. (1984) Antibacterial constituents in the essential oil of Cymbopogon citratus (DC) Stapf. *J. Ethnopharmacol.*, **12**(3), 279–286.

Onawunmi, G. O. (1989) Antifungal activity of lemongrass oil. *Int. J. Crude Drug Res.*, **27**(2), 121–126.

Onawunmi, G. O. and Ogunlana, E. O. (1986) A study of the antibacterial activity of the essential oil of lemongrass (Cymbopogon citratus (DC) Stapf). *Int. J. Crude Drug Res.*, **24**(2), 64–68.

Opdyke, D. L. K. (1976) Inhibition of sensitization reactions induced by certain aldehydes. *Food Cosmet. Toxicol.*, **14**, 197.

Ortiz de Urbina, A. V., Martin, M. L., Montero, M. J. *et al.* (1989) Sedating and antipyretic activity of the essential oil of Calamintha sylvatica subsp. ascendens. *J. Ethnopharmacol.* **25**(2), 165–171.

Osternig, L. R., Robertson, R., Troxel, R. and Hansen, P. (1987) Muscle activation during proprioceptive neuromuscular facilitation (PNF) stretching techniques. *Am. J. Physical Med.*, **66**(5), 298–307.

Osternig, L. R., Robertson, R., Troxel, R. and Hansen, P. (1990) Differential responses to proprioceptive neuromuscular facilitation (PNF) stretch techniques. *Med. Sci. Sports Exercise*, **22**(1), 106–111.

Ottenbacher, K. J., Muller, L., Brandt, D. *et al.* (1987) The effectiveness of tactile stimulation as a form of early intervention: a quantitative evaluation. *J. Devel. Behav. Pediat.*, **8**(2), 68–76.

Panizzi, L., Flamini, G., Cioni, P. L. and Morelli, I. (1993) Composition and antimicrobial properties of essential oils of four Mediterranean Lamiaceae. *J. Ethnopharmacol.*, **39**(3), 167–170.

Park, C. M., Clegg, K. E., Harvey-Clark, C. J. and Hollenberg, M. F. (1992) Improved techniques for successful neonatal rat surgery. *Lab. Anim. Sci.*, **42**(5), 508–513.

Parys, B. T. (1983) Chemical burns resulting from contact with peppermint oil. *Burns Incl. Therm. Inj.*, **995**, 374–375.

Pattison, J. E. (1973) Effects of touch on self-exploration and the therapeutic relationship. *J. Couns. Clin. Psychol.*, **40**, 170–175.

Pauk, J., Kuhn, C. M., Field, T. M. and Schanberg, S. M. (1986) Positive effects of tactile versus kinesthetic or vestibular stimulation on neuroendocrine and ODC activity in maternally-deprived rat pups. *Life Sci.*, **39**(22), 2081–2087.

Payne, M. B. (1989) The use of therapeutic touch with rehabilitation clients. *Rehab. Nurs.*, **14**(2), 69–72.

Peets, J. M. and Pomeranz, B. (1978) CXBK mice deficient in opiate receptors show poor electroacupuncture analgesia. *Nature*, **273**(5664), 675–676.

Peña, E. F. (1962) *Melaleuca alternifola oil. Obs. Gyn.*, **19**(6), 793–795.

Penny, K. S. (1979) Postpartum perceptions of touch received during labor. *Res. Nurs. Health*, **2**(1), 9–16.

Perrucci, S., Mancianti, F., Cioni, P. L. *et al.* (1994) In vitro antifungal activity of essential oils against some isolates of *Microsporum canis* and *Microsporum gypseum* (letter). *Planta Med.*, **60**(2), 184–187.

Perry, J., Jones, M. H. and Thomas, L. (1981) Functional evaluation of Rolfing in cerebral palsy. *Devel. Med. Child Neurol.*, **23**(6), 717–729.

Petersen, L. N., Faurschou, P., Olsen, O. T. and Svendsen, U. G. (1992) Foot zone therapy and bronchial asthma: a controlled clinical trial. *Ugeskr. Laeger*, **154**(30), 2065–2068.

Pietroni, P. C. (1990) *The Greening of Medicine*, Gollancz, London.

Pietroni, P. C. (1992) Alternative medicine: methinks the doctor protests too much and incidentally befuddles the debate. *J. Med. Ethics*, **18**(1), 23–25.

Pohlman, S. and Beardslee, C. (1987) Contact experienced by neonates in intensive care environments. *Matern. Child Nurs. J.*, **16**(3), 207–226.

Pomeranz, B. and Stux, G. (1991). *Scientific Bases of Acupuncture*, Springer Verlag, Berlin.

Powell, L. F. (1974) The effect of stimulation and maternal involvement on the development of low birth-weight infants and on maternal behaviour. *Child Devel.*, **45**, 106–113.

Price, S. (1991) *Aromatherapy for Common Ailments*, Gaia Books, London.

Price, S (1993) *The Aromatherapy Workbook*, Thorsons, London.

Price, S. and Price, L. (1995) *Aromatherapy for Health Professionals*, Churchill Livingstone, Edinburgh.

Puustjarvi, K., Hanninen, O. and Leppåluoto, J. (1986) Effects of massage on endorphin levels and some physiological parameters. *Acta Physiol. Hung.*, **68**, 243.

Rahman, M. N. G., McAll, G. and Chai, K. G. (1987) Massage-related perforation of the sigmoid colon in kelantan. *Med. J. Malaysia*, **42**(1), 56–57.

Ramsey, N. F. and Van Ree, J. M. (1993) Emotional but not physical stress enhances intravenous cocaine self-administration in drug-naive rats. *Brain Res.*, **16**; 608(2), 216–222.

Rangelov, A., Pisanetz, M., Toreva, D. and Kosev, R. (1988) Experimental study of the cholagogic and choleretic actions of some of the basic ingredients of essential oils on laboratory animals. *Folia Med. (Plovdiv)*, **30**(4), 30–38.

Rankin-Box, D. (ed.) (1995a) *The Nurses' Handbook of Complementary Therapies*, Churchill Livingstone, Edinburgh.

Rankin-Box, D. (1995b) Managing change in the workplace, in *The Nurses' Handbook of Complementary Therapies*, (ed. D. Rankin-Box), Churchill Livingstone, Edinburgh.

Rausch, P. B. (1981) Effects of tactile and kinesthetic stimulation on premature neonates. *J. Obs. Gyn. Neonat. Nurs.*, **10**, 34–37.

Ravid, U. and Putievsky, E. (1986). Carvacrol and thymol chemotypes of east Meditarranean wild Labiatae herbs, in *Progress in Essential Oil Research*, (ed. E. J. Brunke), Walter de Gryter, Berlin, p.163–167.

Reed, B. V. and Held, J. M. (1988) Effects of sequential connective tissue massage on autonomic nervous system of middle-aged and elderly adults. *Physical Ther.*, **68**(8), 1231–1234.

Reed, L. and Norfolk, L. (1993) Aromatherapy in midwifery. *Int. J. Altern. Complement. Med.*, **11**(12), 15–17.

Rees, W. D. et al. (1979) Treating irritable bowel syndrome with peppermint oil. *Br. Med. J.*, **ii**, 835–836.

Reilly, D. (1994). Self-healing and complementary medicine. RCCM Conference – Complementary Medicine Research: An International Perspective.

Remmal, A. et al. (1993a) Improved method for the determination of antimicrobial activity of essential oils in agar medium. *J. Essential Oil Res.*, **5**, 179–184.

Remmal, A., Bouchikhi, T., Tantaoui-Elaraki, A. and Ettayebi, M. (1993b) Inhibition of antibacterial activity of essential oils by tween 80 and ethanol in liquid medium. *J. Pharm. Belg.*, **48**(5), 352–356.

Reynolds, P., Boyd, P. T., Blacklow, R. S. et al. (1994) The relationship between social ties and survival among black and white breast cancer patients. National Cancer Institute Black/White Cancer Survival Study Group. *Cancer Epidemiol. Biomarkers Prevent.*, **3**(3), 253–259.

Rice, R. D. (1977) Neurophysical development in premature nenonates following stimulation. *Dev. Psychol.*, **13**, 69–76.

Ries, A. L., Ellis, B. and Hawkins, R. W. (1988) Upper extremity exercise training in chronic obstructive pulmonary disease. *Chest*, **93**(4), 688–692.

Robbins, T. (1991) *Jitterbug Perfume*, Bantam, London.

Rodenburg, J. B., Steenbeek, D., Schiereck, P. and Bar, P. R. (1994) Warm-up, stretching and massage diminish harmful effects of eccentric exercise. *Int. J. Sports Med.*, **15**(7), 414–419.

Roffey, S. J., Walker, R. and Gibson ,G. G. (1990) Hepatic peroxisomal and microsomal enzyme induction by citral and linalool in rats. *Food Chem. Toxicol.*, **28**(6), 403–408.

Rolf, I. P. (1977). *Rolfing: The Integration of Human Structures*, Harper & Row, New York.

Rompelberg, C. J., Verhagen, H. and van Bladeren, P. J. (1993) Effects of the naturally occurring alkenylbenzenes eugenol and trans-anethole on drug-metabolizing enzymes in the rat liver. *Food Chem. Toxicol*, 31(9), 637–645.

Rose, J. E. and Behm, F. M. (1994) Inhalation of vapor from black pepper extract reduces smoking withdrawal symptoms. *Drug Alcohol Dependence*, 34(3), 225–229.

Rose, S., Lewontin, R. C. and Kamin, L. J. (1984a). *Not in Our Genes*, Penguin, Harmondsworth.

Rose, S. A. (1984b) Preterm responses to passive, active and social touch, in *The Many Facets of Touch*. (ed. C. Cardwell-Brown), Johnson & Johnson Baby Products Company, Pediatric Round Table Series.

Rose, S. A. and Bridger, W. H. (1979). Enhancing Visual Recognition Memory in Pre-term Infants, cited in Field, T. (1980) Supplemental stimulation of preterm neonates. *Early Hum. Dev.*, 4, 301–314.

Rosenblatt, J. S. and Lehrman, D. S. (1963) *Maternal behavior of the laboratory rat, in Maternal Behavior in Mammals*, (ed. H. L. Rheingold), John Wiley, New York.

Rossi, T., Melegari, M., Bianchi, A. *et al.* (1988) Sedative, anti-inflammatory and anti-diuretic effects induced in rats by essential oils of varieties of *Anthemis nobilis*: a comparative study. *Pharmacol. Res. Commun.*, 20(Suppl 5), 71–74.

Roth, L. L. and Rosenblatt, J. S. (1965) Mammary glands of pregnant rats: development stimulated by licking. *Science*, 151, 1043–1044.

Ruegamer, W. R. *et al.* (1954) Growth, food utilization and thyroid activity in the albino rat as a function of extra handling. *Science*, 120, 184–185.

Ryman, D. (1984) *The Aromatherapy Handbook*, C. W. Daniel, Saffron Walden.

Sadler, J. (1991) *Aromatherapy*, Ward Lock, London.

Sady, S. P., Wortman, M. and Blanke, D. (1982) Flexibility training: ballistic, static or proprioceptive neuromuscular facilitation? *Arch. Physical Med. Rehab.*, 63(6), 261–263.

Sagan, L. A. (1989) On radiation, paradigms and hormesis. *Science*, 245, 574, 621.

Saller, R., Beschorner, M., Hellenbrecht, D. and Buhrimg, M. (1990) Dose dependency of symptomatic relief of complaints by chamomille steam inhalation in patients with common cold. *Eur. J. Pharm.*, 183, 728–729.

Sanderson, H. and Harrison, J. (1991) *Aromatherapy and Massage for People with Learning Difficulties*, Hands On Publishing, Birmingham.

Scafidi, F. A. *et al.* (1986) Effects of tacktile/kinesthetic stimulation on the clinical course and sleep/wake behaviour of preterm neonates. *Infant Behav. Dev.*, 9, 91–105.

Scafidi, F. A. *et al.* (1990) Massage stimulates growth in preterm infants: a replication. *Infant Behav. Dev.*, 13, 167–188.

Scafidi, F. A., Field, T. and Schanberg, S. M. (1993) Factors that predict which preterm infants benefit most from massage therapy. *J. Develop. Behav. Pediat.*, 14(3), 176–180.

Scarr-Salapatek, S. and Williams, M. L. (1973) The effects of early stimulation on low birthweight infants. *Child Develop.*, 33, 94–101.

Schaeffer Jay, S. (1982) The effects of gentle human touch on mechanically ventilated very short gestation infants. *Matern. Child Nurs. J.*, 11(4), 199–257.

Schäfer, V. D. and Schäfer, W. (1981) Pharmakologische Untersuchungen zur Broncholytischen und sekretolytisch-expektorierenden Wirksamkeit einer Salbe auf Basis von Menthol, Campher und ätherischen Ölen. *Arzneimittelforschung*, **31**(1), 82–86.

Schanberg, S. M., Evoniuk, G. and Kuhn, C. M. (1984) Tactile and nutritional aspects of maternal care: specific regulators of nutritional aspects of neuroendocrine function and cellular development. *Proc. Soc. Exp. Biol. Med.*, **175**, 135.

Schelinger, M. and Yoidfat, Y. (1988) Effect of psychosocial stress on natural killer cell activity. *Cancer Detect. Prevent.*, **12**, 9–14.

Schneirla, T. C., Rosenblatt, J. S. and Tobach, E. (1963). *Maternal behavior in the cat, in Maternal Behavior in Mammals*, (ed. H. L. Rheingold), New York, Wiley.

Schoenhofer, S. O. (1985) Affectational touch in Intensive Care Nursing: a descriptive study. *Heart Lung*, **18**(2), 146–154.

Schulz, H., Stolz, C. and Muller, J. (1994) The effect of valerian extract on sleep polygraphy in poor sleepers: a pilot study. *Pharmacopsychiatry*, **27**(4), 147–151.

Schwartz, D. and Natyncuk, S. (eds) (1990) *Chemical Signals in Vertebrates*, Oxford University Press, Oxford.

Scott, S., Cole, T., Lucas, P. l. and Richards, M. (1983) Weight gain and movement patterns of very low birthweight infants nursed on lambswool. *Lancet*, **ii**, 1014–1016.

Seay, B. M., Hansen, E. W. and Harlow, H. F. (1962) Mother–infant separation in monkeys. *J. Child Psychol. Psychiat.*, **69**, 534–554.

Serby, M. J. and Chobor, K. L. (eds) (1992) *Science of Olfaction*, Springer-Verlag, New York.

Seto, T. A. and Keup, W. (1969) Effects of alkylmethoxybenzene and alkylmethylenedioxybenzene essential oils on pentobarbital and ethanol sleeping time. *Arch. Int. Pharmacodyn. Ther.*, **180**(1), 232–240.

Severini, V. and Venerando, A. (1967) Physiological effects of massage on the cardiovascular system. *Europa Medicophysiol.*, **3**, 165–183.

Shao, X. (1990) Effect of massage and temperature on the permeability of initial lymphatics. *Lymphology*, **23**(1), 48–50.

Sharma, U. (1991). *Complementary Medicine Today: Practitioners and Patients*, Routledge, London.

Shrivastav, P. *et al.* (1988) Suppression of puerperal lactation using jasmine flowers. *Aust. N. Z. J. Obs. Gynaecol.*, **28**, 68–71.

Shwaireb, M. H. (1993) Caraway oil inhibits skin tumors in female BALB/c mice. *Nutr. Cancer*, **19**(3), 321–325.

Silverman, A. F., Pressman, M. E. and Bartel, H. W. (1973) Self-esteem and tactile communication. *Humanistic Psychol.*, **13**, 73–77.

Sims, S. (1986) Slow stroke back massage for cancer patients. *Nurs. Times*, **82**(13), 47–50.

Skoglund, C. R. and Knutsson, E. (1985) Vasomotor changes in human skin elicited by high frequency low amplitude vibration. *Acta Physiol. Scand.*, **125**, 335–336.

Smart, J. L., McMahon, A. C., Massey, R. F. *et al.* (1990) Evidence of non-maternally mediated acceleration of eye-opening in 'enriched' artificially reared rat pups. *Brain Res. Dev.*, **56**(1), 141–143.

Smith, L. L., Keating, M. N., Holbert, D. *et al.* (1994) The effects of athletic massage on delayed onset muscle soreness, creatine kinase, and neutrophil count: a preliminary report. *J. Orthopaed. Sports Physical Ther.*, **19**(2), 93–99.

Smotherman, W. P. (1983) Mother-infant interaction and the modulation of pituitary adrenal activity in rat pups after early stimulation. *Dev Psychobiol.*, **16**(3), 169–176.

Smythe, G. A. and Edwards, S. R. (1992) Suppression of central noradrenergic neuronal activity inhibits hyperglycemia. *Am. J. Physiol.*, **263**(5 Pt 1), E823–827.

Solkoff, N., Yaffe, S., Weintraub, D. and Blase, B. (1969) Effects of handling on the subsequent development of premature infants. *Developmental Psychol.*, **1**, 765–768.

Solkoff, N. and Matuszak, D. (1975) Tactile stimulation and behavioral development among low-birthweight infants. *Child Psychiat. Hum. Dev.*, **6**, 33.

Solomon, G. F., Levine, S. and Kraft, J. K. (1968) Early experiences and immunity. *Nature*, **220**, 821–823.

Somerville, K. W. *et al.* (1985) Stones in the common bile duct: experience with medical dissolution therapy. *Postgrad. Med. J.*, **61**, 313–316.

Speigel, D. *et al.* (1989) Effect of psychosocial treatment on survival of patients with metastatic breast cancer. *Lancet*, **ii**, 888–889.

Stack, D. M. and Muir, D. W. (1992) Adult tactile stimulation during face-to-face interactions modulates five-month-olds' affect and attention. *Child Develop.*, **63**(6), 1509–1525.

Stahl (1986) Chemical composition and variation of the essential oil from the Norwegian *Thymus praecox ssp* arcticus and *Thymus pulegioides, in Progress in Essential Oil Research*, (ed. E. J. Brunke), Walter de Gryter, Berlin, p.157–161.

Stanton, M. E. and Levine, S. (1984) Maternal contact inhibits pituitary-adrenal activity in preweanling rats. *Soc. Neurosci.*, **10**, 86.

Stevensen, C. (1994) The psychophysiological effects of aromatherapy massage following cardiac surgery. *Comp. Ther. Med.*, **2**(1), 27–35.

Stier, D. S. and Hall, J. A. (1984) Gender differences in touch: an empirical and theoretical review. *J. Pers. Soc. Psychol.*, **47**, 440–459.

Sullivan, M. K., Dejulia, J. J. and Worrell, T. W. (1992) Effect of pelvic position and stretching method on hamstring muscle flexibility. *Med. Sci. Sports Exercise*, **24**(12), 1383–1389.

Sullivan, S. J., Williams, L. R., Seaborne, D. E. and Morelli, M. (1991) Effects of massage on alpha motoneuron excitability. *Physical Ther.*, **71**(8), 555–560.

Surburg, P. R. (1979) Interactive effects of resistance and facilitation patterning upon reaction and response times. *Physical Ther.*, **59**(12), 1513–1517.

Suskind, P. (1985) *Perfume: The Story of a Murderer*, Penguin, Harmondsworth.

Tanigawa, M. C. (1972) Comparison of the hold–relax procedure and passive mobilization on increasing muscle length. *Physical Ther.*, **52**, 725–735.

Tappan, F. M. (1978) *Healing Massage Techniques*, Reston Publishing, Virginia.

Taylor, B. A., Luscombe, C. K. and Duthie, H. L. (1983) Inhibitory effect of peppermint oil on gastrointestinal smooth muscle. *Gut*, **24**, A992.

Taylor, B. A., Luscombe, D. K. and Duthie, H. L. (1984) Inhibitory efffect of peppermint and menthol on human isolated coli. *Gut*, **25**, A1168.

Taylor, B. A. *et al.* (1985) Calcium antagonist activity of menthol on gastrointestinal smooth muscle. *Br. J. Clin. Pharmacol.*, **20**, 293P–294P.

Teece, J., Savignas-Brown, J. and Meinbresse, D. (1976) CNV and the distraction–arousal hypothesis. *Electroencephalogr. Clin. Neurophysiol.*, **41**, 277–286.

Thomas, J. G. (1962) Peppermint fibrillation. *Lancet*, **i**, 222.

Thomas, K., Fall, M., Nicholl, J. and Williams, B. (1993). Methodological study to investigate the feasibility of conducting a population-based survey of the use of complementary health care. Unpublished report submitted to the Research Council for Complementary Medicine.

Tisserand, M. (1990) *Aromatherapy for Women*, Thorsons, Wellingborough.

Tisserand, R. (1977) *The Art of Aromatherapy*, C. W. Daniel, Saffron Walden.

Tisserand, R. (1988) *Aromatherapy for Everyone*, Arkana, London.

Tisserand, R. and Balacs, T. (1995) *Essential Oil Safety*, Churchill Livingstone, Edinburgh.

Tobiason, S. J. B. (1981) Touching is for everyone. *Am. J. Nurs.*, **81**, 728–730.

Tomasik, M. (1983) Effect of hydromassage on changes in blood electrolyte and lactic acid levels an haematocrit value after maximal effort. *Acta Physiol. Polon.*, **34**, 257–261.

Tomoda, M., Gonda, R., Ohara, N. *et al.* (1994) A glucan having reticuloendothelial system-potentiating and anti-complementary activities from the tuber of Pinellia ternata. *Biol. Pharmaceut. Bull.*, **17**(6), 859–861.

Tong, M. M., Altman, P. M. and Barnetson, R. S. (1992) Tea tree oil in the treatment of tinea pedis. *Australas. J. Dermatol.*, **33**(3), 145–149.

Torri, S. *et al.* (1991) Contingent negative variation (CNV) and the psychological effects of odour, in *Perfumery: The Psychology and Biology of Fragrance*, (eds S. Van Toller and G. H. Dodd), Chapman & Hall, London.

Trevelyan, J. and Booth, B. (1994) *Complementary Medicine for Nurses, Midwives and Health Visitors*, Macmillan, London.

Triplett, J. L. and Arneson, S. W. (1979) The use of verbal and tactile comfort to alleviate distress in young hospitalized children. *Res. Nurs. Health*, **2**(1), 17–23.

Tubaro, A., Zilli, C., Redaelli, C. and Della Loggia R. (1984) Evaluation of the anti-inflammatory activity of a chamomile extract topical application. *Planta Med.*, **50**(4), 358.

Turton, P. (1989) Touch me, feel me, heal me. *Nurs. Times*, **19**(8), 42–45.

Tyler, D. O., Winslow, E. H., Clark, A. P. and White, K. M. (1990) Effects of a 1-minute back rub on mixed venous oxygen saturation and heart rate in critically ill patients. *Heart Lung*, **19**(5 Pt 2), 562–565.

Tyurin, A. M. (1985) The influence of difference forms of massage on the psycho-emotional state of athletes. *Teoriya I Praktika Fizichekoi Kultury*, **7**, 19–20.

Ueda, W., Katatoka, Y. and Sagara, Y. (1993) Effect of gentle massage on regression of sensory analgesia during epidural block. *Anesth. Analg.*, **76**(4), 783–785.

United Kingdom Central Council for Nursing, Midwifery and Health Visiting (1992). *The Scope of Professional Practice*, UK Central Council for Nursing, Midwifery and Health Visiting, London.

Valnet, J. (1980) *The Practice of Aromatherapy*, C. W. Daniel, Saffron Walden.

Van Bergeijk, J. P., van Herck, H., de Boer, S. F. *et al.* (1990) Effects of group size and gentling on behaviour, selected organ masses and blood constituents in female Rivm: TOX rats. *Z. Versuchstierkd*, **33**(2), 85–90.

Van Toller. S. (1979) *The Nervous Body: An Introduction to the Autonomic Nervous System and Behaviour*, John Wiley, Chichester.

Van Toller, S., Dodd, G. H. and Billing, A. (1985). *Ageing and the Sense of Smell*, Charles C. Thomas, Springfield, IL.

Van Toller, S. and Dodd, G. H. (eds) (1991) *Perfumery: The Psychology and Biology of Fragrance*, Chapman & Hall, London.

Van Toller, S. and Dodd, G. H. (eds) (1992). *Fragrance: The Psychology and Biology of Perfume*, Elsevier, Barking.

Vickers, A. J. (1993) *Complementary Medicine and Disability*, Chapman & Hall, London.

Vickers, A. J. (1994a) Complementary medicine, intermediate medicine and the degree of intervention. *Complement. Ther. Med.*, **2**(3), 123–127.

Vickers, A. J. (1994b) *Health Options: Complementary Therapies for Cerebral Palsy and Related Conditions*, Element Books, Shaftesbury, in association with the Spastics Society.

Vickers, A. J. (1995) Critical appraisal: how to read a clinical research paper. *Complement. Ther. Med.*, **3**, 158–166.

Villar, D., Knight, M. J., Hansen, S. R. and Buck, W. B. (1994) Toxicity of melaleuca oil and related essential oils applied topically on dogs and cats. *Vet. Hum. Toxicol.*, **36**(2), 139–142.

Vincent, C. A. (1989) A controlled trial of the treatment of migraine by acupuncture. *Clin. J. Pain*, **5**(4), 305–312.

Vormbrock, J. K. and Grossberg, J. M. (1988) Cardiovascular effects of human–pet dog interactions. *J. Behav. Med.*, **11**(5), 509–517.

Wade, A. E. *et al.* (1968) Alteration of drug metabolism in rats and mice by an environment of cedarwood. *Pharmacology*, **1**, 317–328.

Wafer, M. (1994) Finding the formula to enhance care. Guidelines for the use of complementary therapies in nursing practice. *Professional Nurse*, **9**(6), 414, 416–417.

Wakim, K. G., Martin, G. M. and Krusen, F. H. (1955) Influence of centripetal rhythmic compression on localized edema of an extremity. *Arch. Physical Med.*, **36**, 98–103.

Wakim, K. G., Martin, G. M., Terrier, J. C. *et al.* (1949) The effects of massage on the circulation in normal and palaysed extremities. *Arch. Physical Med.*, **30**, 135–144.

Waldman, C. S., Tseng, P., Meulman, P. and Whittet. H. B. (1993) Aromatherapy in the intensive care unit. *Care Crit. Ill.*, **9**(4), 170–174.

Wang, R. Y. (1994) Effect of proprioceptive neuromuscular facilitation on the gait of patients with hemiplegia of long and short duration. *Physical Ther.*, **74**(12), 1108–1115.

Warm, J. S., Dember, W. N. and Parasuraman, R. (1990) Effects of fragrance on vigilance performance and stress. *Perfumer Flavorist*, **15**, 15–18.

Warm, J. S., Dember, W. N. and Parasuraman, R. (1991) Effects of olfactory stimulation on performance and stress in a visual sustained attention task. *J. Soc Cosmet. Chem.*, **42**, 1999–2100.

Warrenburg, S. and Schwartz, G. E. (1990) A psychophysiological study of 3 odorants. *Chem. Senses*, **13**, 744.

Watson, W. H. (1975) The meanings of touch: geriatric nursing. *J. Commun.*, **25**(3), 104–112.

Weber, M. D., Servedio, F. J. and Woodall, W. R. (1994) The effects of three modalities on delayed onset muscle soreness. *J. Orthopaed. Sports Physical Ther.*, **20**(5), 236–242.

Weinberg, R. E., Jackson, A. and Kolodny, K. (1988) The relationship of massage and exercise to mood enhancement. *Sports Psychologist*, **2**, 202–211.

Weininger, O. (1953) Mortality of rats under stress as a function of early handling. *Can J. Psychol.*, **7**, 111–114.

Weinrich, S. P. and Weinrich, M. C. (1990) The effect of massage on pain in cancer patients. *Appl. Nurs. Res.*, **3**(4), 140–145.

Weiss, S. J. (1984). Parental touch and the child's body image, in *The Many Facets of Touch*. (ed. C. Cardwell-Brown), Johnson & Johnson Baby Products Company, Pediatric Round Table Series.

Weiss, S. J. (1992) Psychophysiologic and bevhavioral effects of tactile stimulation on infants with congenital heart disease. *Res. Nurs. Health*, **15**(2), 93–101.

Weiss, S. J. (1986) Psychophysiologic effects of caregiver touch on incidence of cardiac dysrhythmia. *Heart Lung*, **15**(5), 495–506.

Weller, L. and Weller, A. (1993) Human menstrual synchrony: a critical assessment. *Neurosci. Biobehav. Rev.*, **17**:427–439.

Wells, M. E. and Smith, D. W. (1983) Reduction of self-injurious behavior of mentally retarded persons using sensory-integrative techniques. *Am. J. Mental Deficiency*, **87**, 664–666.

Wenos, J. Z., Brilla, L. R. and Morrison, M. J. (1990) Effect of massage on delaued onset muscle soreness. *Med. Sci. Sports Exercise*, **22**, S34.

Westland, G. (1993) Massage as a therapeutic tool: Part 2. *Br. J. Occup. Ther.*, **56**(5), 177–180.

Wheeden, A., Scafidi, F. A., Field, T. *et al.* (1993) Massage effects on cocaine-exposed preterm neonates. *J. Develop. Behav. Pediat.*, **14**(5), 318–322.

Whitcher, S. J. and Fisher, J. D (1979). Multidimensional reaction to therapeutic touch in a hospital setting. *J. Personality Soc. Psychol.*, **37**(1), 87–96.

White, J. and Day, K. (1992) *Aromatherapy for Scentual Awareness*, Nacson & Sons, New South Wales.

White, J. L. and Labarda, R. C. (1976) The effects of tactile and kinesthetic stimulation on premature infants. *Dev. Psychobiol.*, **9**, 569.

White-Traut, R. C. and Goldman, M. B. (1988) Premature infant massage: is it safe?. *Pediat. Nurs.*, **14**(4), 285–289.

White-Traut, R. C. and Nelson, M. N. (1988) Maternally administered tactile, auditory, visual, and vestibular stimulation: relationship to later interactions between mothers and premature infants. *Res. Nurs. Health*, **11**(1), 31–39.

White-Traut, R. C. and Tubeszewski, K. (1986) Multimodal stimulation of the premature infant. *J. Pediat. Nurs.*, **1**, 90–95.

Wiktorsson-Möller, M., Öberg, B., Erkstrand, J. and Gillquist, J. (1983) Effects of warming up, massage, and stretching on range of motion and muscle strength in the lower extremity. *Am. J. Sports Med.*, **11**, 249–252.

Wildwood, C. (1992) *Holistic Aromatherapy*, Thorsons, London.

Wilkes, E. (1992) Complementary therapy in hospice and palliative care. Unpublished study available from Trent Palliative Care Centre, Abbey Lane, Sheffield S11 9NE, UK.

Wilkinson, S. (1995) Aromatherapy and massage in palliative care. *Int. J. Palliative Nurs.*, **1**(1), 21–30.

Williams, H. E., Drury, B. J. and Bierman, W. (1961) The influence of cyclomassage on physical activity. *J. Ass. Physical Mental Rehab.*, **15**, 41.

Wood, E. C. and Becker, P. D. (1981) *Beard's Massage*, W. B. Saunders. Philadelphia, PA.

Wooten, S. (1994) Rosen method. *Int. J. Alt. Complement. Med.*, **12**(8), 9–14.

Worwood, V. A. (1991) *The Fragrant Pharmacy*, Bantam, London.

Worwood, V. A. (1987) *Aromantics*, Pan Books, London.

Yamada, K., Mimaki, Y. and Sashida, Y. (1994) Anticonvulsive effects of inhaling lavender oil vapour. *Biol. Pharmaceut. Bull.*, **17**(2), 359–360.

Yeo, T. C., Choo, M. H. and Tay, M. B. (1994) Massive haematoma from digital massage in an anticoagulated patient: a case report. *Singapore Med. J.*, **35**(3), 319–320.

Zani, F., Massimo, G., Benvenuti, S. *et al.* (1991) Studies on the genotoxic properties of essential oils with *Bacillus subtilis* rec-assay and Salmonella/microsome reversion assay. *Planta Med.*, **57**(3), 237–241.

Zelikovski, A., Kaye, C. L., Fink, G. *et al.* (1993) The effects of the modified intermittent sequential pneumatic device (MISPD) on exercise performance following an exhaustive exercise bout. *Br. J. Sports Med.*, **27**(4), 255–259

Author index

1 kg = 2-2 lB

Subject index